Atlas of Infections in
Dermatology

Atlas of Infections in
Dermatology

SECOND EDITION

Archana Singal MD FAMS
Director-Professor and Head
Department of Dermatology and STD
University College of Medical Sciences and GTB Hospital
New Delhi, India

Chander Grover MD DNB FAMS FIAD
Director-Professor
Department of Dermatology and STD
University College of Medical Sciences and GTB Hospital
New Delhi, India

Foreword

Bhushan Kumar

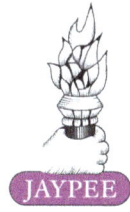

JAYPEE

JAYPEE BROTHERS MEDICAL PUBLISHERS
The Health Sciences Publisher
New Delhi | London

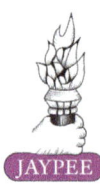

Jaypee Brothers Medical Publishers (P) Ltd

Headquarters
EMCA House
23/23-B, Ansari Road, Daryaganj
New Delhi 110 002, India
Landline: +91-11-23272143, +91-11-23272703
+91-11-23282021, +91-11-23245672
E-mail: jaypee@jaypeebrothers.com

Corporate Office
Jaypee Brothers Medical Publishers (P) Ltd.
4838/24, Ansari Road, Daryaganj
New Delhi 110 002, India
Phone: +91-11-43574357
Fax: +91-11-43574314
E-mail: jaypee@jaypeebrothers.com

Overseas Office
JP Medical Ltd.
83, Victoria Street, London
SW1H 0HW (UK)
Phone: +44-20 3170 8910
E-mail: info@jpmedpub.com

EU GPSR Authorised Representative
Logos Europe, 9 rue Nicolas Poussin
17000, La Rochelle, France
Phone: +33 (0) 6 67 93 73 78
E-mail: Contact@logoseurope.eu

Website: www.jaypeebrothers.com
Website: www.jaypeedigital.com

© 2025, Jaypee Brothers Medical Publishers

The views and opinions expressed in this book are solely those of the original contributor(s)/author(s) and do not necessarily represent those of editor(s) or publisher of the book.

All rights reserved. No part of this publication may be reproduced, stored or transmitted in any form or by any means, electronic, mechanical, photocopying, recording or otherwise, without the prior permission in writing of the publishers.

All brand names and product names used in this book are trade names, service marks, trademarks or registered trademarks of their respective owners. The publisher is not associated with any product or vendor mentioned in this book.

Medical knowledge and practice change constantly. This book is designed to provide accurate, authoritative information about the subject matter in question. However, readers are advised to check the most current information available on procedures included and check information from the manufacturer of each product to be administered, to verify the recommended dose, formula, method and duration of administration, adverse effects and contraindications. It is the responsibility of the practitioner to take all appropriate safety precautions. Neither the publisher nor the author(s)/editor(s) assume any liability for any injury and/or damage to persons or property arising from or related to use of material in this book.

This book is sold on the understanding that the publisher is not engaged in providing professional medical services. If such advice or services are required, the services of a competent medical professional should be sought.

Every effort has been made where necessary to contact holders of copyright to obtain permission to reproduce copyright material. If any have been inadvertently overlooked, the publisher will be pleased to make the necessary arrangements at the first opportunity.

Inquiries for bulk sales may be solicited at: jaypee@jaypeebrothers.com

Atlas of Infections in Dermatology / **Archana Singal, Chander Grover**

First Edition: 2019
Second Edition: **2025**
ISBN: 978-93-5696-810-3

Dedications

I dedicate this book to all my patients who have taught me the art of practicing dermatology by presenting challenging problems to me in nearly four decades. They have taught me to be patient, empathetic, and curious to know more and keep me updated in the sea of knowledge pertaining to dermatology.

—**Archana Singal**

I would wish to thank my parents, Smt Shanno Devi Grover and Shri Shiv Kumar Grover, as well as my parents-in-law, Smt Anita Kubba and Shri Manmohan Kubba, for their constant and unflinching support. Many thanks go to my children, Samira and Bhavya, for putting up with their mother's crazy work schedule. Last but not least, I wish to thank my husband, Dr Samir Kubba, who has been my pillar of strength, best friend, mentor, and guide, all rolled into one!

—**Chander Grover**

Foreword

Having read this new version, I realize the extra value it provides over and above the bestselling older version of the handbook and textbook by the same authors. The authors have done a great balancing act to respect limitations of space and address the need to cover the entire subject in its completeness. In addition, they have included the emerging infections in the last one decade, notably Coronavirus infections and its cutaneous manifestations, recalcitrant dermatophytosis, and likewise. The utility of the office diagnostic tool—dermatoscope—has been highlighted with appropriate images. The treatment modalities have been updated as per the current practices and protocols. The addition of a few good-quality clinical images is welcome. This book will most certainly provide a concise and ready reference in situations when general physicians in primary healthcare facilities and private clinics would need consolidated, relevant, and practical information.

Much like the previous edition, the new edition strives to enable every medical personnel to access information on all aspects of infection, recognize an unusual clinical presentation, and investigate and isolate not so common pathogens and find their drug sensitivity patterns. The book systematically provides all the required information about clinical presentations and various pathogens (known, opportunistic, or nonpathogenic, which become invasive). As the immunosuppressed states—human immunodeficiency virus (HIV)—related or due to other reasons would continue to be a problem of significant magnitude, this book will act as a ready reckoner. The book provides the essential information for the dermatologist, infectious disease specialist, and microbiologist.

For one of the elaborate, illustrated, and accomplished books on the subject, it is a pleasure and a privilege for me to write this foreword and to compliment Director Professors Archana Singal and Chander Grover for their hard work to produce this second edition to spread knowledge of commonly encountered dermatoses, an area often neglected by specialists and general physicians alike. I am sure this book will remain a useful resource on the subject as was the earlier edition.

Bhushan Kumar
MD FRCP(Edinburgh) FRCP(London)
Former Professor and Head
Department of Skin, STD, and Leprosy
Postgraduate Institute of Medical Education and Research
Chandigarh, India

Preface

Infections contribute significantly to morbidity and mortality worldwide, particularly in the developing world. Despite the global availability of antimicrobial drugs, advances in the development of newer agents, and dedicated healthcare endeavors to improve sanitation, the management of infections remains a daunting task. Given the climactic conditions of tropical countries like India, such as high temperature, humidity, and overcrowding, dermatological infections tend to be rampant. As management of skin infections contributes to a large chunk of dermatologic, pediatric, and general physicians' practice, a need for a concise guide is always felt. This book, like its previous version and predecessor *"Comprehensive Approach to Infections in Dermatology,"* aims at compiling relevant information about infections and their management, but in a concise format.

Infections constitute the bulk of dermatologic practice in most areas. In areas where they are not common, they tend to be "exotic" and thus even more difficult to identify or diagnose. This text aims to be a valuable tool for the practicing physicians.

The novelty and exclusivity of this handbook stem from its presentation of an Indian perspective, where infections are seen quite commonly. The book exhaustively covers all important and relevant skin infections—bacterial, mycobacterial (including tuberculosis and leprosy), fungal, viral, protozoal, parasitic infestations, and sexually transmitted infections as well as emerging dermatoses in the last one decade. The book seeks to provide a critical, yet practical approach to treatment. The most effective and safest remedies that have been time-tested and also backed by high-quality evidence are presented. The liberal use of tables, graphics, and clinical photographs, with less text, make this book a reader-friendly must-have manual for dermatologists, pediatricians, physicians, and general practitioners alike.

A wholehearted and sincere attempt has been made to eliminate any errors in the text. We welcome readers' criticism and suggestions, which will help improve and refine this further. Please feel free to communicate with us and give your suggestions.

Archana Singal
Chander Grover

Acknowledgments

We wish to acknowledge the encouragement we received from our readers for our first edition. We felt the need to update this concise version and a ready-reference book after almost a decade.

This book continues to contain the concise, super-relevant information but updated information in a ready-to-use table-top format for busy practitioners. The wealth of images is enriched by the addition of few new high-quality images that have been displayed in a large frame to enhance the visual appeal.

We would again like to express our immense gratitude toward our patients who have taught us so much over the years. No amount of written material or internet searches can yield the wealth of information or the gift of satisfaction we have received by interacting and treating them.

We thank our department and institution for the academic freedom and support and our students for constantly inspiring us to learn more and more. We thank the authors from the parent textbook and our publishers, Jaypee Brothers Medical Publishers (P) Ltd, for bringing out this book. We also thank Dr Pratibha Gupta MD DNB, for carefully proofreading the final version of the book.

Last but not least, we wish to thank our families and friends, who have stood with us through thick and thin, put up graciously with our long working hours, and gave us their unconditional emotional support and love.

Archana Singal
Chander Grover

Acknowledgments

We sincerely acknowledge the help received from our dermatologist colleagues.

- Aditi Jha
- Ambresh Badad
- Amrita Upadhyaya
- Anupam Varshney
- Archana Singal
- Arun C Inamdar
- Asit Mittal
- Biju Vasudevan
- Chander Grover
- Deepashree Daulatabad
- Deepika Pandhi
- Devinder M Thappa
- Divya Gupta
- Divya Seshadri
- Gomathy Sethuraman
- Hemanta K Kar
- Kabir Sardana
- Keshavmurthy A Adya
- KS Prasanna
- Manas Chatterjee
- Minty Jambhore
- Namrata Chhabra
- Pratibha Gupta
- Pravesh Yadav
- Rahul Mahajan
- Raj K Singh
- Richa Chaudhary
- Sacchidanand A Sarvajna Murthy
- Shilpa Garg
- Sidharth Sonthalia
- SR Narahari
- Sumedha Ballal
- Sunil Dogra
- Suruchi Vohra
- Sharad Mehta
- Tarang Goyal
- Taru Garg
- Vikram K Mahajan
- Vinay Gopalani
- Vishalakshi Viswanath
- V Ramesh

Contents

CHAPTER 1:	Cutaneous Gram-positive Bacterial Infections	1
CHAPTER 2:	Gram-negative Bacterial Infections	18
CHAPTER 3:	Superficial Fungal Infections	25
CHAPTER 4:	Subcutaneous Mycoses	56
CHAPTER 5:	Deep Fungal Infections	66
CHAPTER 6:	Herpes Virus Infections	76
CHAPTER 7:	Human Papillomavirus	89
CHAPTER 8:	Pox, Rubella, Coxsackie, and Other Viral Cutaneous Disorders	100
CHAPTER 9:	Leprosy	114
CHAPTER 10:	Cutaneous Tuberculosis	124
CHAPTER 11:	Nontuberculous Mycobacteria	135
CHAPTER 12:	Human Helminthic Infections (Nematodes, Cestodes, and Trematodes)	139
CHAPTER 13:	Leishmaniasis	147
CHAPTER 14:	Infestations	154
CHAPTER 15:	Bites and Stings	161
CHAPTER 16:	Sexually Transmitted Infections	165
CHAPTER 17:	Human Immunodeficiency Virus and Related Infections	182
CHAPTER 18:	Cutaneous Manifestations of Coronavirus Disease 2019	192

Index   197

CHAPTER 1

Cutaneous Gram-positive Bacterial Infections

Introduction

Bacterial infections, also known as pyodermas, constitute a sizable proportion of cases in dermatology outpatients in India. The main predisposing factors are hot and humid climate, poor hygiene, malnutrition, diabetes, and other systemic diseases including immunodeficiency states. Most of the gram-positive bacterial infections of the skin and its appendages are caused by *Staphylococci* and *Streptococci* and can be divided into three main categories as listed here:
1. Primary pyoderma
2. Secondary pyoderma (infection of a primary disease, e.g., eczema and atopic dermatitis)
3. Skin manifestations due to bacterial toxins

Table 1 lists the various cutaneous gram-positive bacterial infections.

Gram-positive bacterial infections can also be classified as purulent and nonpurulent infections **(Table 2)**. Purulent infections are generally caused by *staphylococci* and nonpurulent by *streptococci*.

Impetigo

Impetigo is a contagious superficial skin infection. There are two main clinical forms including nonbullous impetigo (impetigo contagiosa) and bullous impetigo.

Nonbullous impetigo is caused mainly by *Staphylococcus aureus*, less often by *streptococci*, or by a

TABLE 1: Major cutaneous infections caused by *staphylococci* and *streptococci*.			
	Direct infection (Primary pyoderma)	**Secondary infection (Secondary pyoderma)**	**Cutaneous disease due to bacterial toxins**
Staphylococcal infections	• Impetigo • Ecthyma • Folliculitis • Sycosis • Furunculosis • Carbuncle • Abscess • Cellulitis (occasional) • Acute paronychia • Botryomycosis	• Eczema • Infestations • Ulcers	• Staphylococcal scalded skin syndrome • Toxic shock syndrome • Recurrent toxin-mediated perineal erythema
Streptococcal infections	• Impetigo • Ecthyma • Erysipelas • Cellulitis • Perineal streptococcal dermatitis • Streptococcal intertrigo • Blistering distal dactylitis	• Eczema • Infestations • Ulcers	• Scarlet fever • Toxic-shock-like syndrome • Recurrent toxin-mediated perineal erythema

CHAPTER 1: Cutaneous Gram-positive Bacterial Infections

TABLE 2: Purulent and nonpurulent infections.	
Purulent infections	**Nonpurulent infections**
• Folliculitis • Furuncle • Carbuncle • Abscess • Purulent cellulitis	• Impetigo • Ecthyma • Erysipelas • Classical (nonpurulent) cellulitis

combination of both. In cases with streptococcal impetigo, *Streptococcus pyogenes* is the most common causative agent implicated. Impetigo contagiosa represents about three-fourths of all cases of impetigo, with peak incidence at 2–6 years of age. It is highly contagious both by direct contact and fomites. Often rapid dissemination occurs in day-care centers and schools.

Bullous impetigo is almost always caused by *S. aureus*, Group II, phage type 71. The exfoliative (epidermolytic) toxins A and B produced by this species act as trypsin-like serine proteases and cleave desmoglein-1 in the desmosomes in stratum granulosum. Bullous impetigo is often less contagious than nonbullous impetigo. It usually occurs sporadically. The lesions are localized due to a local production of the toxin, whereas lesions in staphylococcal scalded skin syndrome (SSSS) are generalized as the toxin is disseminated hematogenously. The organism can generally be cultured from the blister fluid.

Clinical Features

Impetigo Contagiosa

The initial lesion is a thin-walled vesicle on an erythematous base. It is seldom seen as it rapidly ruptures, leaving a superficial erosion covered with purulent discharge. The discharge dries up forming the characteristic honey-colored crusts resembling "glued-on cornflakes" **(Figs. 1 and 2)**. The crusts tend to be thicker and dirtier in the streptococcal form **(Fig. 3)**. Lesions are about 1–2 cm in size and grow centrifugally. They are generally asymptomatic except for mild itching. Satellite lesions, caused by self-inoculation, are frequent and a linear distribution of lesions can be seen at sites of scratching **(Fig. 4)**. There is predominant involvement of exposed areas, i.e., the limbs and face, particularly around the nose and mouth where the lesions tend to be extensive **(Fig. 5)**. Regional lymphadenopathy is common, but fever is rare.

Bullous Impetigo

The vesicles progressively enlarge up to 1–2 cm in size and persist for 2–3 days instead of rupturing rapidly. The blister fluid, initially clear **(Fig. 6)**, becomes frank purulent

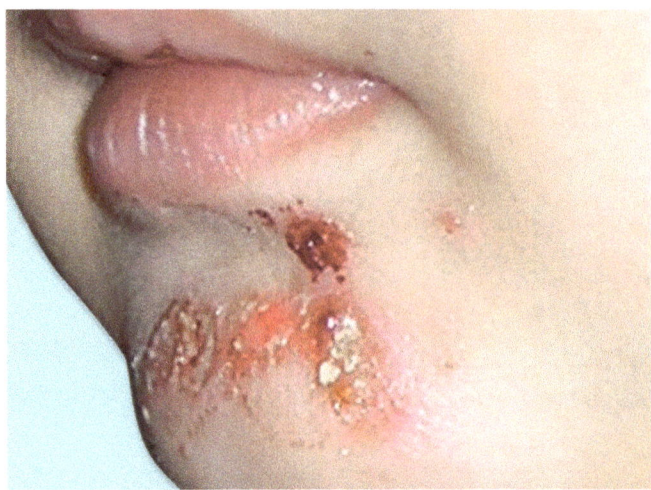

FIG. 1: Localized lesion of impetigo contagiosum (nonbullous impetigo). Superficial erosions with honey-colored crusts are seen.

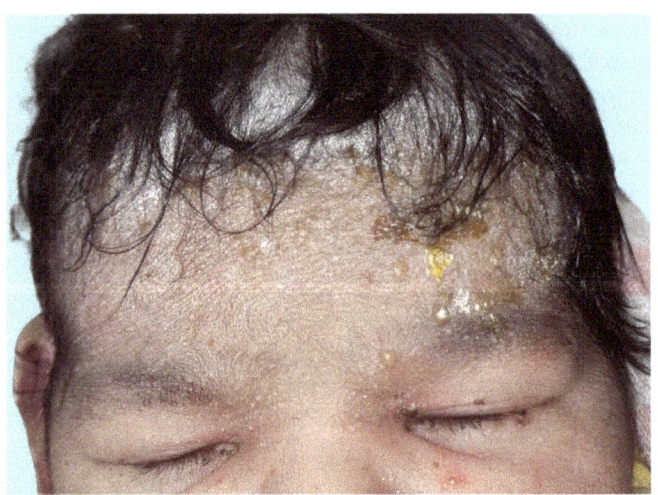

FIG. 2: Honey-colored crusts in a neonate suggestive of impetigo.

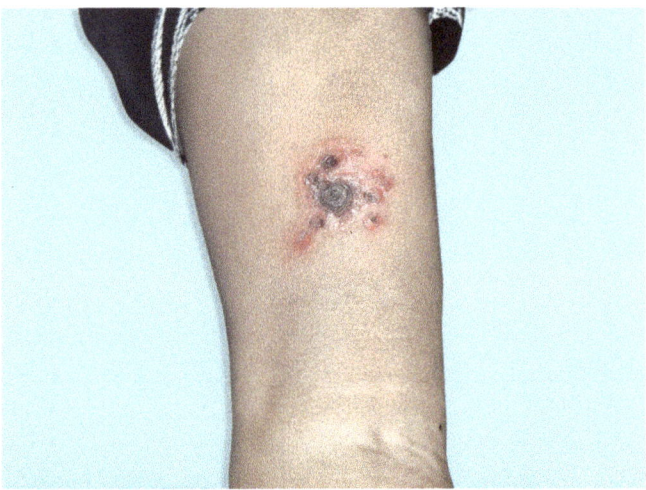

FIG. 3: Localized nonbullous impetigo on the leg in a young child with hemorrhagic crusting.

CHAPTER 1: Cutaneous Gram-positive Bacterial Infections

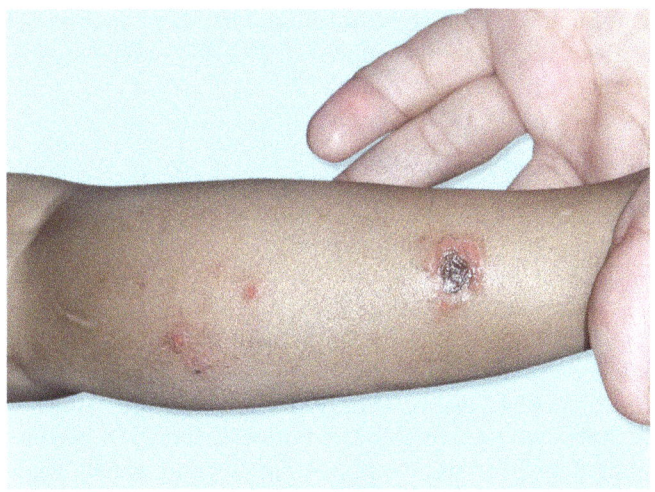

FIG. 4: Linearly distributed lesions of impetigo on the arm in a young child.

later **(Fig. 7)**. On blister rupture, an erythematous, shiny wet base is seen covered by flat, brownish crusts. Circinate lesions and polycyclic figures are commonly seen due to the confluence of lesions, central healing, and peripheral extension. Bullous impetigo often involves the intertriginous regions, such as the diaper area, axillae **(Fig. 8)**, and neck. The face is less often affected. Scalp involvement is common in children with tinea capitis. The buccal mucosa may also be involved. Regional lymphadenopathy is usually absent.

Course

Impetigo contagiosa tends to resolve spontaneously over 2–3 weeks without any scarring. Temporary postinflammatory pigmentary changes (hypo or hyperpigmentation) may be seen in darker individuals.

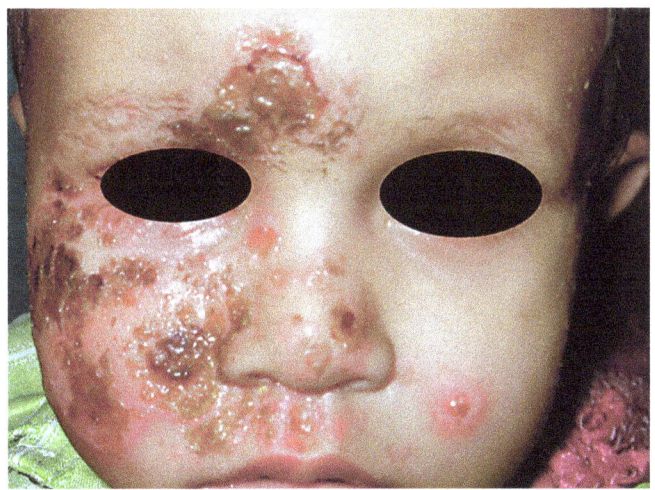

FIG. 5: Extensive lesions of impetigo with characteristic honey-colored crusts, in a malnourished child.

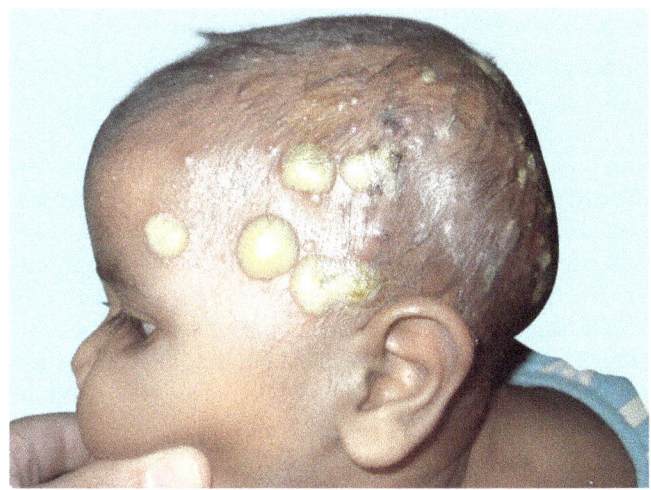

FIG. 7: Extensive purulent lesions of bullous impetigo in an infant.

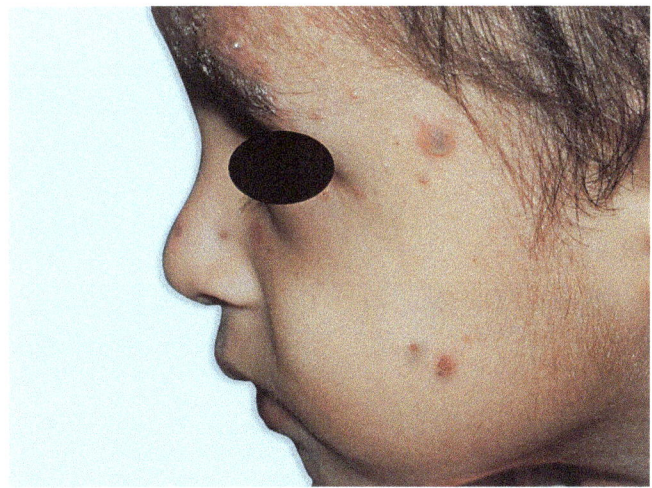

FIG. 6: Lesions of bullous impetigo involving the face in a young child.

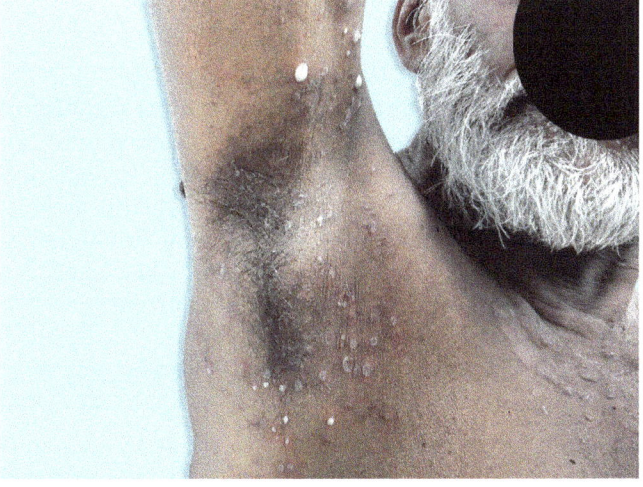

FIG. 8: Extensive lesions of bullous impetigo involving the axillae in an adult.

CHAPTER 1: Cutaneous Gram-positive Bacterial Infections

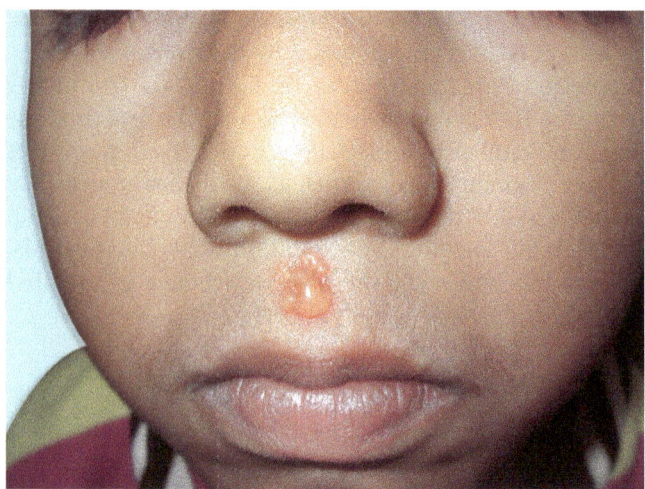

FIG. 9: Bullous impetigo (early-stage clear fluid) in a child involving the "dangerous area of the face."

Complications

Impetigo may progress to deeper infections including cellulitis, especially in the streptococcal form, in the setting of malnutrition, or underlying systemic disease. Other rare potential complications include sepsis, osteomyelitis, arthritis, endocarditis, lymphangitis or lymphadenitis, guttate psoriasis, and toxic shock syndrome. Involvement of the centrofacial part including the upper lip (dangerous area of the face) is associated with a potential risk of ascending infection and cavernous sinus thrombosis **(Fig. 9)**. Acute poststreptococcal glomerulonephritis is a serious complication that affects 1–5% cases of nonbullous impetigo.

Differential Diagnosis

- Herpes simplex infection
- Bullous scabies
- Bullous tinea pedis/manuum

Investigations

The diagnosis of impetigo is made mainly on clinical grounds. Gram-stained smears of the blister content can help identify the etiologic organism, both *staphylococci* and *streptococci*. Pus culture and sensitivity are not routinely done; however, may be pertinent if methicillin-resistant *Staphylococcus aureus* (MRSA) is suspected, the infection is resistant to treatment or is recurrent.

Ecthyma

Ecthyma is a cutaneous bacterial infection that extends into the dermis and heals with scarring. It can be caused by both *streptococci* and *staphylococci*, either alone or in combination. Predisposing factors include poor hygiene, malnutrition, tropical climate, and other dermatoses, particularly scabies.

Clinical Features

The defining lesion of ecthyma is an erythematous plaque, 2–3 cm in diameter, which develops overlying vesiculation or pustulation. It rapidly ruptures resulting in the formation of hard, thick, adherent crusts over an underlying area of ulceration with an indurated and violaceous margin **(Figs. 10 and 11)**. Often there are multiple such lesions **(Fig. 12)**. Common sites affected include feet, legs, thighs, and buttocks. It may be accompanied by fever and lymphadenopathy and usually heals with scarring.

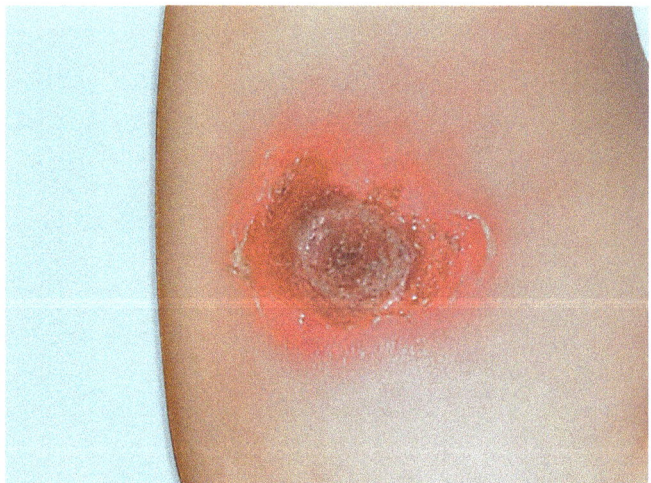

FIG. 10: Ecthyma with thick adherent crust.

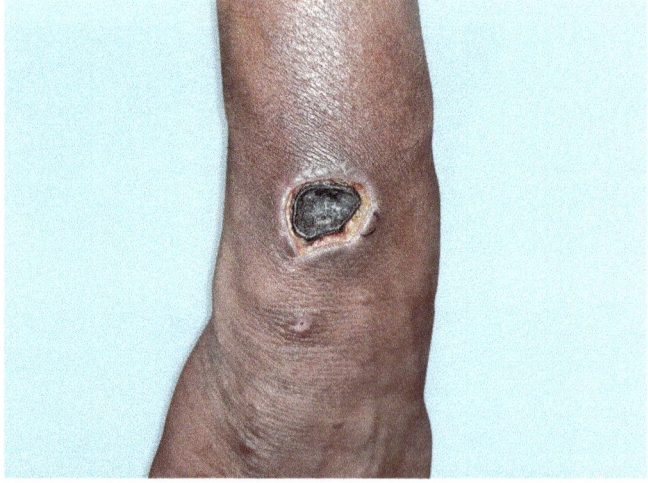

FIG. 11: Thick adherent eschar in a typical lesion of ecthyma over the lower leg.

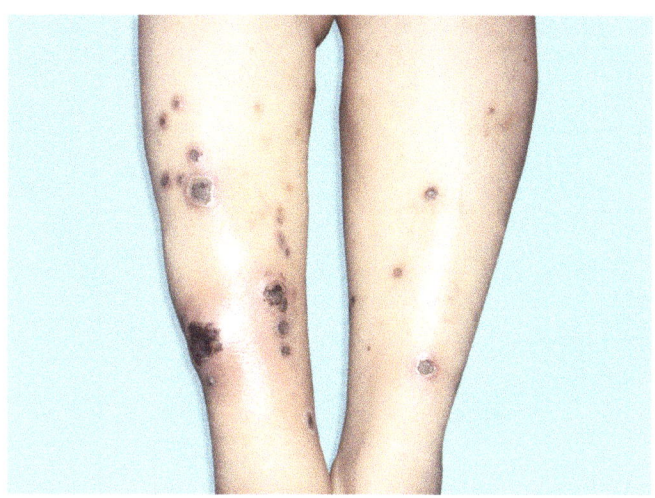

FIG. 12: Multiple lesions of ecthyma involving both legs in a young male.

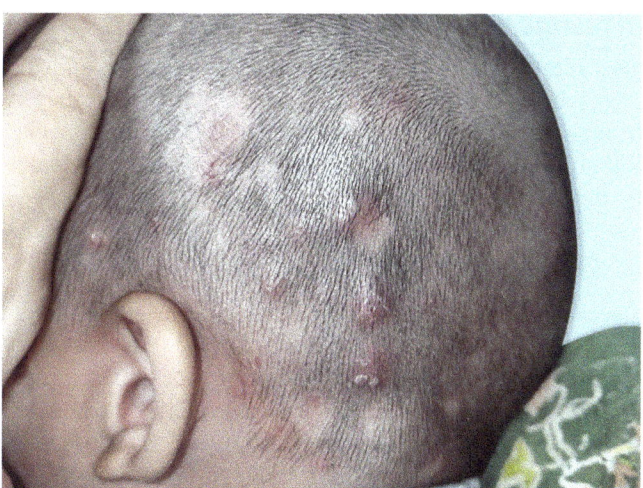

FIG. 13: Multiple lesions of scalp folliculitis in an infant.

Diagnosis

Ecthyma is a clinical diagnosis. Partial removal of the crust, followed by Gram-stained smears from the ulcer base can help confirm the etiology. The same methodology can be used for collecting specimens for pus culture and sensitivity, if the need arises (as detailed further).

Differential Diagnosis

Other conditions which may present similarly include arthropod bites, stasis ulcers, leishmaniasis, and atypical mycobacterial infection. Gram-staining and culture of pus or exudates can help to confirm the diagnosis.

Folliculitis

Folliculitis is an inflammatory disorder of the hair follicle. *S. aureus* is the most frequent cause of bacterial folliculitis. Other implicated pathogens include *Streptococcus*, *Pseudomonas* (hot tub folliculitis), *Proteus*, and coliform bacteria. Various types of folliculitis caused by *S. aureus* include superficial folliculitis (Bockhart's impetigo) and deep folliculitis (sycosis).

Superficial Folliculitis (Bockhart's Impetigo)

Bockhart's impetigo occurs worldwide at all ages, though it is most common in childhood. Inflammatory changes are confined to the follicular infundibulum/orifice. Predisposing factors include nasal carriage of *S. aureus*, occlusion, hot and humid temperature, any itchy skin diseases (e.g., scabies and eczema), diabetes mellitus, obesity, frequent shaving, or vigorous application of topical corticosteroids.

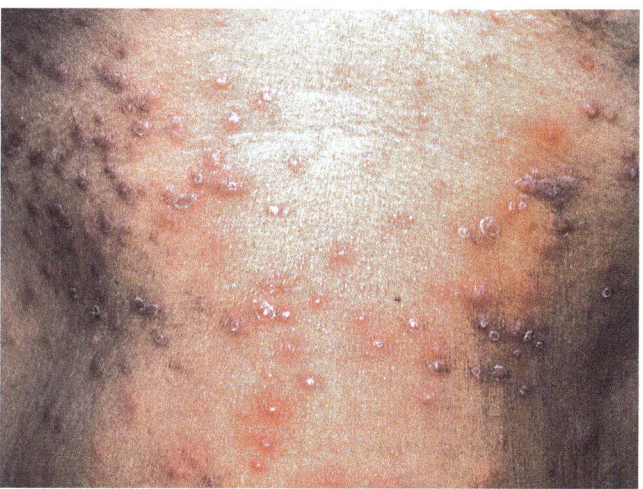

FIG. 14: Folliculitis of the beard region.

Clinical Features

There are dome-shaped, yellow pustules, sometimes surrounded by a narrow, red areola **(Fig. 13)**. The pustules develop in crops, become crusted, and heal within 7–10 days, without scarring. Lesions are often itchy, but pain is rare. A hair shaft can frequently be seen in the center of the pustule. It can affect any hair-bearing area including face **(Fig. 14)**, scalp, buttocks, or axillae in children, or legs in adolescent girls and boys. Occasionally, the follicular pustules may develop into furuncles.

Differential Diagnosis
- Miliaria pustulosa
- Subcorneal pustular dermatosis
- Dermatophytosis
- Herpetic folliculitis

Investigations

Gram stain of the pus can help in confirming the diagnosis. Potassium hydroxide scrapings help to rule out any fungal etiology. A Tzanck smear is useful in case herpetic folliculitis is suspected. Pus culture and sensitivity may be done if MRSA is suspected.

■ Deep Folliculitis (Sycosis)

Deep folliculitis refers to inflammation of the entire follicle or its deeper portion (isthmus and below). It is caused by *S. aureus*. This condition affects males after puberty; most commonly in the third or fourth decade of life. The affected individuals often tend to have lesions on the seborrheic area, with greasy skin, and chronic blepharitis.

Clinical Features

The disease usually affects the upper lip and beard area; hence, the term sycosis barbae **(Fig. 15)**. Individual lesions are edematous, red, follicular papules or pustules **(Fig. 16)**. These may be discrete or coalesce to form a plaque studded with pustules, resembling the appearance of a ripe fig **(Fig. 17)**. There is usually some crusting and scaling. However, the hair is retained and there is no evident scarring. Commonly, it is a subacute process with exacerbations of varying duration, occurring at irregular intervals over months or years. In more chronic forms, scarring may occur, destroying the follicles **(Fig. 18)**. Active papules and pustules are seen at the advancing margin around a pink atrophic scar (lupoid sycosis).

Differential Diagnosis

Pseudofolliculitis caused by ingrowing hairs, tinea barbae, and kerion (fungal infections) of the beard area are the common differentials.

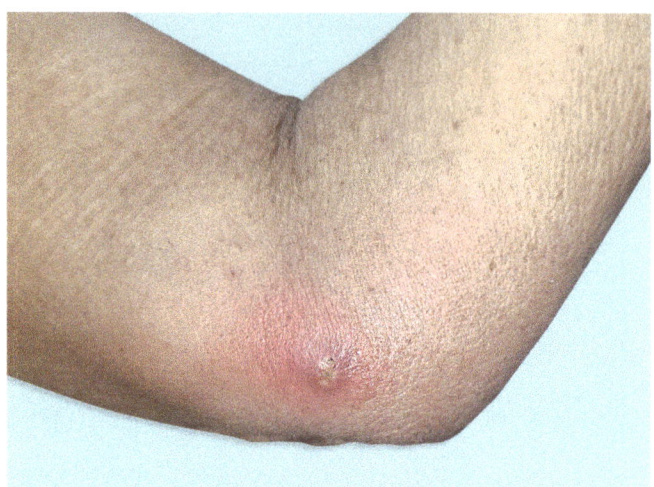

FIG. 16: Lesion of deep folliculitis near the elbow.

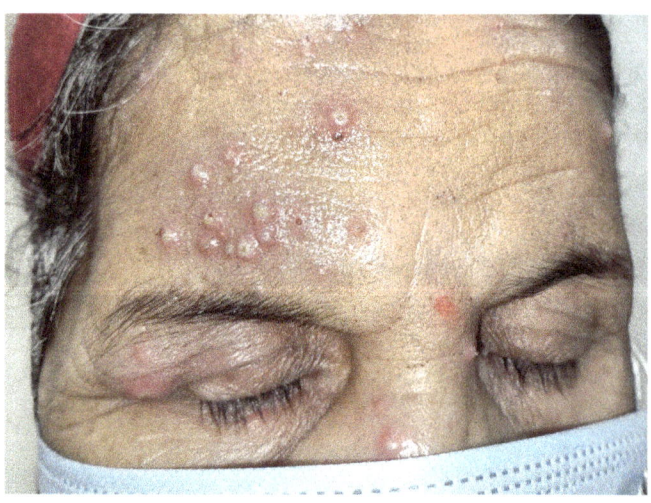

FIG. 17: Multiple lesions of folliculitis over the forehead.

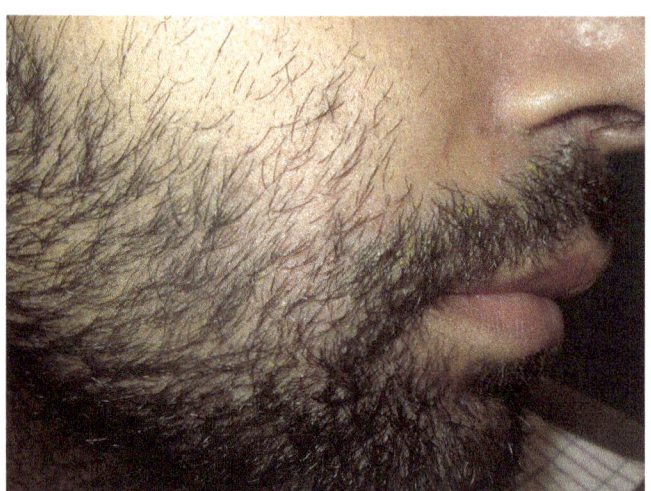

FIG. 15: Sycosis barbae in an adult male.

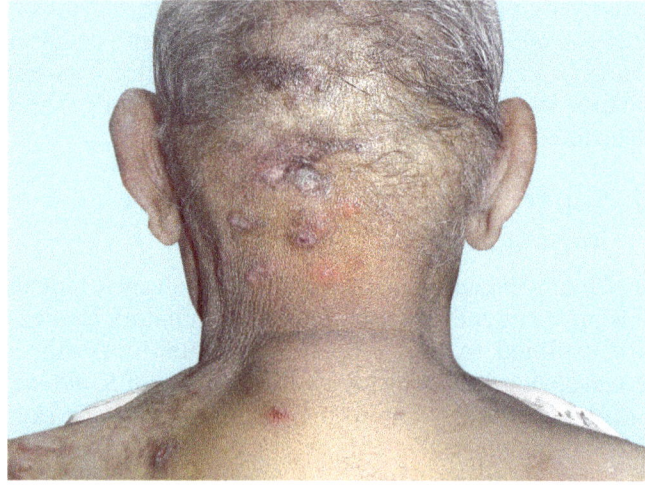

FIG. 18: Folliculitis involving the occipital area in an elderly male.

Investigations

Diagnosis may be confirmed with Gram-stained smears. Bacterial culture and sensitivity can help in resistant cases.

Furuncles (Boil)

A furuncle is an abscess involving a hair follicle (usually, vellus hair) along with the perifollicular tissue. It results in necrosis and destruction of the follicle.

Clinical Features

A furuncle begins as a small, follicular, erythematous, firm nodule, which develops into a fluctuant mass. It eventually opens onto the skin surface, allowing the purulent contents to drain **(Figs. 19A and B)**. Once the necrotic contents are discharged, it heals to leave a violaceous macule and, ultimately, a permanent scar. Furuncles may be single or multiple and tend to appear in crops. Body areas exposed to friction and heavy sweating are favored sites. Lesions commonly arise on the face, neck, arms, buttocks, and anogenital region. These are always tender with larger lesions developing throbbing pain. Fever and mild constitutional symptoms may be present. Furuncles in certain areas such as the nose and external ear canal can be severely painful.

Complications

Patients with recurrent furunculosis may keep on developing crops of new lesions for many months. Malnourished and immunocompromised patients may develop septicemia as a complication. Cavernous sinus thrombosis is a rare and dangerous complication seen with lesions on the upper lip and cheek (a dangerous area of the face).

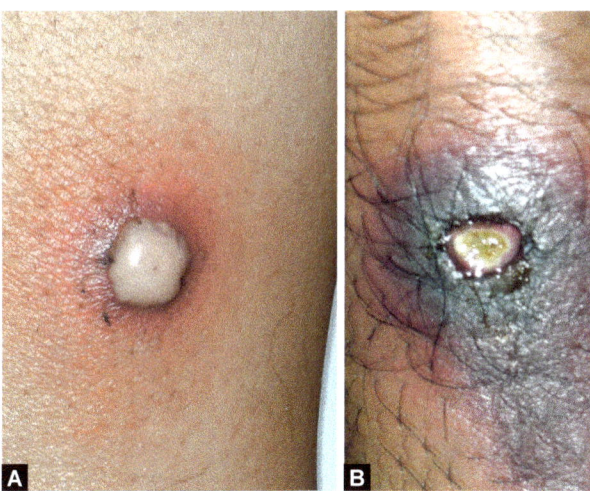

FIGS. 19A AND B: Classical lesion of furuncle on the leg.

Differential Diagnosis

- Folliculitis
- Disseminated herpes simplex
- Nodulocystic acne
- Pilonidal cyst
- Cutaneous myiasis

Investigations

The diagnosis is mostly made clinically, though Gram-stained smears from the deeper lesion can help confirm. Pus culture sensitivity may be required in cases with poor response. In cases with recurrent furunculosis, nasal swabs should be taken to rule out staphylococcal carriage.

Carbuncle

Carbuncle is a deep infection involving multiple contiguous hair follicles and the intervening tissue including subcutaneous fat. This type is almost always caused by *S. aureus*. Carbuncle is commoner in middle- or old-aged men, in the setting of diabetes, malnutrition, cardiac failure, drug addiction, severe generalized dermatoses (erythroderma or pemphigus), and during prolonged steroid therapy. It is less often seen in apparently healthy people.

Clinical Features

The lesion begins as a smooth, dome-shaped painful hard lump. Over a few days, it enlarges into a broad, swollen, erythematous, deep, and painful mass (3–10 cm or more), discharging pus through multiple follicular orifices. Necrosis of the intervening skin leaves a yellow slough surmounting a crateriform nodule **(Figs. 20 and 21)**. Lesions are usually solitary and most commonly involve the back of the neck, especially in diabetics. Other common sites include the shoulders, hips, and thighs. The lesion has been likened to a red-hot coal **(Fig. 22)**. Constitutional symptoms, including fever and malaise, are commonly associated.

Diagnosis

Gram-stained smears and pus culture with sensitivity are recommended to confirm the diagnosis.

Differential Diagnosis

Anthrax should be considered. It can be differentiated by the presence of hemorrhagic crust and vesicular margin.

CHAPTER 1: Cutaneous Gram-positive Bacterial Infections

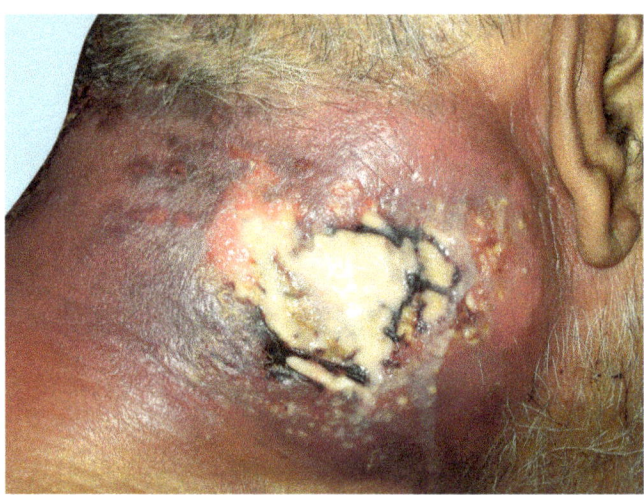

FIG. 20: Carbuncle of the neck in an uncontrolled diabetic.

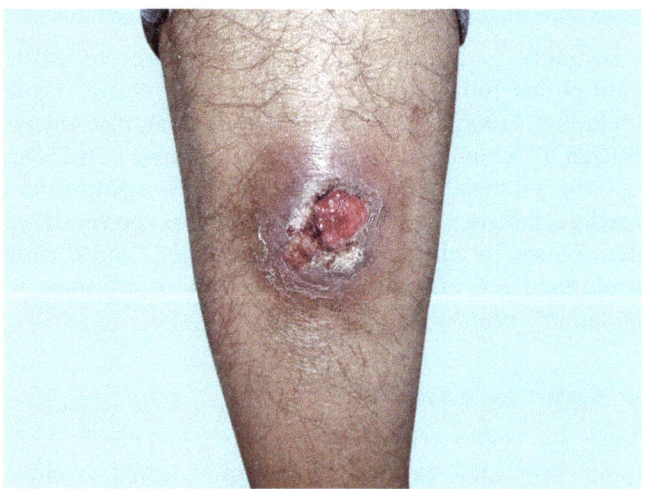

FIG. 21: Carbuncle over leg in an adult diabetic male.

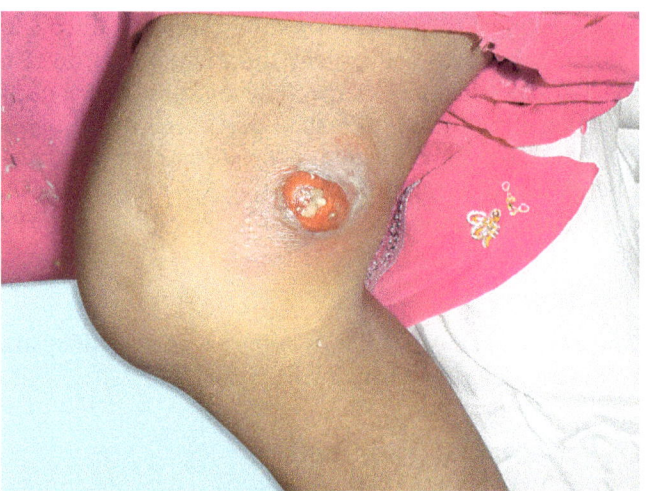

FIG. 22: A carbuncle appearing like a "red-hot coal" in a human immunodeficiency virus (HIV)-positive patient.

Cutaneous Abscess

It refers to a collection of pus within the dermis and deeper skin tissues. The vast majority of cases are caused by *S. aureus*, especially MRSA. However, lesions adjacent to a mucous membrane (perioral, vulvovaginal, or perirectal) or those associated with injection drug use, may be polymicrobial in etiology.

Clinical Features

A cutaneous abscess presents as a painful, swollen, red, tender, and fluctuant mass **(Fig. 23)**, often surmounted by a pustule and encircled by a rim of erythematous swelling **(Fig. 24)**. The common sites of involvement are the extremities and trunk. The abscess can be associated with surrounding cellulitis. Abscesses that extend deeper

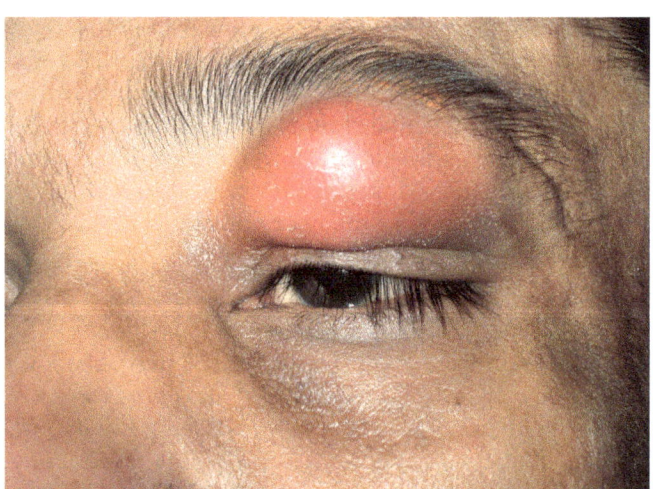

FIG. 23: Fluctuant abscess over left upper eyelid.

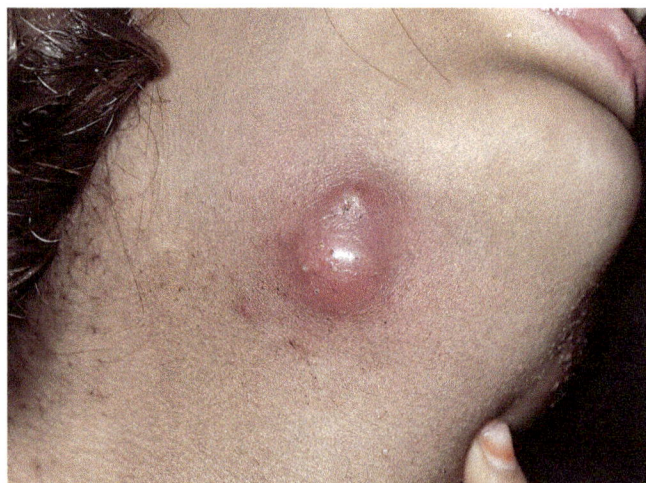

FIG. 24: Abscess involving the neck and surmounted by a pustule.

CHAPTER 1: Cutaneous Gram-positive Bacterial Infections

into the dermis and subcutaneous tissue, especially those associated with extensive cellulitis, may be more difficult to diagnose because overlying tissue edema and induration may prevent fluctuance from being observed.

Differential Diagnosis

These include an inflamed epidermoid cyst, or hidradenitis suppurativa (in the axillae and perineum).

Investigations

The diagnosis is usually clinical. If there is confusion with cellulitis, needle aspiration is used to differentiate the two. Aspirated pus confirms the presence of an abscess. High-resolution ultrasonography is a highly sensitive tool to accurately differentiate an abscess from cellulitis. Gram-stained smears and pus culture and sensitivity from the aspirated pus should be done, especially in cases with systemic symptoms.

Staphylococcal Scalded Skin Syndrome (Ritter's Disease)

Staphylococcal scalded skin syndrome is caused by *S. aureus* phage type II. The pathogenesis is similar to that of bullous impetigo; however, in SSSS, the staphylococcal exfoliative toxin (ET) is disseminated hematogenously. Exfoliative toxin (ETA) and exfoliative toxin B (ETB) (more virulent) are the two exotoxins linked to SSSS.

Clinical Features

Staphylococcal scalded skin syndrome is generally seen in children < 5 years of age, though adults may be rarely affected, particularly in the setting of renal failure, malignancy, immunosuppression, or alcohol abuse. Predilection for newborns and young children is attributed to decreased renal clearance of ET and/or the lack of antitoxin antibodies. The trigger is usually a localized staphylococcal infection (skin or a distant/occult site such as otitis, conjunctivitis, pneumonia, or urinary tract). There is a prodrome of fever, irritability, and malaise, followed by the development of skin tenderness. An initial complaint may even be a "tummy ache" due to tender skin over the abdomen. Mild erythema involving the flexures may be seen **(Fig. 25)**. Even before the initial eruption, the child may show positive Nikolsky's sign (skin erosion upon tangential pressure). This is followed by faint, erythematous, tender patches, which become well-demarcated over a few hours. The lesions coalesce into a widespread erythematous eruption and progress rapidly to blistering, with large sheets of epidermal detachment **(Fig. 26)**, beginning on the face, axillae, groin, and neck.

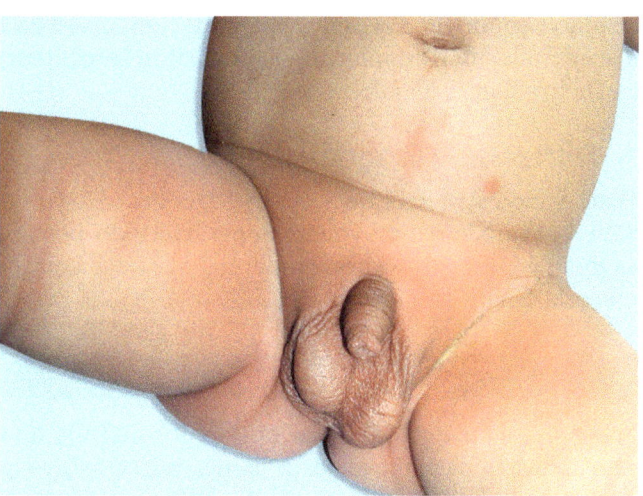

FIG. 25: Faint tender erythema of groin; the beginning of staphylococcal scalded skin syndrome (SSSS) in an infant.

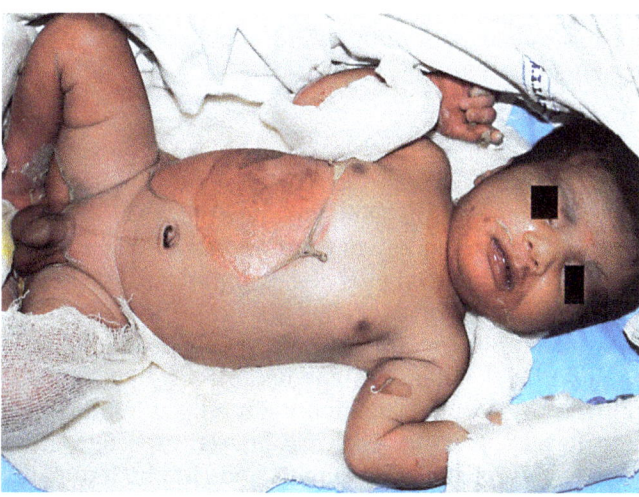

FIG. 26: Sheet of epidermal detachment in staphylococcal scalded skin syndrome (SSSS).

This leads to extremely painful moist, raw, red areas that appear scalded. Within 2 weeks the skin generally heals without scarring.

Complications

The prognosis is usually good in children (mortality < 5% in treated children). However, in adults, mortality up to 63% has been reported, possibly due to underlying comorbidities. Acute skin failure may be accompanied by fluid and electrolyte imbalance, temperature dysregulation, and secondary infection necessitating intensive care and prompt management.

Diagnosis

The diagnosis is mostly clinical as skin swabs and culture of blister fluid will not grow the organism. However, the results of culture and sensitivity patterns from blood and the original site of staphylococcal infection (if evident) can help in better management.

■ Differential Diagnosis

Toxic epidermal necrolysis is a close differential. However, SSSS is characterized by more superficial skin peeling as there is no full-thickness epidermal necrosis. Lack of mucosal lesions also favors SSSS.

Erysipelas

Erysipelas is a bacterial infection of the dermis and sometimes, upper subcutaneous tissue, caused by Group A beta-hemolytic *Streptococcus*. It is often seen in very young or very old patients. Predisposing factors include disruption of the cutaneous barrier (by wounds, fissured toe-web, intertrigo, pressure ulcers, venous insufficiency, local surgical operations), and subclinical lymphatic dysfunction of the legs.

■ Clinical Features

It is characterized by an abrupt onset of a single, erythematous, warm, painful plaque with a well-defined, clearly demarcated, raised edge, and advancing margin. The well-defined edge is the hallmark of erysipelas, distinguishing it from cellulitis **(Fig. 27)**. The skin surface may resemble an orange peel (peau d'orange) due to superficial cutaneous edema surrounding the hair follicles. Blistering is common. Superficial hemorrhage into the blisters or intact skin may be seen, especially in the elderly. Associated lymphangitis and lymphadenopathy are frequent. The most commonly affected site is the leg, followed by the face **(Fig. 28)**. In newborns, the

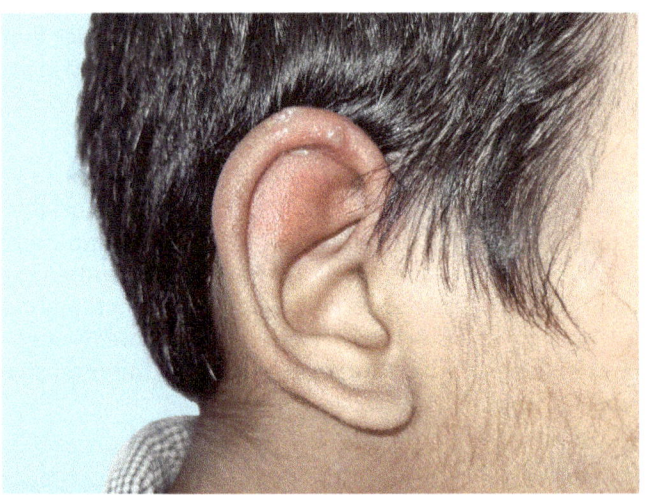

FIG. 27: Erysipelas involving the ear in a boy. The well-defined margin of inflammation is seen.

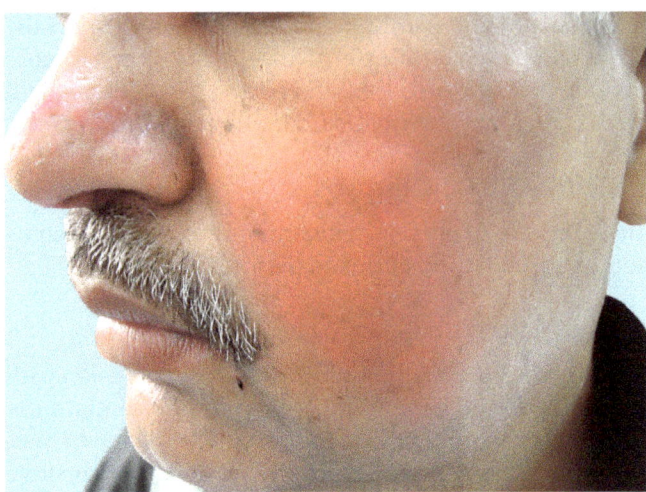

FIG. 28: Erysipelas involving the face in an adult male.

periumbilical area is often affected. Bilateral facial infection may occasionally occur. Associated systemic symptoms such as fever, malaise, and vomiting can be quite severe. The response to treatment is quite rapid as compared to cellulitis.

■ Complications

Recurrent erysipelas occurs in about 20% of cases. It most frequently involves the legs, possibly due to damage to lymphatics. If the treatment is delayed in an acute stage, an infection may extend deeper, progressing to necrotizing fasciitis and septicemia. Poststreptococcal glomerulonephritis is also a potential complication.

■ Differential Diagnosis

- Cellulitis
- Necrotizing fasciitis
- Contact dermatitis
- Deep vein thrombosis

■ Diagnosis

Erysipelas can be diagnosed clinically. Blood counts usually show slight leukocytosis and a raised erythrocyte sedimentation rate. Blood cultures are usually negative. Histopathology shows a neutrophil-rich interstitial infiltrate, within a markedly edematous dermis with dilated lymphatics and capillaries. Giemsa or Gram stain may show the presence of streptococci within the tissue and lymphatics.

Cellulitis

Cellulitis is a common, rapidly spreading infection of the dermis and subcutaneous tissues. The predisposing factors are similar to those for erysipelas. In addition, obesity, a prior episode of cellulitis, and diabetes mellitus (specifically linked to purulent cellulitis) may predispose. The majority of cases are caused by *streptococci*, especially in immunocompetent patients. *S. aureus* (alone or together with streptococcus) is implicated at times, especially in cases with purulent cellulitis. *Haemophilus influenzae* type B is an important cause of facial cellulitis in young children < 2 years of age, often associated with otitis media.

Clinical Features

Cellulitis presents with a recent onset of pain, redness, warmth, and swelling of the involved area, with poorly demarcated borders **(Fig. 29)**. Constitutional symptoms may be present. The most commonly affected sites are the lower limbs **(Fig. 30)**, though upper limbs, trunk, perineum, or head and neck may also be involved. Commonly there is a history of a predisposing condition. There may be associated blistering, with superficial blisters filled with clear fluid. Petechiae and ecchymoses may develop resulting in hemorrhagic cellulitis. Associated lymphangitis and lymphadenopathy are less frequent.

Complications

Severe cellulitis can progress to dermal necrosis **(Fig. 31)**. If not treated promptly, cellulitis can lead to serious complications including fasciitis, myositis, subcutaneous abscesses, and septicemia. Periorbital and orbital cellulitis may be complicated by cavernous sinus thrombosis, orbital, subperiosteal or cerebral abscess formation, or meningitis.

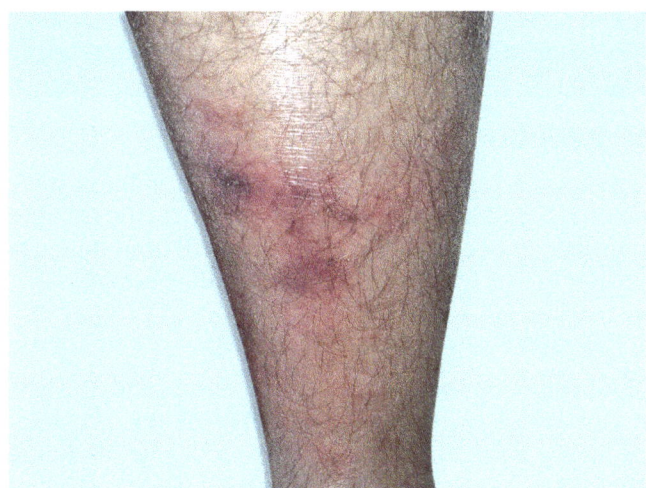

FIG. 30: Early lesion of cellulitis in an adult male.

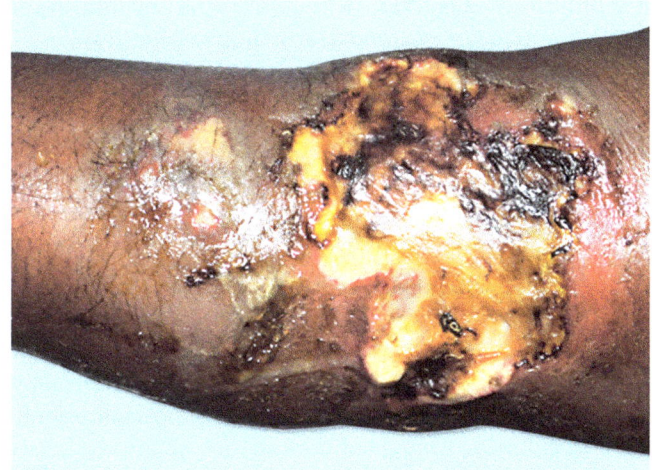

FIG. 31: Purulent cellulitis involving the leg with dermal necrosis in a diabetic man.

The response to treatment can be quick in early and superficial cases; however, it usually takes several days of parenteral antibiotics before significant improvement occurs. Recurrences are common. Lymphedema, venous insufficiency, chronic postcellulitic edema, tinea pedis, and obesity predispose to frequent recurrences.

Differential Diagnosis

Cellulitis is differentiated from necrotizing fasciitis, which is a life-threatening infection requiring immediate surgical intervention. Warning signs for necrotizing fasciitis include purple blisters, necrosis, ecchymosis, very severe pain, marked edema extending beyond the limits of erythema, woody hard induration, crepitus, cutaneous anesthesia, and marked systemic toxicity including hypotension, tachycardia, body temperature below 35°C, or above 40°C, and confusion.

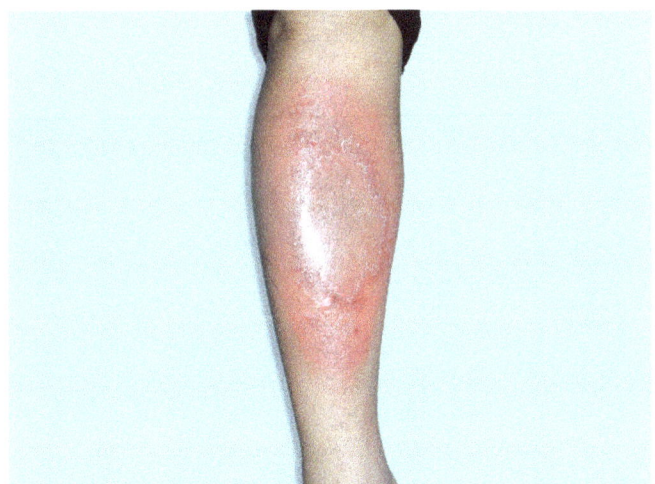

FIG. 29: Cellulitis involving the leg in an adult male. Note the ill-defined border with marked erythema and swelling.

CHAPTER 1: Cutaneous Gram-positive Bacterial Infections

Other Gram-positive Infections Caused by Staphylococci and Streptococci

Periporitis Staphylogenes

This results from secondary infection of miliaria by *S. aureus* **(Fig. 32)**. It is often seen in children in the summer months. It needs to be differentiated from miliaria pustulosa which is characterized by sterile pustules.

Acute Paronychia

This is most commonly caused by *S. aureus* and presents as a painful erythematous swelling of the proximal or lateral nailfold. It is associated with pus discharge **(Fig. 33)**. The swelling soon becomes fluctuant, producing a nailfold abscess which may assume a horse-shoe shape **(Fig. 34)**. It may even extend to the distal nailfold uncommonly **(Fig. 35)**. If fluctuant, paronychia often needs drainage in addition to systemic antibiotics.

Botryomycosis

This is a granulomatous and suppurative infection caused by *S. aureus*. It presents as crusted plaques, ulcers, and sinus tracts draining purulent material. It is commonly seen to involve the legs and feet.

Blistering Distal Dactylitis

It is typically considered to be a streptococcal infection; however, it is often caused by staphylococci, especially when multiple bullae are seen as well. It is most commonly seen in children, though adults can also be affected. It is characterized by a large tense bulla on an erythematous base, containing thin, seropurulent fluid. It usually arises on the palmar pad of the distal digital phalanx. The blister

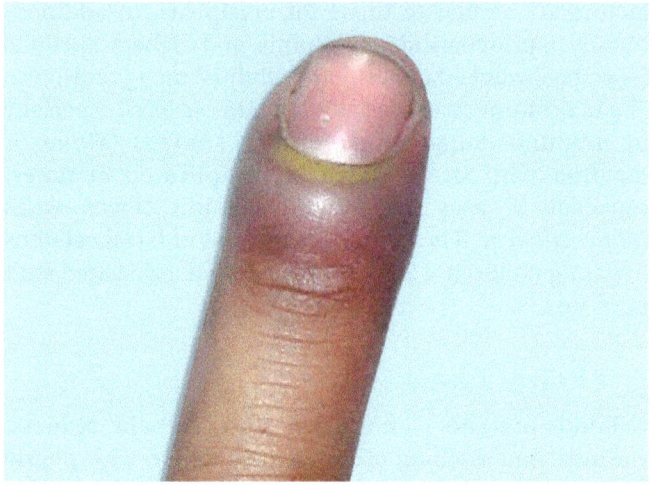

FIG. 33: Acute paronychia.

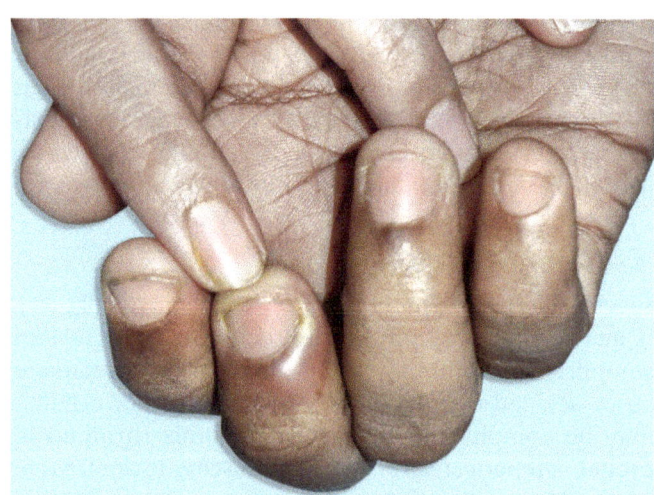

FIG. 34: Acute paronychia with pus tracking along the lateral nailfold.

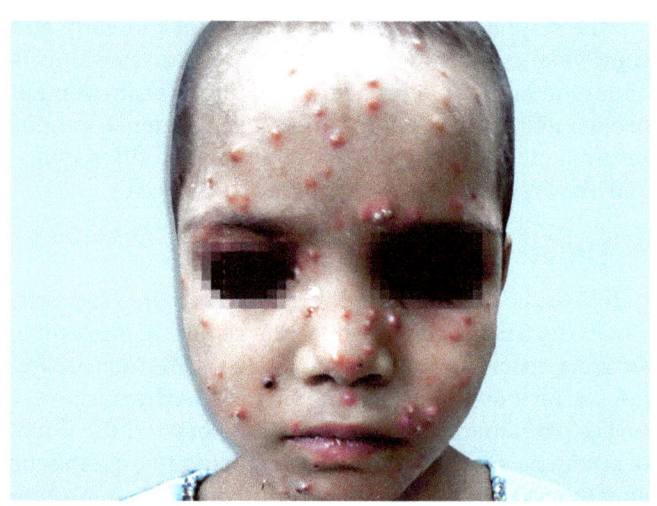

FIG. 32: Periporitis staphylogenes.

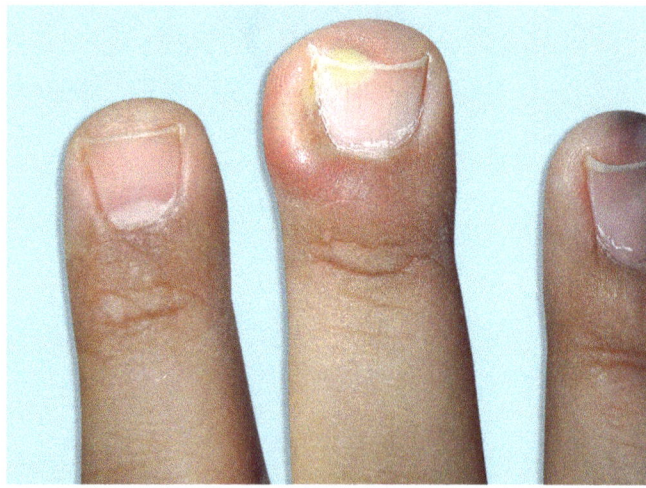

FIG. 35: Severe acute paronychia with pus tracking along the lateral nailfold and pointing towards the distal nailfold and distal nail bed.

may rupture forming erosions. Etiological organisms can be cultured from blister fluid. Apart from systemic antibiotics, blister drainage is required.

Secondary Pyodermas

Secondary pyodermas are very common and may produce diagnostic difficulty. These are associated with a variety of underlying conditions that alter the integrity of the cutaneous barrier to infections. These include atopic dermatitis **(Fig. 36)**; eczemas of other causes including seborrheic dermatitis or stasis eczema; infestations including scabies and pediculosis **(Fig. 37)**; fungal infections including tinea capitis and cruris **(Fig. 38)**; bullous disorders, e.g., pemphigus **(Fig. 39)**; mechanical conditions including ingrown nail **(Fig. 40)**, etc. Correspondingly, it is important to understand that unless

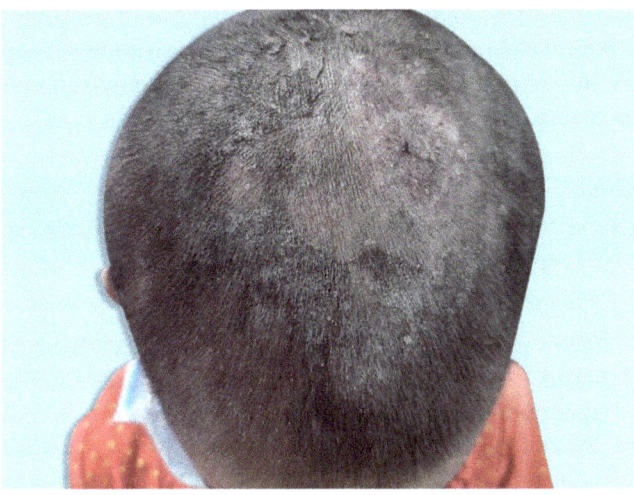

FIG. 38: A child with tinea capitis with scaling and crusting suggestive of secondary bacterial infection.

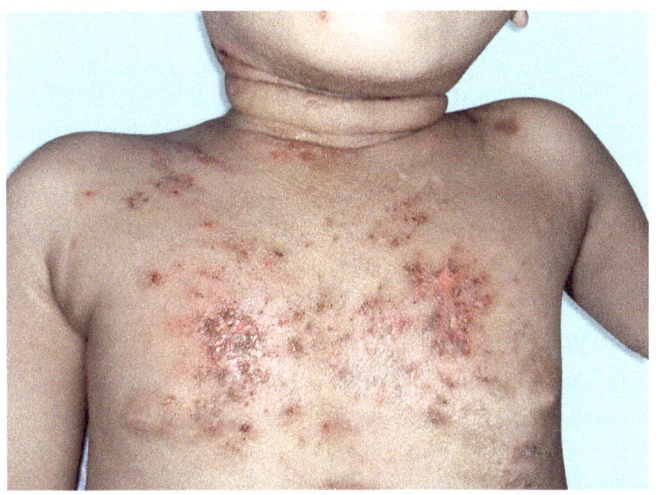

FIG. 36: Extensive impetiginization in a child with atopic dermatitis.

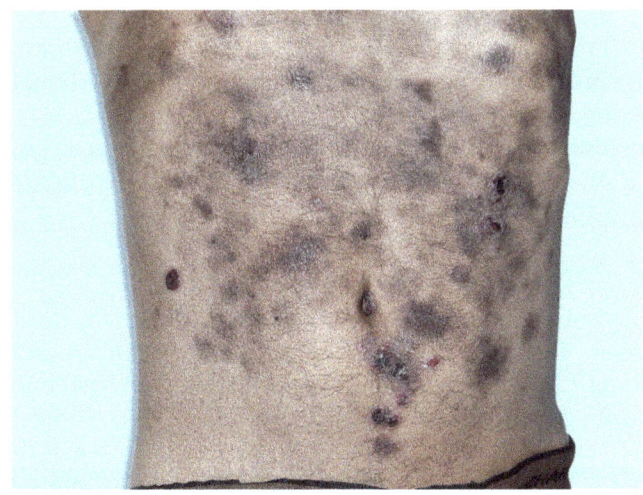

FIG. 39: An adult male with pemphigus vulgaris, on treatment with steroids, showing secondary infection and crusting of lesions.

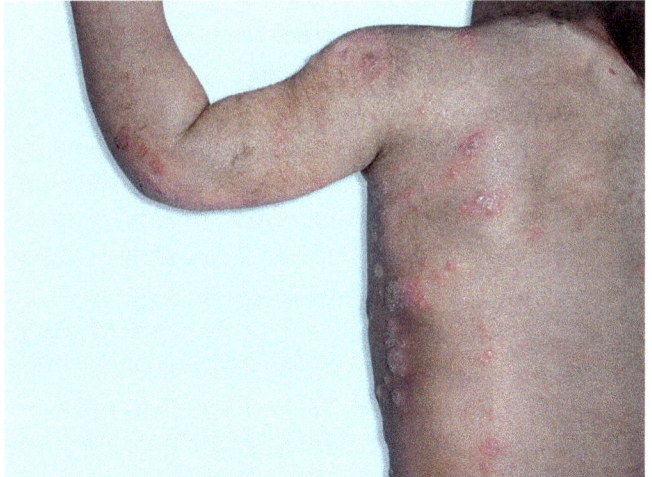

FIG. 37: Impetiginized lesions of scabies in an infant.

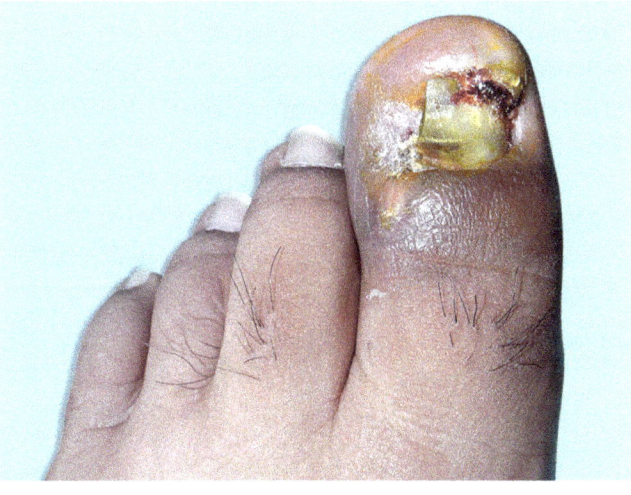

FIG. 40: Ingrown toenail with secondary infection of the nailfold.

the underlying condition is identified and appropriate therapy is instituted for that condition, the pyoderma may be only partially responsive to therapy and may keep on recurring.

Treatment of Infections Caused by Staphylococci and Streptococci

General Measures

- Strict hygiene practices include regular washing of hands and separate towels/clothes to prevent the spread of infection among family members.
- Regular bathing and cleaning of the lesions with common soap and water is recommended. Soaps containing antiseptic substances, such as triclosan and chlorhexidine may be used.
- Crusts should be removed gently after application of a greasy emollient to soften the area.
- Predisposing factors such as diabetes, malnutrition, and underlying causes of immunosuppression should be addressed.
- Underlying dermatoses including scabies, pediculosis, or eczema need to be treated in cases with secondary pyodermas.

Topical Antibiotic Therapy

Topical antibiotics are the treatment of choice for most cases. These may be used either alone (localized and superficial infections) or in combination with systemic antibiotics (deeper or extensive infections). Topical antibiotics need to be applied twice daily till the lesion heals. The following commonly used agents are effective against staphylococcal and streptococcal infections.

- Fusidic acid 2%
- Mupirocin 1%
- Retapamulin 1%
- Nadifloxacin 1% cream

Systemic Antibiotic Therapy

Systemic antibiotics are indicated for:
- Widespread/extensive lesions in bullous or nonbullous impetigo.
- Deeper infections such as folliculitis, ecthyma, erysipelas, cellulitis, and abscesses.
- Toxin-mediated disease, such as SSSS.
- In cases with constitutional symptoms, such as fever and lymphadenopathy.
- Infections near the oral cavity or scalp.

Ideally, the choice of antibiotic should be guided by culture and sensitivity results. However, pus culture and sensitivity are not routinely resorted to. Empirical therapy involves the use of agents active against staphylococci and streptococci **(Table 3)**. Unless cultures yield streptococci alone, antimicrobial therapy should be active against both *S. aureus* and streptococci.

Severe Infections with Significant Systemic Symptoms

The Infectious Diseases Society recommendations include a similar treatment approach for cutaneous abscesses,

TABLE 3: Oral antibiotics.

Agents covering MSSA + streptococci	Adult dosage	Child dosage
Dicloxacillin	250–500 mg QID	25 mg/kg/day, 6 hourly
Cephalexin	250–500 mg QID	25–50 mg/kg/day in three to four divided doses
Erythromycin	250 mg QID	40 mg/kg/day in three to four divided doses
Clindamycin	150–300 mg QID	20 mg/kg/day in three divided doses
Amoxicillin-clavulanate	• 500/125 mg TDS • 875/125 mg BD	25 mg/kg/day of amoxicillin component in two divided doses
If MRSA is suspected or confirmed		
Cotrimoxazole	800/160 mg DS tablets BD	TMP 4–6 mg/kg/dose BD
Clindamycin	150–300 mg QID	10–13 mg/kg/dose 6–8 hourly, not more than 40 mg/kg/day
Doxycycline	100 mg BD	Above 8 years If <45 kg 2 mg/kg/dose BD
Minocycline	200 mg stat followed by 100 mg BD	If <45 kg 4 mg/kg stat followed by 2 mg/kg BD (above 8 years)
Linezolid	600 mg BD	10 mg/kg/dose BD, not to exceed 600 mg/dose

(BD: twice a day; MRSA: methicillin-resistant *Staphylococcus aureus*; MSSA: methicillin-susceptible *Staphylococcus aureus*; QID: four times a day; TDS: thrice a day; TMP: trimethoprim)

furuncles, and carbuncles. Additional measures to be decided on a case-to-case basis include:
- *Incision and drainage with antibiotic therapy*: This may be recommended for paronychia, abscess, etc.
- *Surgical inspection/debridement*: This is of paramount importance if deeper infections, especially necrotizing fasciitis, are suspected.
- *Intravenous antibiotics*: These are recommended for patients with severe infections, comorbidities, suspected poor bioavailability, poor response to oral antibiotics, or multiple recurrences. Antibiotics targeting MRSA include vancomycin (30 mg/kg/day in two divided doses); piperacillin/tazobactam (4 g piperacillin/0.5 g tazobactam given every 8 hours); amikacin (15 mg/kg/day divided IV/IM every 8–12 hours) or linezolid (10 mg/kg every 8–12 hours) should be initiated for 7–14 days.
- Culture and sensitivity should be promptly sent (pus and blood) to guide further treatment.
- Adequate coverage from gram-negative and anaerobic organisms should be added in suspected cases of polymicrobial infections.

Diseases Caused by Coryneform Bacteria

Coryneform bacteria are gram-positive, nonsporing, rod-shaped organisms commonly referred to as diphtheroids. Many different strains of aerobic coryneform bacteria are part of the normal flora of human skin. However, the overgrowth of some of these organisms can cause chronic superficial skin infections, as covered in this section.

Erythrasma

Erythrasma is a mild, chronic superficial skin infection of the tropics caused by *Corynebacterium minutissimum*, a collective term used for a group of closely related aerobic coryneform bacteria. It is more common in overweight and obese patients, elderly, and diabetics.

Clinical Features

The sites involved include the inguinal, interdigital, intergluteal, and crural folds, as well as the submammary areas **(Fig. 41)**. It is characterized by well-circumscribed, irregular, red-brown plaques and patches, present discretely **(Fig. 42)**. The initial red color later becomes brown. New lesions are smooth, but older lesions tend to be finely creased. In temperate climates, most lesions are asymptomatic but, in the tropics, irritation and pruritus may lead to scratching and lichenification, especially in the groins.

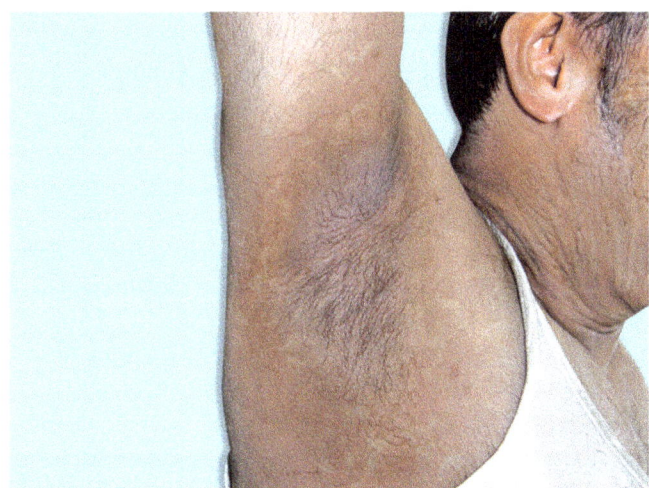

FIG. 41: Erythrasma involving axillae.

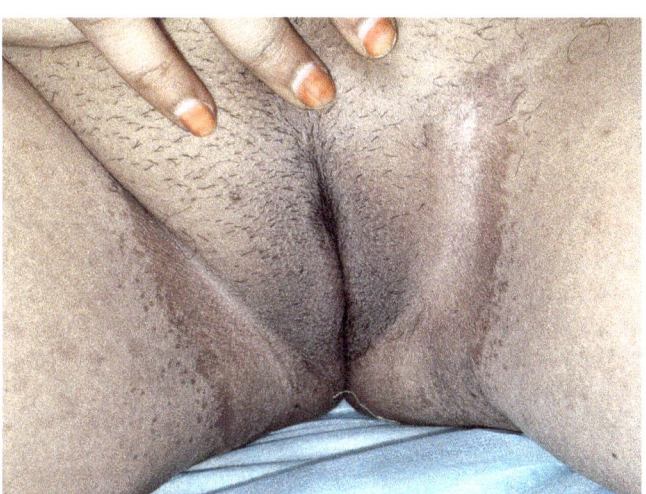

FIG. 42: Erythrasma in an adult female, involving the crural area.

Diagnosis

Wood's lamp often reveals bright purple-red (coral red) fluorescence attributable to the presence of coproporphyrin III in the lesions. Skin scrapings from the affected skin may show bacteria and fine filaments, visible on Gram stain, Giemsa stain, and even potassium hydroxide (KOH) mounts.

Differential Diagnosis

- Superficial dermatophytosis (differentiated by relative lack of inflammation, complete absence of vesiculation, and absence of satellite lesions).
- Pityriasis versicolor (differentiated by color changes).
- Candidiasis (absence of satellite lesions points against *Candida*).

- Flexural psoriasis (often associated with psoriasis elsewhere).
- Acanthosis nigricans (velvety skin thickening).

Treatment

- Erythromycin (250 mg four times daily for 2 weeks) is the treatment of choice.
- Erythrasma responds well to most topical azole antifungals, such as miconazole 2% or clotrimazole 1% cream.
- Oral tetracyclines and 2% fusidic acid for topical use are also recommended.

Trichobacteriosis (Trichomycosis Axillaris)

It is an asymptomatic superficial bacterial infection of the hair shaft involving large skin folds. The etiological agent is *Corynebacterium* species and *Serratia marcescens*. It occurs in both temperate and tropical climates and is not limited to any race or sex. Predisposing factors include a warm and moist environment and poor hygiene.

Clinical Features

It is usually asymptomatic, and the patient is often unaware of its presence. It is characterized by pale yellowish (even red to black) adherent, small, granular nodules, or fine sheaths, encasing the hair shafts. The yellow type is the most common **(Fig. 43)**, while the black type is the rarest. These nodules consist of a bacterial biofilm and are found involving axillary or (less commonly) pubic hair. The axillary sweat may turn yellow, black, or red according to the color of the concretions, staining the clothing.

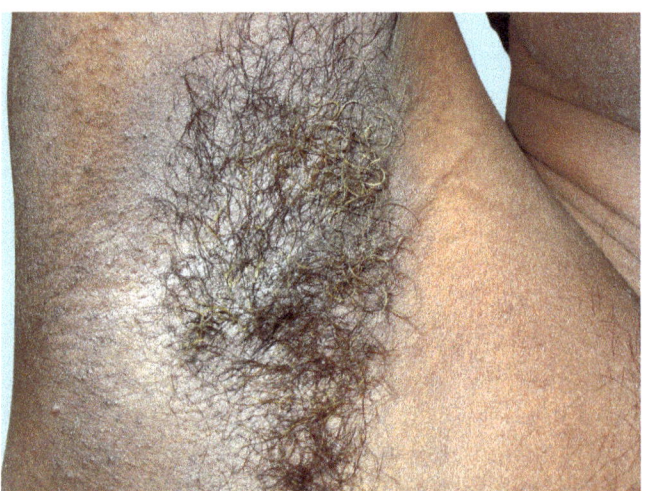

FIG. 43: Yellowish concretions of trichomycosis involving axillary hair.

Diagnosis

The diagnosis is usually clinical. Wood's lamp examination reveals a pale-yellowish fluorescence. Gram-stain and KOH examination can help confirm the diagnosis.

Differential Diagnosis

- Pediculosis
- Piedra

Treatment

- Clipping or shaving the axillary and pubic hair is recommended.
- Application of topical antimicrobials (benzoic acid compound ointment, erythromycin, clindamycin lotions, or imidazole creams) can help in resolution.
- Antiperspirants, e.g., anhydrous aluminum chloride, helps resolution and prevention of recurrence.
- Rubbing the hairs while bathing helps disrupt the biofilm, making the bacteria more accessible to topical antiseptic treatment.

Pitted Keratolysis

It is a chronic, noninflammatory, superficial bacterial infection of the skin, confined to the stratum corneum. It is caused by gram-positive cocci *Micrococcus sedentarius*, *Corynebacterium species*, or both. These bacteria can invade keratin softened by sweat.

Pitted keratolysis is common in tropical regions, in individuals who walk barefoot. In the Western population, the risk factors include occlusive shoes, maceration, and poor hygiene. It appears more frequently in farmers, military personnel, and some athletes. Adult males with sweaty feet are most susceptible. It is most common during summer and the rainy season.

Clinical Features

The disease usually affects the soles; palmar involvement is seen less often. The most frequent sites of involvement are pressure-bearing areas **(Fig. 44)** such as the ventral aspect of the toe, the ball of the foot, and the heel. In extensive cases, the whole of the sole **(Fig. 45)** and even palms may be involved **(Fig. 46)**. The lesions are composed of numerous conspicuous, discrete, shallow, circular, punched-out, small pits or craters. These may coalesce in places to produce irregular erosions, ranging from 0.5 to 7.0 mm in diameter and 1–2 mm in depth. Soaking the feet in water accentuates the lesions due to swelling of the horny layer. Irritation is minimal; hence, most patients

CHAPTER 1: Cutaneous Gram-positive Bacterial Infections

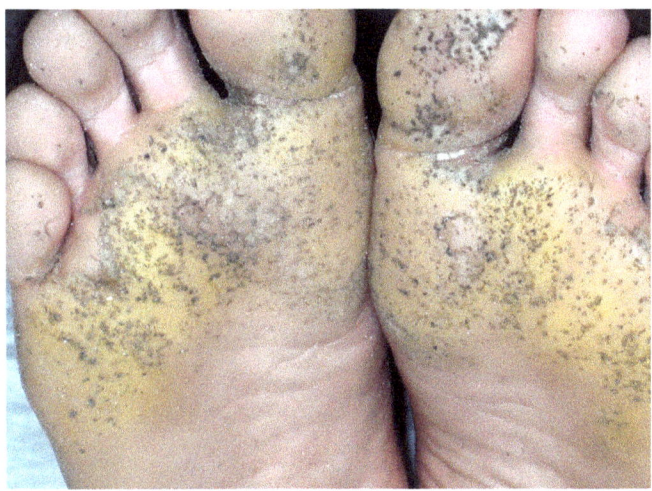

FIG. 44: Pitted keratolysis of both soles.

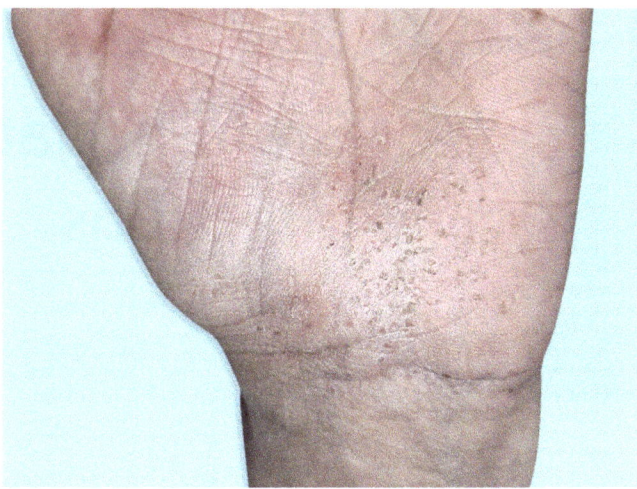

FIG. 46: The same patient showing involvement of the palm as well.

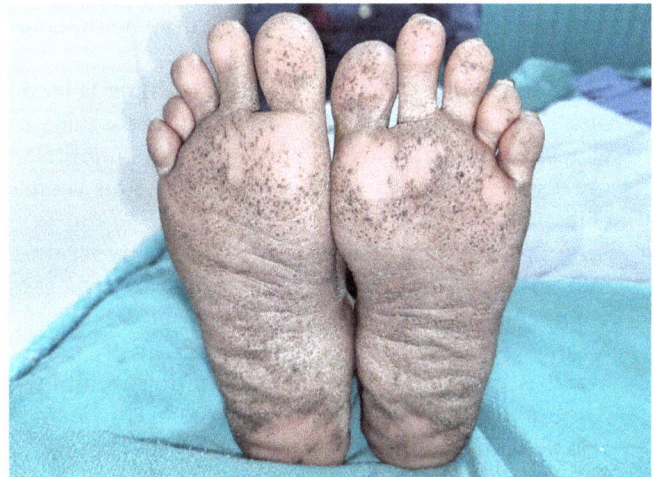

FIG. 45: Extensive pitted keratolysis extending even to the nonpressure bearing areas.

are unaware of the condition. Hyperhidrosis is often associated, sometimes with maceration, stickiness, and foul smell.

Differential Diagnosis
- Plantar warts
- Tinea pedis
- Punctate palmoplantar keratoderma

Diagnosis
The diagnosis is mainly clinical. Gram stain of skin scraps and KOH mounts can help detect organisms.

Treatment
- Maintaining appropriate hygiene is important.
- Controlling hyperhidrosis with the use of open footwear, topical aluminum hydroxide, or botulinum toxin is helpful.
- Socks should be changed regularly and washed at 60°C temperature to inactivate the corynebacteria.
- Oral and/or topical erythromycin are considered the first line of treatment.
- Other options include imidazole, clindamycin, mupirocin, and fusidic acid creams.

CHAPTER 2: Gram-negative Bacterial Infections

Introduction

Gram-negative bacteria are so named because of their inability to retain the primary stain (crystal violet) during the Gram staining procedure; hence, they appear pink in smears. This is due to the lack of a thick peptidoglycan layer in their cell wall. They are much more resistant to antibiotics due to the presence of an additional lipid layer known as the "bacterial outer membrane." Unlike their gram-positive counterparts, gram-negative bacteria do not release exotoxins. Their virulence is mediated by their lipopolysaccharide (endotoxin) layer, and some other components of their cell membrane, making them efficiently capable of producing septicemia much more frequently.

Most of the cutaneous lesions associated with gram-negative infections are manifestations of systemic infection, rather than being skin and soft tissue infections; however, some of them are capable of producing primary cutaneous infections as well, which may later systematize. The important gram-negative infections with cutaneous features are summarized in this chapter.

Meningococcal Infections

These are infections caused by *Neisseria meningitidis*. Meningococcal asymptomatic nasopharyngeal carriage is the most common infection. Predisposing factors for clinically manifest meningococcemia include immunosuppression, asplenia, deficiency of terminal complement components, and components of the properdin pathway.

Clinical Features

Meningococcemia can manifest as an acute or chronic disease as well as postmeningococcal reactive disease.

Acute Meningococcemia

- It is characterized by fever, meningitis, and purpuric skin rash, which in the early stages may be indistinguishable from a viral exanthema.
- Later the lesions may progress to bullous **(Fig. 1)** or hemorrhagic lesions (purpura fulminans) due to widespread microvascular occlusion and endothelial necrosis involving dermal and subcutaneous vessels **(Figs. 2A and B)**.
- Angulated cutaneous infarcts with hyperemic margins and a "gun-metal" gray center are typical of meningococcemia.
- Associated pneumonia, pyogenic arthritis, osteomyelitis, purulent pericarditis, endophthalmitis, conjunctivitis, primary peritonitis, or urethritis may also be seen.
- The fatality rate is about 7%, the highest among infants younger than 1 year of age. Morbidity is also

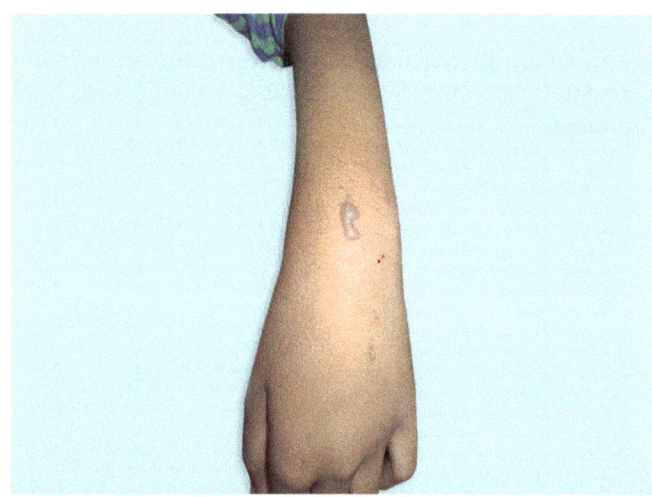

FIG. 1: Bullous lesions appearing on the dorsae of hands in a septicemic child with meningitis.

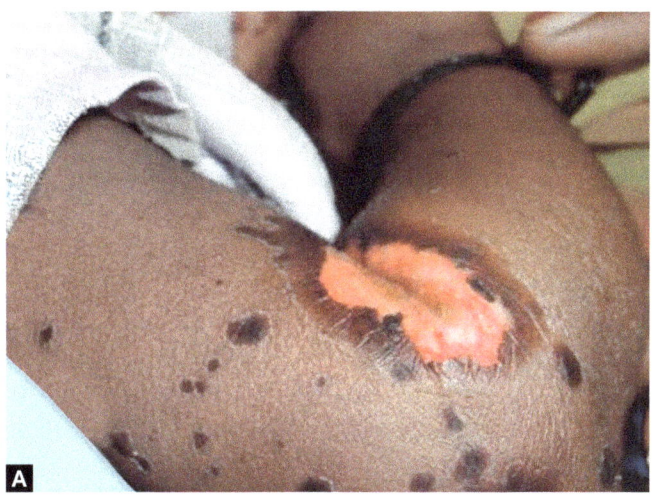 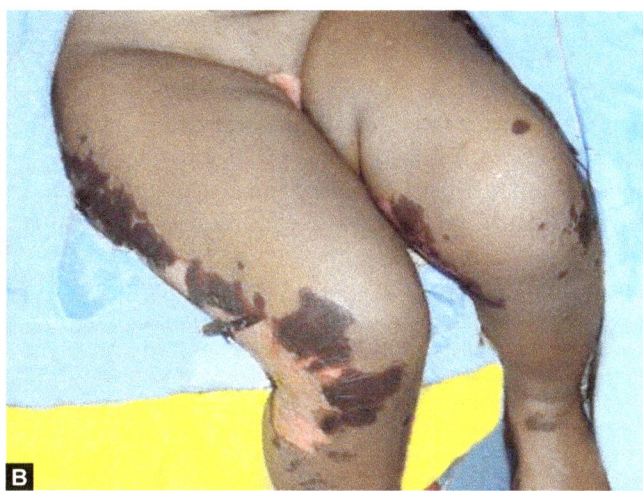

FIGS. 2A AND B: Acute meningococcemia in a child.

high. Around 9–11% of patients may have sequelae (neurologic disability, limb loss, and hearing loss).

Postmeningococcal Reactive Disease
- This is an immune complex-mediated disease, which may develop in some patients 4–10 days after the onset of meningococcal infection.
- It manifests as fever, maculopapular or vasculitic rash, arthritis, iritis, pericarditis, and/or polyserositis.

Chronic Meningococcemia
- It is rare and is characterized by recurrent episodes of fever (lasting for 12 hours) associated with arthralgia/arthritis, and splenomegaly.
- Skin lesions in the form of erythematous macules, vesiculopustular lesions, or purpuric lesions similar to those seen in acute disease, may develop 12–24 hours after the onset of fever.
- Fever and rash tend to resolve concurrently without treatment only to recur over the next 1–4 days.

Diagnosis
- The diagnosis of meningococcal disease is mainly clinical. In clinically suspicious cases, treatment should be instituted without waiting for diagnostic confirmation.
- Organisms can be demonstrated by Gram-stained smears of the skin lesions in about 70% of cases.
- Definitive diagnosis is based on the isolation of the organism from blood, cerebrospinal fluid (CSF), and skin lesion cultures. These are positive in acute disease.
- Molecular diagnosis using polymerase chain reaction (PCR) from blood or CSF samples has better sensitivity and specificity.
- Histopathology of the rash demonstrates leukocytoclastic vasculitis and microvascular thromboses. It may show the organisms within the endothelium.

Treatment
- Prophylaxis with polyvalent meningococcal vaccine is recommended for high-risk groups.
- Prophylaxis of close family contacts is recommended. Rifampicin (10 mg/kg every 12 hours for 2 days) is recommended, with close clinical surveillance. They should be clinically followed up.

Acute Meningococcemia
- Treatment of choice is high-dose intravenous penicillin (penicillin G 300,000 U/kg/day up to 24 MU/day for 10–14 days).
- Third-generation cephalosporins, e.g., ceftriaxone [75–100 mg/kg per day (maximum, 4 g/day) in one or two divided intravenous doses] or cefotaxime [200 mg/kg/day (maximum, 8 g/day) in four divided intravenous doses] may be used empirically to cover other (potentially penicillin-resistant) bacteria that may produce an indistinguishable clinical syndrome.
- A single dose of ciprofloxacin 500 mg should be given after the initial course of antibiotics to clear nasal carriage.

Chronic Meningococcemia
- It should be treated similarly with lower dosages.
- Close contacts should receive prophylactic treatment with rifampicin.

Postmeningococcal Reactive Disease
- It requires only symptomatic treatment as the condition resolves spontaneously without any after-effects.

CHAPTER 2: Gram-negative Bacterial Infections

Pseudomonas Infections

Pseudomonas aeruginosa is mainly responsible for hospital-acquired infections as it is a frequent contaminant of bedpans, showers, sinks, urine bottles, polythene sheeting, and the hands of caregivers. It is ubiquitous and thrives in moist environmental conditions. It frequently colonizes burn wounds, chronic venous ulcers, and other chronic moist lesions. It is also the most common cause of Gram-negative bacteremia among neutropenic patients.

Clinical Features

The spectrum of pseudomonal infections includes:
- Ecthyma gangrenosum
- Otitis externa—swimmer's ear
- Malignant otitis externa (necrotizing otitis externa)
- Green nail syndrome
- *Pseudomonas* folliculitis
- *Pseudomonas* hot-foot syndrome
- Noma neonatorum
- Toe-web infection
- Blastomycosis-like pyoderma

Ecthyma Gangrenosum

Patients with pseudomonal septicemia may develop erythematous macules, developing into tense hemorrhagic vesicles with a typical violaceous margin. The bullae rupture to form ulcers covered with a necrotic eschar **(Fig. 3)**. These distinctive skin lesions generally develop in the setting of pseudomonal septicemia in immunocompromised hosts. It may be commonly seen in old and debilitated individuals with leukemia, severe burns, pancytopenia or neutropenia, terminal carcinoma, those on ventilators, broad-spectrum antibiotics, or cytotoxic drugs. Anogenital area and extremities are frequently involved sites **(Figs. 4 and 5)**. In some instances, such as human immunodeficiency virus (HIV) infection, premature infants, and other immunocompromised states, the lesions may occur at the site of inoculation without accompanying bacteremia.

Malignant Otitis Externa (Necrotizing Otitis Externa)

It is a serious, potentially life-threatening condition caused by *P. aeruginosa*. It is classically described in elderly uncontrolled diabetics, and also seen in HIV/acquired immunodeficiency syndrome (AIDS) patients. Initial symptoms are decreased hearing with lancinating ear pain. The external ear becomes red, swollen, and tender. The ear canal shows inflammation, exudation,

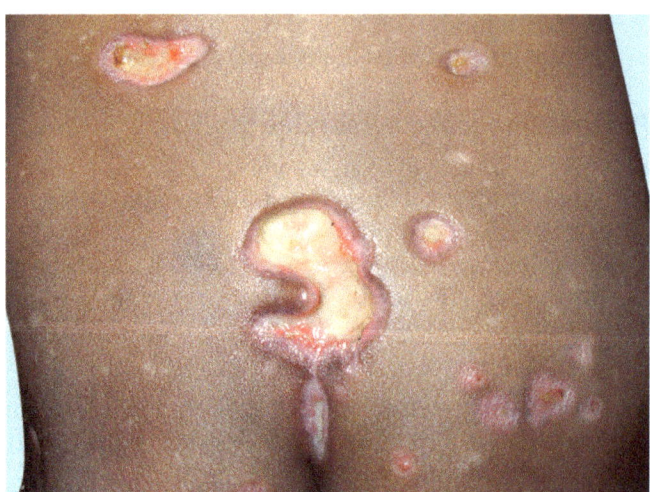

FIG. 4: Involvement in the anogenital area and buttocks.

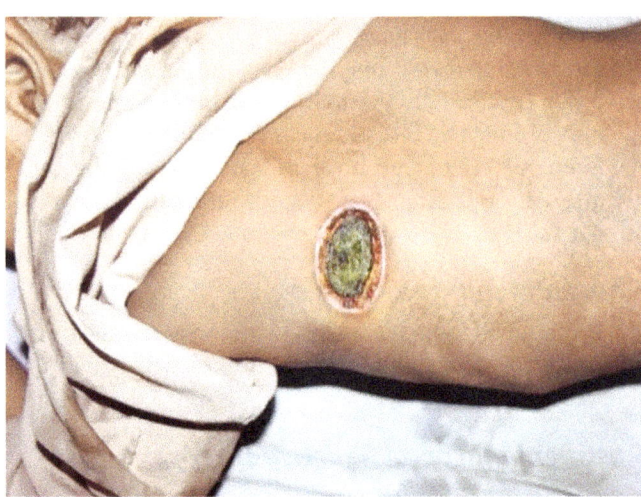

FIG. 3: Ecthyma gangrenosum.

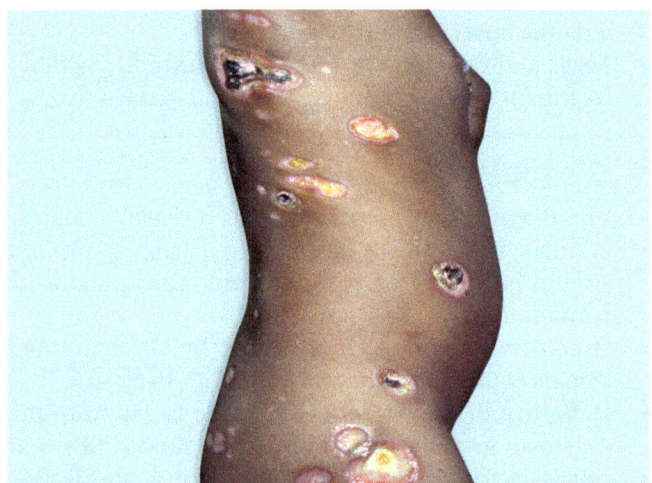

FIG. 5: Extensive areas of deep necrotic ulceration covered with thick eschar in a 3-year-old, malnourished child with *Pseudomonas* septicemia.

and granulation tissue at the junction of the bony and the cartilaginous part. Invasion of cartilage, bone, nerve, and soft tissue can occur resulting in osteomyelitis, facial palsy, mastoiditis, sepsis, and sigmoid sinus thrombosis.

Chloronychia/Green Nail Syndrome (Goldman–Fox Syndrome)

It is characterized by excessive colonization of the nail unit by *P. aeruginosa*. The predisposing factors include prolonged exposure to water, use of detergents, nail trauma, paronychia, onycholysis, etc. The affected nail appears greenish-blue or greenish-black due to the production of pyocyanin pigment by the organism **(Fig. 6)**.

Pseudomonas Folliculitis

It is associated with bathing in hot tubs, whirlpools, and swimming pools in public places. With the rise in water temperature, the growth of *P. aeruginosa* is enhanced leading to "hot tub folliculitis." Lesions appear within 8–48 hours of contact. They are localized mostly on the trunk and flexures, and areas in contact with diving suits colonized by *Pseudomonas*. There may be erythematous macules, pruritic papules, or follicular pustules which resolve spontaneously within a week. Some patients have associated fever, sore throat, eye/earache, etc.

Diagnosis

- Gram-stained smears from lesion exudate may show the organism.
- *Blood culture*: *P. aeruginosa* readily grows on blood agar and MacConkey agar.
- Biopsy and histopathology show epidermal and upper dermal necrosis, with hemorrhage extending into the dermis. A mixed inflammatory infiltrate with necrotizing vasculitis may be seen. Organisms may be visualized within the media and adventitia of the deeper vessels, with characteristic sparing of vessel intima.
- Technetium-99m bone scan is the "Gold standard" for diagnosis in patients with otitis externa.

Treatment

Treatment for suspected pseudomonas septicemia should be instituted empirically, without diagnostic delay.

- *Non-neutropenic patients*: Monotherapy with ceftazidime or cefepime; or combination therapy with piperacillin/tazobactam; or imipenem/meropenem/doripenem with amikacin are recommended.
- *Neutropenic patients*: Cefepime or all other agents (except doripenem) mentioned above are recommended. Granulocyte-macrophage colony-stimulating factor (GM-CSF) may be used adjunctively.
- For malignant otitis externa, cefepime or ceftazidime are used at the same dosages as for bacteremia.
- Ciprofloxacin is recommended for typically longer duration (up to 6 weeks).

Prevention

- Standard precautions should be followed to reduce nosocomial transmission.
- Pseudomonas in burns patients may be eradicated by twice daily application of nadifloxacin 1% cream or silver nitrate (0.5%).

Rickettsial Infections

Rickettsiae are obligate intracellular gram-negative bacteria that naturally reside in blood-sucking arthropods. Human infections are incidental, occurring through bites of such arthropods. The organisms primarily infect the endothelium, leading to vascular infarcts, fluid loss into the interstitium, and disseminated intravascular coagulation. Rickettsial infections are reemerging and prevalent throughout the world. These are grouped as the typhus group, spotted fever group, and rickettsialpox.

Clinical Features

Typhus Group

This group includes epidemic typhus, endemic typhus, and scrub typhus **(Table 1)**. These infections are principally transmitted by scratching or rubbing the fecal matter

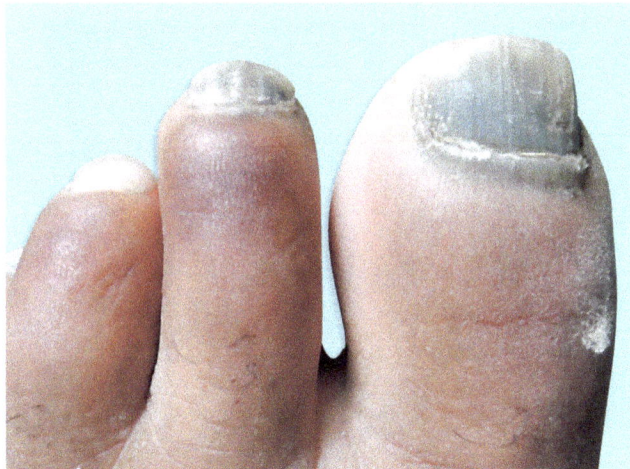

FIG. 6: *Pseudomonas* green nail syndrome.

CHAPTER 2: Gram-negative Bacterial Infections

TABLE 1: Rickettsial infections (typhus group).		
Disease	Causative organism	Vector
Epidemic typhus	*Rickettsia prowazekii*	*Pediculus humanus* var. *corporis*
Endemic typhus	*Rickettsia typhi*	• *Xenopsylla cheopis* (rat flea) • *Ctenocephalides felis* (cat flea)
Scrub typhus	*Rickettsia tsutsugamushi*	• *Tokunagayusurika akamushi* • *Trombicula deliensis* (rodent infesting mites)

of body lice or fleas containing the organism, which are deposited onto the skin during their bite.

Epidemic Typhus (Brill–Zinsser Disease)
- After an incubation period of 7–14 days, an acute febrile illness develops, characterized by fever, headache, prostration with severe myalgia, and cough.
- On the 5th day, an erythematous macular or maculopapular rash develops initially on the trunk and then the entire body except the face, palms, and soles **(Figs. 7A to C)**. The rash may later progress to petechial and purpuric lesions.
- The lesions are accompanied by severe conjunctival injection and photophobia.
- Severe cases may develop cutaneous necrosis leading to gangrene of the extremities and pneumonia.
- Untreated patients may develop renal insufficiency and multiorgan failure with prominent neurological symptoms.

Endemic Typhus
- Clinical manifestations are similar to epidemic typhus except that skin lesions occur in 13–20% of cases.
- A careful examination of axillae and inner surfaces of upper extremities may reveal a rash that is similar to epidemic typhus; however, petechial and purpuric lesions are very uncommon, and gangrene never occurs.
- Pulmonary involvement is prominent.

Scrub Typhus
- It is the most common rickettsial infection in India.
- After an incubation period of 1–2 weeks, an acute fever with chills, headache, myalgia, gastrointestinal symptoms, and pneumonitis develops.
- This is uncommonly accompanied by a maculopapular skin rash, appearing on the trunk and spreading centrifugally. It resolves spontaneously.
- Indurated papulonodules topped with a blister develop at the site of the mite bite, which later breaks down to form an ulcer with eschar. This may be seen in less than half of the cases.

Spotted Fever Group

Rickettsiae causing this group of diseases are transmitted vertically from generation to generation in their reservoirs, through infected ova. In humans, the organisms are injected along with the saliva during the arthropod bites. Rocky Mountain spotted fever, Mediterranean spotted fever, and other spotted fevers in this group, are named after the geographic region in which they are prevalent **(Table 2)**.

This group includes diseases caused by spotted fever group *Rickettsia,* which spread through the bite of infected mites and ticks. The early lesion is mostly an eschar at the site of the tick or mite bite. It develops a few days to a week following the bite of an infected tick or mite.

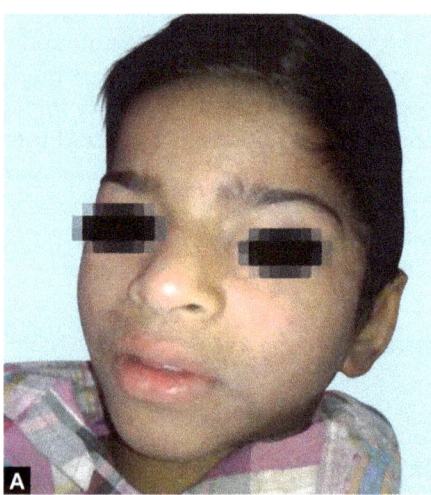
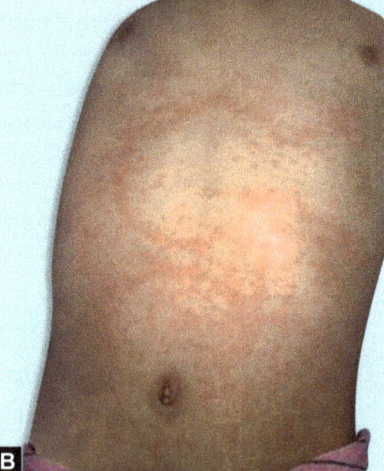
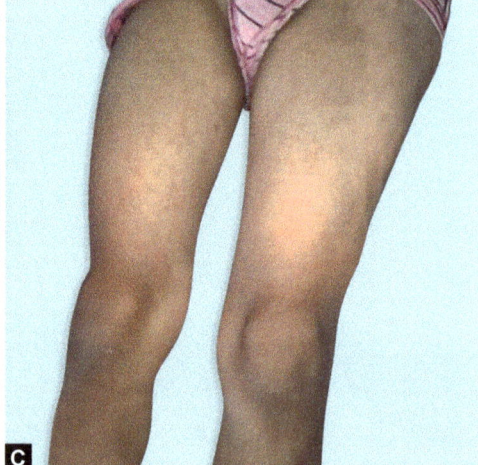

FIGS. 7A TO C: Rickettsial fever with rash.

CHAPTER 2: Gram-negative Bacterial Infections

TABLE 2: Rickettsial infections (spotted fever group).		
Disease	**Organism**	**Vector**
Rocky Mountain spotted fever	*Rickettsia rickettsii*	• *Dermacentor andersoni* (wood tick) • *Dermacentor variabilis* and *Rhipicephalus sanguineus* (dog ticks) • *Amblyomma americanum* (lone star tick)
Mediterranean spotted fever	*Rickettsia conorii*	*R. sanguineus* (brown dog tick)
North Asian tick-borne rickettsiosis	*Rickettsia sibirica*	Tick
Queensland tick typhus	*Rickettsia australis*	Tick
African tick bite fever	*Rickettsia africae*	• *Amblyomma hebraeum* • *Amblyomma variegatum*
Flinders Island spotted fever	*Rickettsia honei*	Tick
Yucatan spotted fever	*Rickettsia felis*	*Ctenocephalides felis* (cat flea)
Japanese spotted fever	*Rickettsia japonica*	Tick
Russian vesicular rickettsiosis	*Rickettsia akari*	Tick

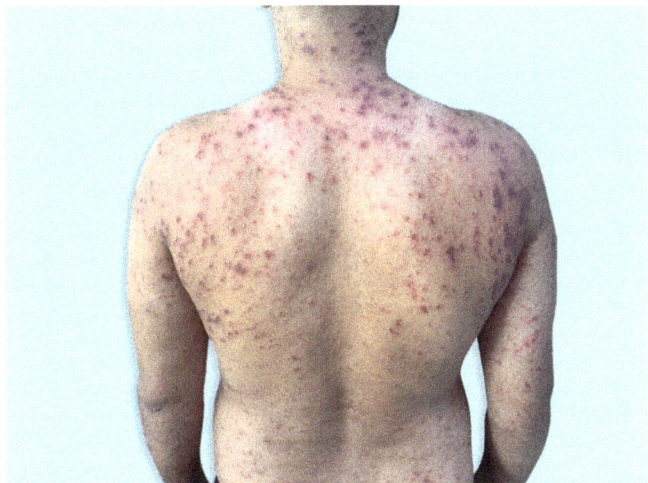

FIG. 8: Generalized hemorrhagic and petechial rash in a young male with suspected spotted fever.

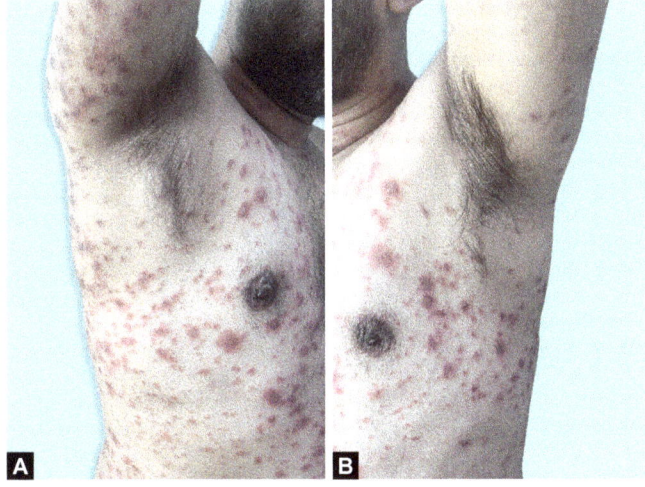

FIGS. 9A AND B: Extensive involvement in the same patient.

Several days later other signs and symptoms develop including fever, headache (very common in up to 90% of cases), generalized rash **(Fig. 8)**, and severe myalgia. The spotted fevers tend to be difficult to distinguish based on the rash. The rash, which usually becomes apparent after 3–5 days of onset of symptoms, is initially pink, blanching, discrete macules, subsequently evolving to maculopapular, petechial, or hemorrhagic rash **(Figs. 9A and B)**. The localization around the wrist and ankles is suggestive **(Fig. 10)**.

Other noticeable features reported include facial edema, anasarca, nausea or vomiting, respiratory symptoms, meningeal signs, altered sensorium, seizure, conjunctival effusion, myalgia, arthralgia, jaundice, abdominal pain, and bleeding manifestations. Less commonly the rash may be vesicular.

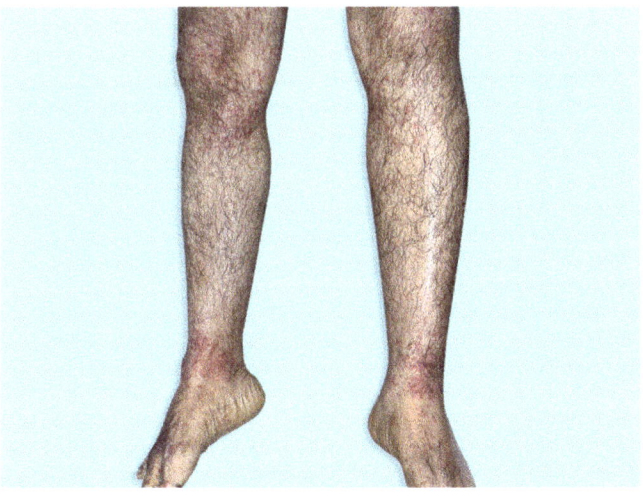

FIG. 10: Rash is localized around bilateral ankles.

Rickettsialpox

Rickettsialpox is caused by *Rickettsia akari,* transmitted by the rodent mite *Allodermanyssus sanguineus* that naturally infects house mice (*Mus musculus*).

The initial lesion is an oval or round tense vesicle developing at the site of the mite bite, which heals in about 2–4 weeks. After about a week, a remittent fever sets in, lasting for about a week. It is associated with sweating, headache, and backache. A macular rash appears 2–6 days after the onset of fever which sequentially evolves into papules, vesicles, and crusts resembling varicella. The rash heals without scarring.

Diagnosis

- The diagnosis of rickettsial infections can be established by serologic tests, including indirect fluorescent antibody testing, PCR, or western blot techniques. These become positive after about 10 days, 2 weeks, and 3 weeks in epidemic typhus, endemic typhus, and Rocky Mountain spotted fever, respectively.
- The Weil–Felix test (heterophile agglutination test) is based on the fact that antibodies produced against the rickettsiae cross-react with those of *Proteus vulgaris*. However, this test lacks both sensitivity and specificity.

Treatment

- Treatment may be started empirically if the suspicion is strong based on the characteristics of the rash.
- Various useful antibiotics are tetracyclines (doxycycline is the drug of choice), chloramphenicol, macrolides, and fluoroquinolones.

CHAPTER 3

Superficial Fungal Infections

Introduction

Infections caused by pathogenic fungi which are limited to the stratum corneum are known as superficial fungal infections. These infections are prevalent worldwide. The common superficial mycoses are as follows:
- *Dermatophytosis*: Infections caused by dermatophytes [three genera: (1) *Trichophyton*, (2) *Epidermophyton*, and (3) *Microsporum*].
- *Pityriasis versicolor*: Infections caused by *Malassezia furfur* (*Pityrosporum orbiculare*).
- *Candidiasis*: Infections caused by the yeast *Candida*.

Dermatophytosis

- All types of dermatophyte infections are more common in regions with hot and humid climates where they are the major source of skin infections.
- In India, tinea corporis is the most common type followed by tinea cruris. Tinea capitis is more commonly seen in children.
- The incidence and prevalence have been on the rise in recent years, possibly due to rising temperatures, the use of occlusive clothing, the universality of closed footwear, and overcrowding.
- Not only are dermatophytic infections becoming more common, but they are also increasingly becoming recalcitrant with poor treatment responses and longer durations of treatment being required. Recalcitrant dermatophytosis refers to the relapse, recurrence, reinfection, persistence, and possibly microbiological resistance of dermatophytosis.
- Over the past decade, cutaneous dermatophytoses have assumed epidemic proportions with much more severe and extensive fungal infections that are treatment-resistant. We are seeing atypical and extensive disease presentations. There has been an increase in chronic, relapsing, and recurrent cases.

A few important terms to understand in the context of superficial dermatophytosis include:
- *Chronic dermatophytosis*: Patient suffering from the disease for more than 6 months to 1 year, with or without recurrence, despite being treated.
- *Recurrent dermatophytosis*: Recurrence of the dermatophyte infection within 6 weeks of stopping adequate antifungal treatment, with at least two such episodes in the last 6 months.
- *Recalcitrant dermatophytosis*: This unifying umbrella term encompasses both chronic and recurrent dermatophytosis.

Traditionally, dermatophytoses are classified based on the body site involved. Owing to the unique characteristics afforded by the different sites involved, the clinical manifestations vary.

Tinea Corporis

This refers to dermatophyte infection of the glabrous skin except for palms, soles, and groins. The causative organisms are *Trichophyton rubrum, Trichophyton mentagrophytes, Microsporum canis,* and *Microsporum tonsurans.* It can occur in all age groups but is more common in adults.
- Less inflammatory cases have characteristic annular plaques with raised erythematous borders **(Fig. 1)**.
- Central clearing may not always be present.
- Scales can be appreciated at the erythematous border.
- With severe inflammation, vesicles and pustules may be seen at the margin, instead of scales. Rarely, bulla formation (especially with *T. rubrum*).

CHAPTER 3: Superficial Fungal Infections

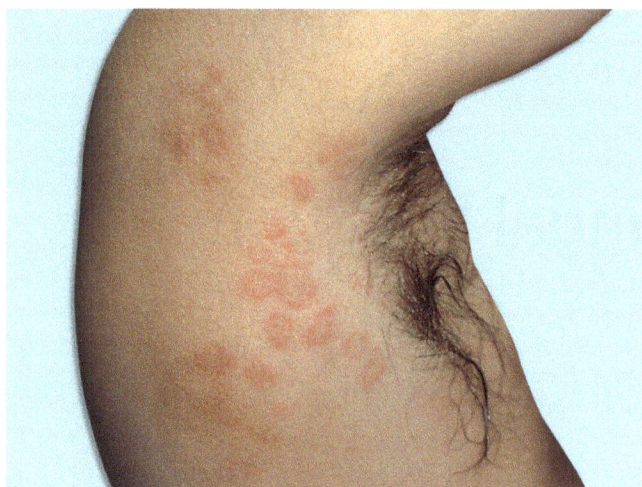

FIG. 1: Annular plaques of tinea corporis.

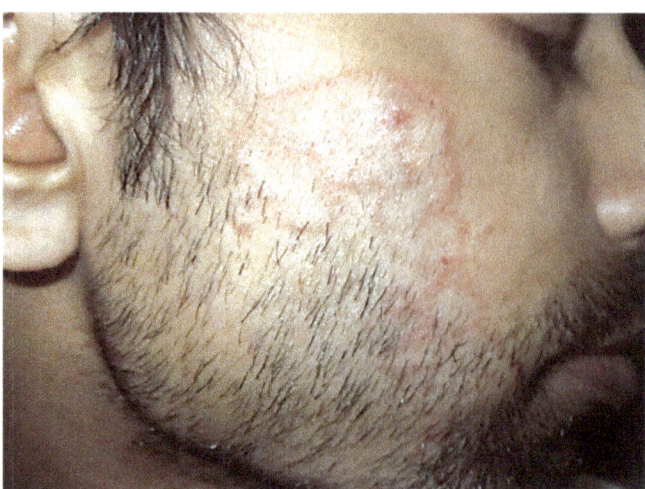

FIG. 2: Large annular plaque of tinea faciei.

- More chronic lesions may present with a psoriasiform presentation with prominent scale overlying thickened plaques.

Differential Diagnosis
- Seborrheic dermatitis
- Psoriasis
- Annular erythema
- Pityriasis versicolor
- Pityriasis rosea
- Secondary syphilis
- Subacute lupus erythematosus

Tinea Faciei

It is a dermatophytic Infection of the facial skin. Its causative organisms are mostly *T. rubrum* and *T. mentagrophytes*.
- Annular plaques with central clearing over the face **(Fig. 2)**.
- Apart from itching, a patient may complain of a burning sensation on sun exposure.
- These lesions are frequently modified by topical corticosteroid application **(Fig. 3)**.
- Minimal to absent scaling or inflammation.

Tinea Incognito

This is also known as tinea modified by topical or systemic corticosteroids. Its causative organisms are generally the same as tinea corporis. It is generally a result of suppression of inflammation.
- It may be difficult to recognize due to the absence of raised margins and scales **(Fig. 3)**.
- The lesions tend to have indistinct margins and may go undetected for a long time.

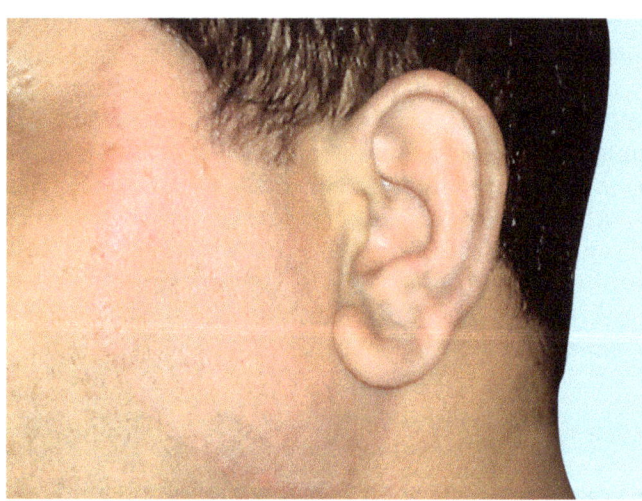

FIG. 3: Atypical lesion of tinea faciei due to steroid modification.

Tinea Indecisiva

Long-term cyclical therapy with topical antifungals and corticosteroids may produce this manifestation due to similar underlying mechanisms of immunosuppression with topical corticosteroids and reinfection due to early discontinuation of topical antifungals. This presentation closely mimics Tinea imbricata caused by *Trichophyton concentricum*. It is also known as *Tinea pseudoimbricata*.
- *Causative organism*: Commonly *T. mentagrophytes* and *Trichophyton tonsurans*.
- Seen as erythematous annular plaques with multiple concentric rings within the plaque resembling tinea imbricata **(Fig. 4)**.
- In these days of topical steroid abuse, extensive lesions over the trunk can be seen.
- The affected patients generally have a history of incomplete and episodic application of creams (antifungals or steroid combinations).

CHAPTER 3: Superficial Fungal Infections

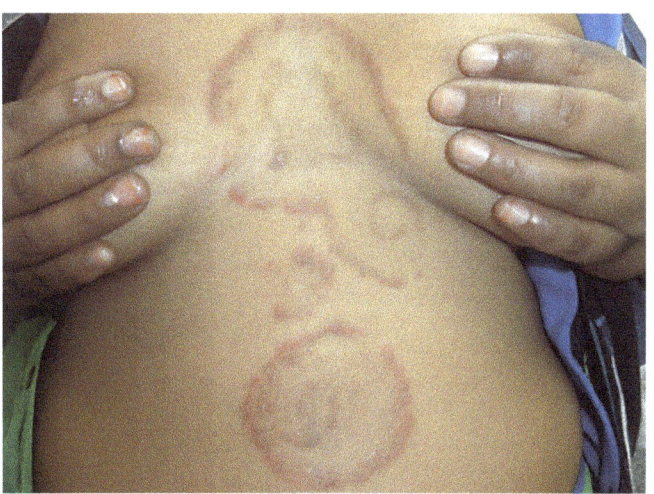

FIG. 4: Concentric rings of tinea due to long-term but inadequate therapy.

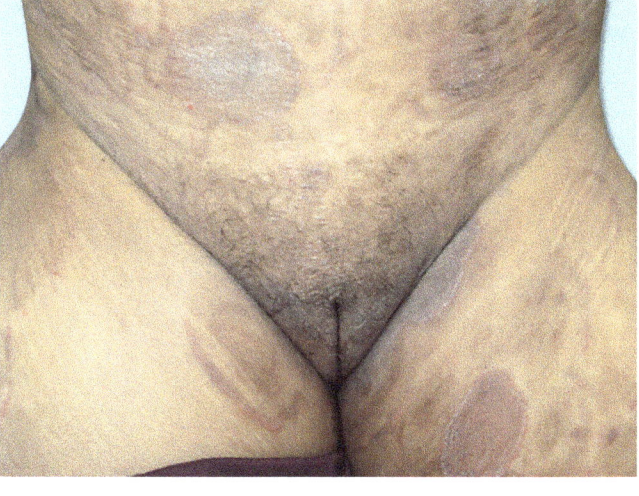

FIG. 6: Extensive tinea cruris involving thighs, and lower abdomen.

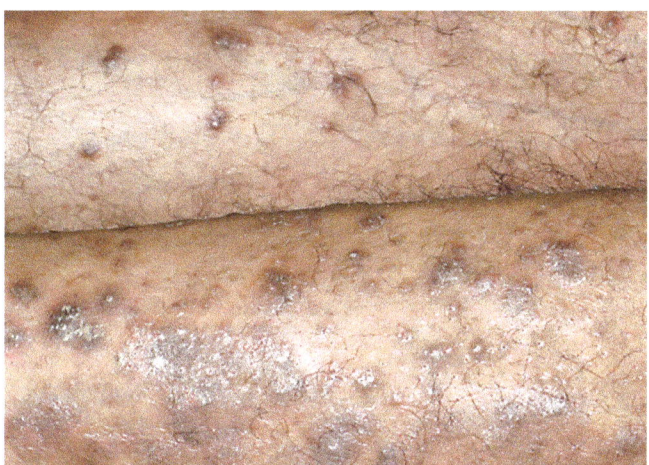

FIG. 5: Perifollicular pustules and nodules due to tinea infection.

- More common in summer months, with increased sweating and heavy manual work.
- Morphology is similar to tinea corporis, but maceration is a more prominent feature.
- Superadded bacterial infection may also develop.
- The lesions are highly pruritic.
- Infection with *T. rubrum* may spread from groins to thighs, lower abdomen, back, and buttocks **(Fig. 6)**. *E. floccosum* is generally associated with fungal infection of the foot, while *T. mentagrophytes var. interdigitale* presents with more inflammation, vesicles, and pustule formation at the margins.

Differential Diagnosis
- Candidal intertrigo
- Erythrasma
- Pityriasis versicolor
- Flexural psoriasis
- Seborrheic dermatitis

Majocchi's Granuloma

It is a type of deep fungal folliculitis. The causative organism is mostly *T. rubrum*.
- Most commonly seen in the women who regularly shave their hair.
- It presents as perifollicular pustules and nodules with surrounding erythema **(Fig. 5)**.
- Large inflammatory plaques may be seen.

Tinea Cruris or Dhobi Itch

- Infection of the groins, perianal, and perineal areas caused by dermatophytes.
- *Causative organisms*: *Trichophyton rubrum* most commonly; less often, *T. mentagrophytes var. interdigitale*, and *Epidermophyton floccosum* could be responsible.

Tinea Barbae

- This is a tinea infection of the beard and moustache area, thus, seen only in males.
- *Causative organism*: Mostly *Trichophyton mentagrophytes* and *Trichophyton verrucosum* (zoophilic species) and occasionally, other species, such as *Microsporum canis*, *Trichophyton violaceum*, and *Trichophyton schoenleinii*.
- More common in adult males in rural areas due to contact with livestock.
- It can also be transmitted through barbers who use shared razors.
- Seen as multiple folliculocentric papules and pustules with surrounding erythema **(Fig. 7)**.

CHAPTER 3: Superficial Fungal Infections

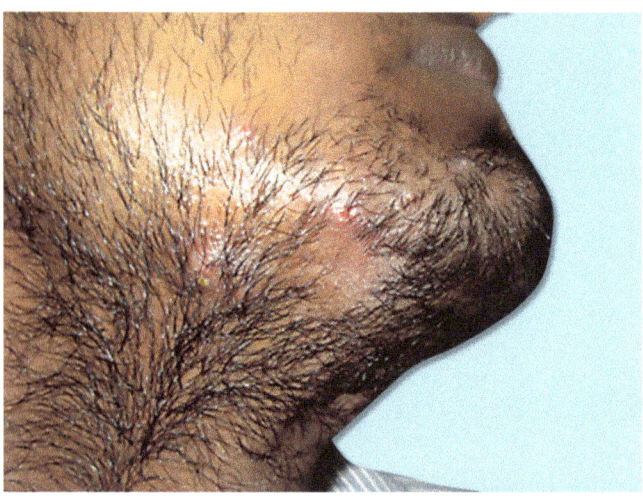

FIG. 7: Multiple folliculocentric papules and pustules in the beard area, leading to hair loss and scarring.

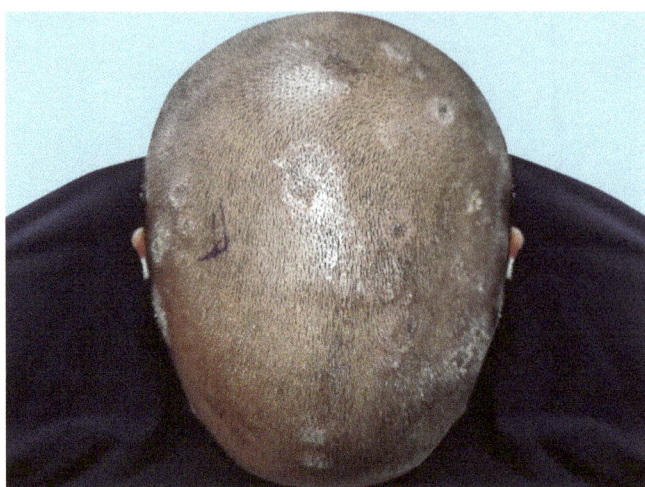

FIG. 8: Gray patch tinea capitis presenting with scaly patches of hair loss.

- Associated exudation and crusting resemble kerion.
- Hair in the area is easily pluckable.
- Chronic cases present with abscess and sinus formation, ultimately leading to scarring.
- An important source of transmission is the shared razors and blades. These should be avoided.

Differential Diagnosis
- Sycosis barbae
- Acne vulgaris
- Rosacea
- Perioral dermatitis

Tinea Capitis (Tinea Tonsurans)
- It is a dermatophytic infection of the scalp hair follicles.
- *Causative organisms*: The predominant species causing tinea capitis varies from region to region and from time to time. The most common species worldwide is *M. canis,* though, recently there has been an increase in *T. tonsurans* prevalence. In India, *T. violaceum* is the most common species isolated.
- It commonly occurs in the preadolescent age group, though, rarely adults can also be affected.
- It is common in school-going children and households with overcrowding.
- *Clinical presentations* vary greatly from noninflammatory types (gray patch) to severe inflammatory variants (kerion).
- Inflammatory variants are associated with cervical or occipital lymphadenopathy.
- The common clinical presentation is partial hair loss.

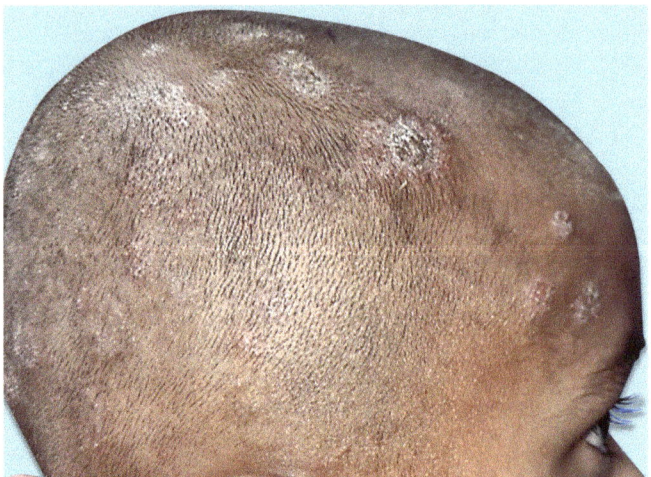

FIG. 9: Gray patch tinea capitis in a young girl.

Clinical Types
Noninflammatory Tinea Capitis
- *Gray patch tinea capitis*:
  - Seen as well-circumscribed round patches of non-cicatricial alopecia, with multiple broken stumps of gray, lusterless hair, and mild scaling **(Figs. 8 and 9)**.
  - The arthroconidia coating the hair gives rise to a gray appearance.
- *Black dot tinea capitis*:
  - This is characterized by grouped black dots (swollen hair shafts) with diffuse scaling **(Fig. 10)**.
  - The lesions are usually multiple and have angulated borders unlike gray patches **(Fig. 11)**.
  - Oftentimes, both these morphologies may coexist **(Fig. 12)**.

CHAPTER 3: Superficial Fungal Infections

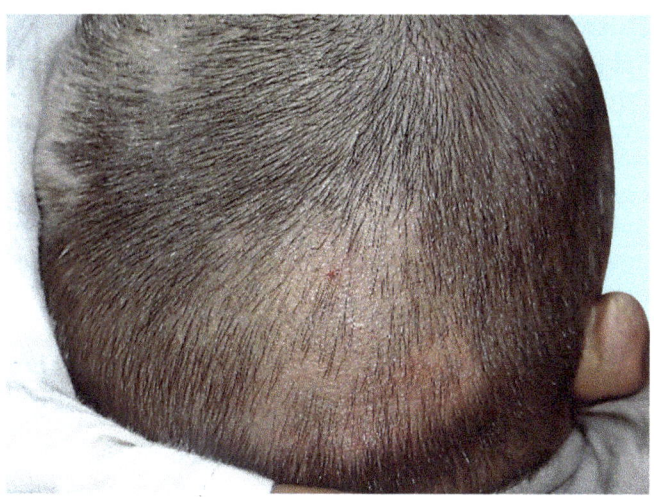

FIG. 10: Black dot tinea capitis. The broken hair shafts at the surface of the scalp give rise to the "black dot morphology."

Inflammatory Tinea Capitis
- It is characterized by a hypersensitivity response to the invading fungus.
- The clinical presentation may vary from follicular pustules (**Fig. 13**) to frank kerion.
- *Kerion*: It is an inflammatory, painful boggy swelling studded with follicular pustules) associated with lymphadenopathy (**Figs. 14 and 15**).
    - Scarring is usual.
- *Favus*:
    - This is caused by *T. schoenleinii*, and occurs sporadically, mainly in South African countries, the Middle East, and Pakistan.
    - It is a long-standing infection that extends over years and is characterized by yellow-colored scutulum around the hair follicles, which may become confluent to form yellow crusts.

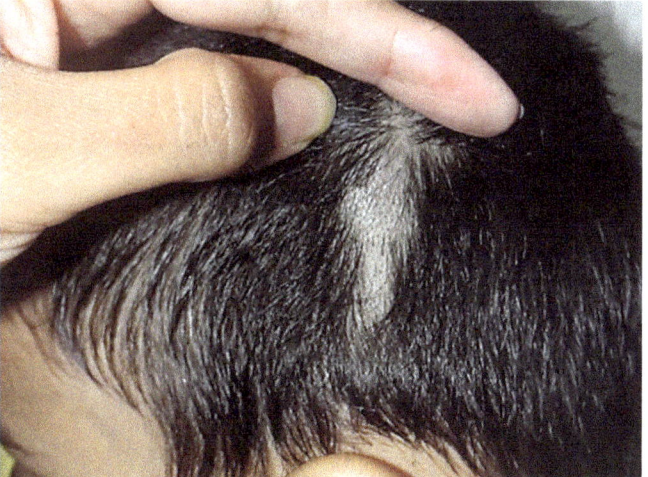

FIG. 11: A linear patch of black dot tinea capitis.

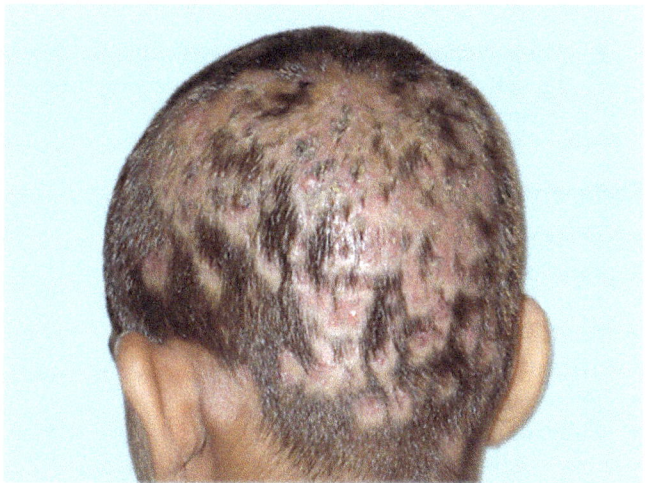

FIG. 13: Inflammatory tinea capitis with extensive scarring and hair loss.

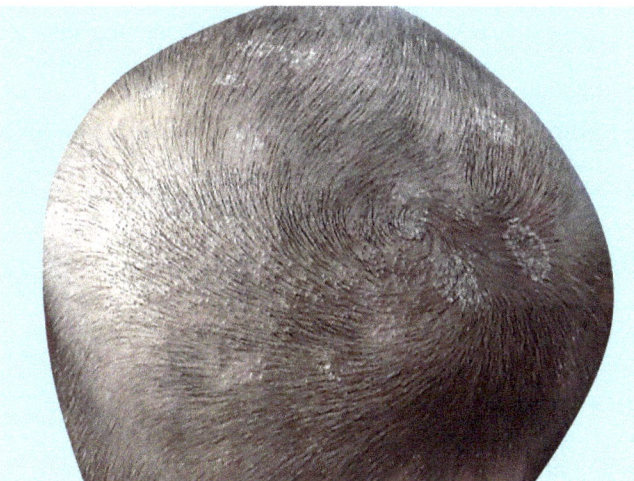

FIG. 12: Coexistent patches of gray patch and black dot tinea capitis in the same child.

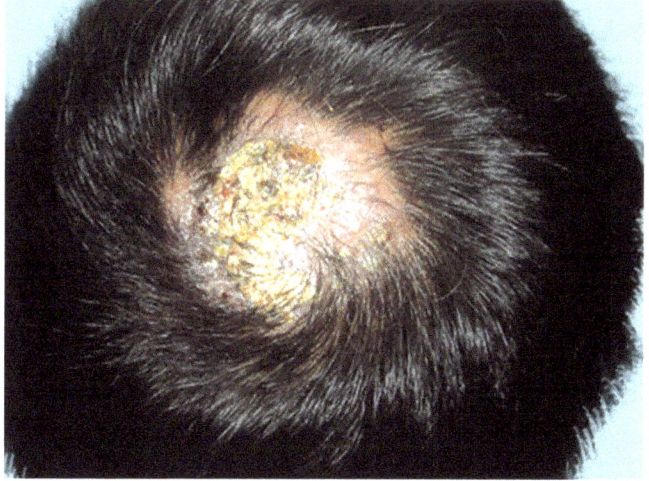

FIG. 14: Kerion presenting as a boggy swelling with deep-seated pustules and overlying thick crusts. This variant generally results in cicatricial hair loss.

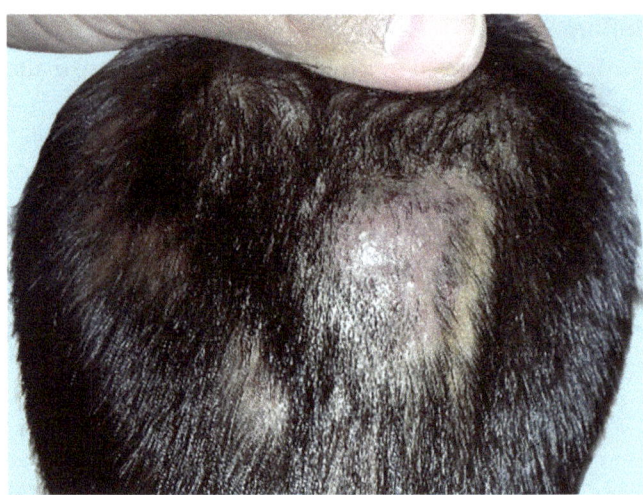

FIG. 15: Boggy swelling in the occipital area with scarring and hair loss.

- o The infection is usually chronic with little tendency for self-resolution and with risk of development of cicatricial alopecia.

Differential Diagnosis

- Seborrheic dermatitis
- Psoriasis
- Atopic dermatitis
- Alopecia areata
- Trichotillomania
- Bacterial folliculitis or impetigo
- Folliculitis decalvans

Management Considerations

Tinea Corporis/Cruris/Faciei

For localized disease, especially in children, topical antifungals like miconazole, clotrimazole, terbinafine, and tolnaftate may be sufficient. They need to be applied twice daily for approximately 4-6 weeks.

However, for most cases, systemic treatment with terbinafine or itraconazole in standard doses is usually recommended. Oral griseofulvin and fluconazole are also effective but require a longer treatment period.

Details of antifungal therapy are summarized in the following text:

Tinea Barbae

Tinea barbae, being an extensive hair infection, needs to be treated with oral antifungals only. The usual time period for continuation of therapy is 4-6 weeks.

Tinea Capitis or Tinea Tonsurans

Systemic antifungals are the mainstay of therapy. Topicals can only help reduce spore shedding but do not cure. Antifungal shampoos (containing ketoconazole or selenium sulfide) reduce spore shedding, preventing transmission to close contacts. Scalp hygiene and avoiding the sharing of combs and pillowcases also reduce the potential of transmission. The various systemic therapies used are

Griseofulvin

The most common oral antifungal used is griseofulvin (standard therapy for tinea capitis). It is the only antifungal approved by the Food and Drug Administration (US FDA) in children with tinea capitis. The dose depends on the formulation being used.
- *Ultramicronized form*: 10 mg/kg/day
- *Micronized form*: Up to 20 mg/kg/day
- Given for a period of 6-8 weeks

Fluconazole

Fluconazole (5 mg/kg/day for 4-6 weeks) is effective against *Trichophyton* species.

Itraconazole

Itraconazole (3-5 mg/kg/day for 4-6 weeks) is reported to be effective.

Terbinafine

Terbinafine (3-6 mg/kg/day for 2-4 weeks) is effective against *T. violaceum* and *T. tonsurans* species.

Tinea Unguium

- This condition is characterized by invasion of the nail plate by dermatophyte molds.
- Causative organisms are *T. rubrum, T. mentagrophytes var. interdigitale, Epidermophyton floccosum* (1.2%), and *Microsporum* species.
- More common in adults, especially males, due to a higher risk of trauma.
- Main clinical types are summarized in **Table 1**.

Differential Diagnosis

- Nail psoriasis
- Chronic eczema
- Nail lichen planus
- Pachyonychia congenita
- Congenital or acquired leukonychia
- Nondermatophytic mold onychomycosis (OM)
- Candidal onychomycosis

CHAPTER 3: Superficial Fungal Infections

TABLE 1: Different clinical types of onychomycosis.

Clinical type	Most common species	Site of invasion	Clinical features	Special considerations
DLSO (Fig. 16)	*Trichophyton rubrum*	Hyponychium and distal nail bed. The infection progresses proximally	Thickening and yellow or brown discoloration of the nail plate, distal onycholysis, and subungual hyperkeratosis	The most common clinical type. Affects toenails more than fingernails; usually accompanied by *Tinea pedis* and *Tinea manuum*
PSO (Fig. 17)	*T. rubrum*	Proximal nail bed and matrix	Proximal onycholysis, subungual hyperkeratosis, and destruction of the proximal nail plate	In AIDS patients; periungual inflammation can also occur
SWO (Fig. 18)	*T. mentagrophytes var. interdigitale*	Dorsal surface of the nail plate	Patches of leukonychia from which powdery material can be scrapped off	Toenails are more commonly involved than fingernails; AIDS patients are more affected; Rare variant may be caused by NDM, such as *Acremonium*, *Aspergillus*, and *Fusarium*
Endonyx (Fig. 19)	• *Trichophyton soudanense* • *Trichophyton violaceum*	The nail plate with the fungus growing between the lamellas	Milky white patches with pits. Nail plate surface and bed remains normal	–
TDO (Fig. 20)	Any of these	Any	End result of severe nail infection with the nail becoming thickened and crumbling down	Difficult to treat

(AIDS: acquired immunodeficiency syndrome; DLSO: distal and lateral subungual onychomycosis; NDM: nondermatophytic mold; PSO: proximal subungual onychomycosis; SWO: superficial white onychomycosis; TDO: total dystrophic onychomycosis)

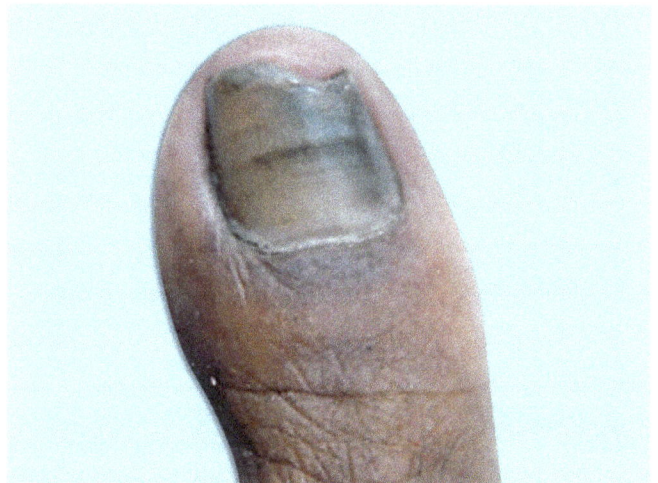

FIG. 16: Distal and lateral subungual onychomycosis involving the toenail.

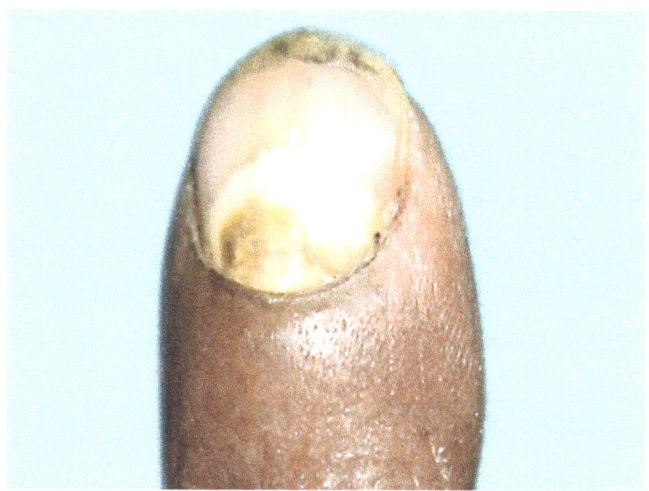

FIG. 17: Proximal subungual onychomycosis.

Management Considerations

- Due to the limited drug penetration as well as the slow rate of nail growth, tinea unguium requires long-term treatment with oral antifungals. The choice of treatment depends on the type of nail invasion and the species involved
- Topical treatment options are also available with enhanced drug delivery systems but are recommended in less severe cases.
- Topical and systemic therapies can also be combined to hasten the cure and ensure broader-spectrum coverage.

CHAPTER 3: Superficial Fungal Infections

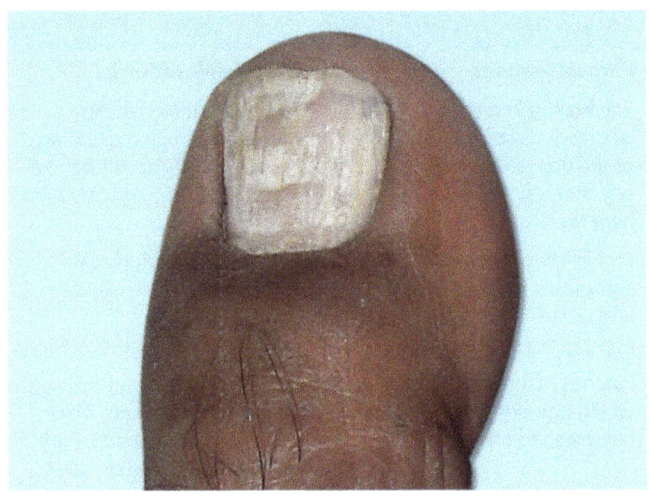

FIG. 18: Superficial white onychomycosis. Note the rough nail plate.

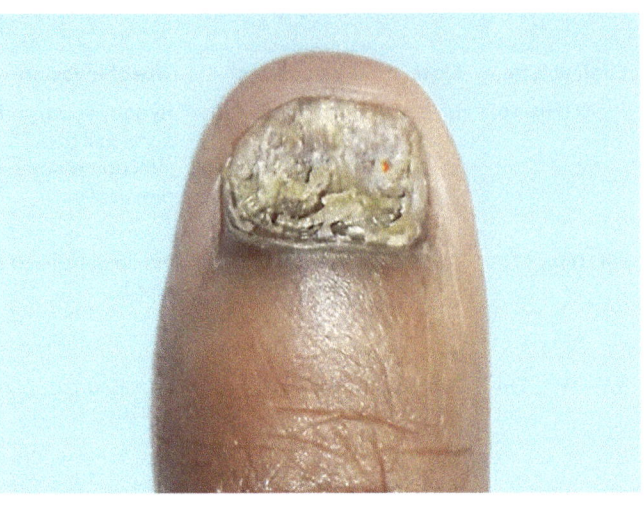

FIG. 20: Total dystrophic onychomycosis.

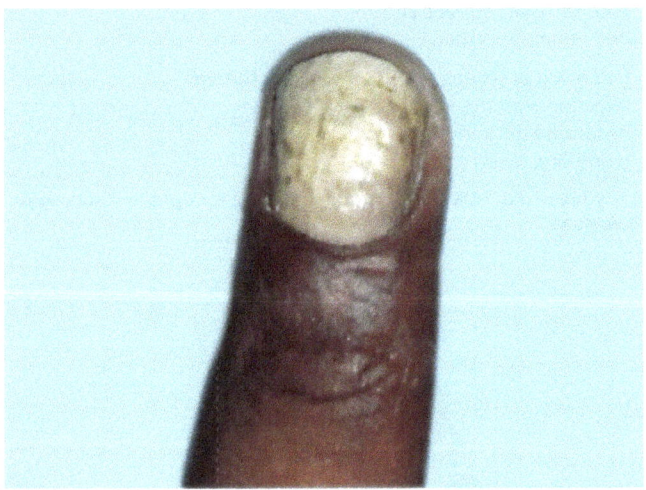

FIG. 19: Endonyx onychomycosis. The nail bed is uninvolved with a thickened and discolored nail plate and smooth surface.

Further details are summarized in the following text:

Tinea Pedis or Athlete's Foot
- Superficial fungal infection of the foot and toes, caused by dermatophytes.
- Causative organisms: *T. rubrum*, *T. mentagrophytes var. interdigitale* and *E. floccosum*.
- Can present as one of the three clinical variants or as a combined infection **(Table 2)**.

Tinea Manuum
- Dermatophyte infection of the skin of the hands.
- On the dorsum of the hand, a presentation may be similar to tinea corporis.

TABLE 2: Clinical variants of tinea pedis.		
Clinical type	Implicated species	Clinical features
Chronic interdigital tinea pedis **(Figs. 21 and 22)**	• *Trichophyton rubrum* • *Trichophyton mentagrophyte var. interdigitale* • *Epidermophyton floccosum*	Erythema, maceration, and erosion of the toe cleft may extend to involve the undersurface of the foot
Chronic hyperkeratotic type or mocassin type of tinea pedis **(Figs. 23 and 24)**	*T. rubrum*	• Diffuse scaling of the sole extending to involve the medial and lateral surface of the foot; erythema variable, involvement often bilateral • Involvement of one hand and two feet is known as "one hand and two feet syndrome"
Vesiculobullous type of tinea pedis **(Figs. 25 and 26)**	*T. mentagrophytes var. interdigitale*	• Multiple tense vesicles or vesicopustules on the sole and periplantar region rupture to leave behind collarette of scale; bullae may also form • Spontaneous resolution can occur

- Palmar infection shows diffuse scaling accentuated at the creases **(Fig. 27)**.
- Most of the cases are unilateral.
- Commonly there is "one hand, two feet involvement" with dermatophytes **(Fig. 28)**.

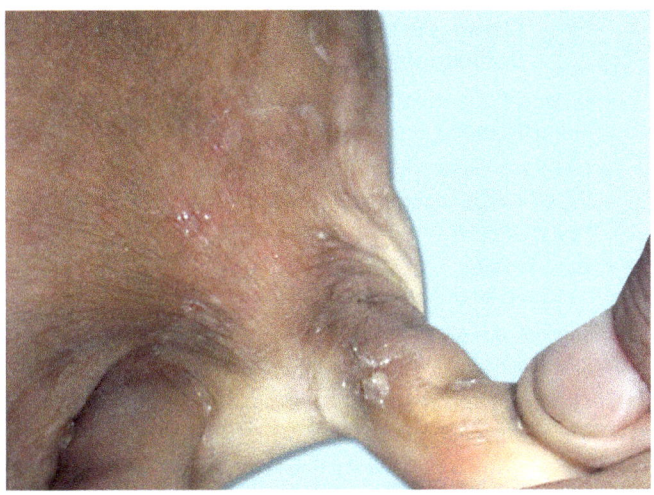

FIG. 21: Interdigital tinea pedis. The erythematous scaly plaque involves the last interdigital cleft and area of predilection.

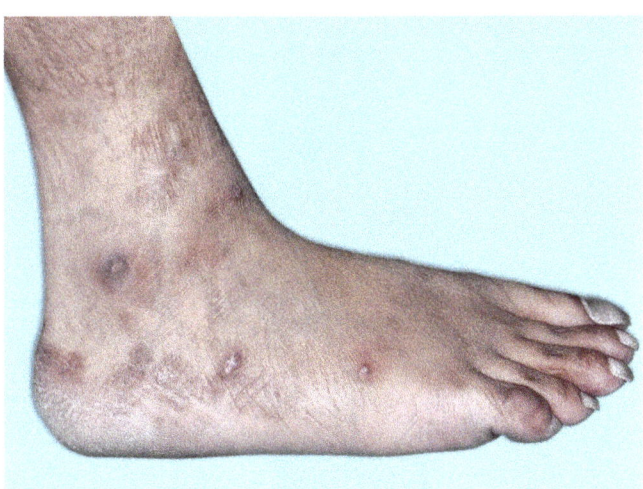

FIG. 24: Moccasin-type tinea pedis involving the posterior lateral border of the foot.

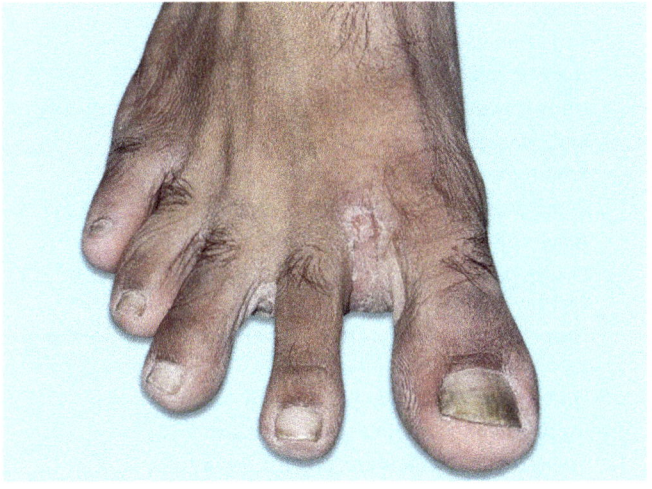

FIG. 22: Interdigital tinea pedis involving the first toe-cleft.

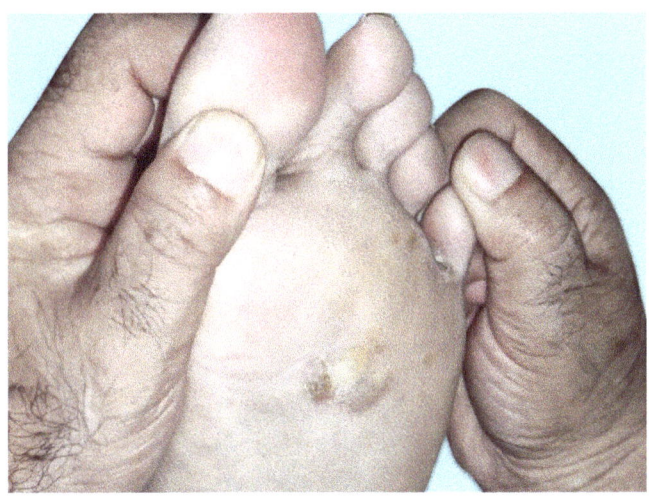

FIG. 25: Bullous tinea pedis involving the plantar aspect. A thick-walled bulla is seen.

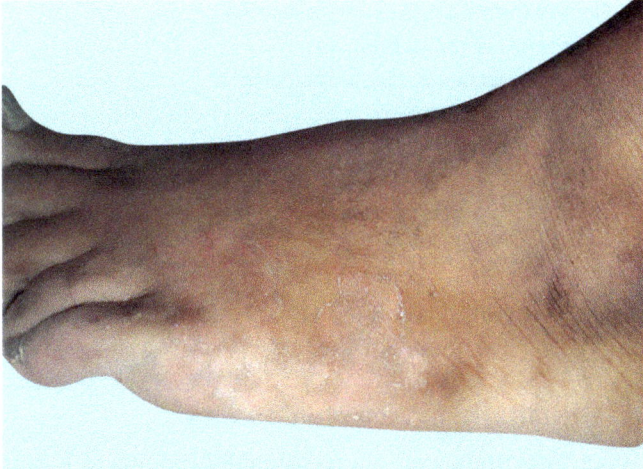

FIG. 23: Moccasin-type tinea pedis or chronic hyperkeratotic tinea pedis. Note the extension of erythema and scaling from the plantar aspect, along the lateral border of the foot.

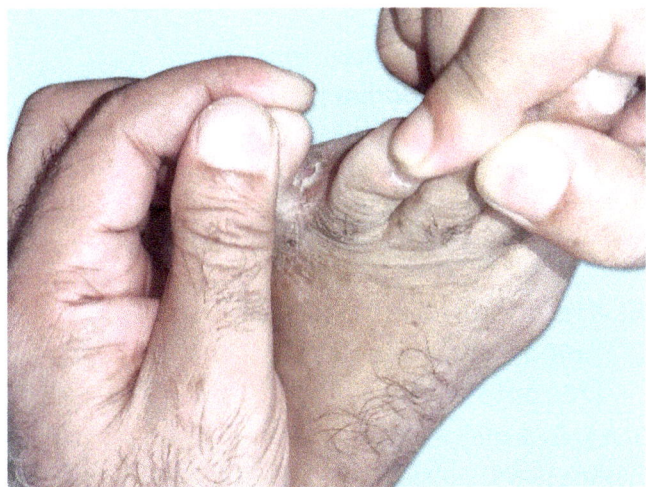

FIG. 26: Dorsal aspect of foot in the same patient, showing interdigital involvement.

CHAPTER 3: Superficial Fungal Infections

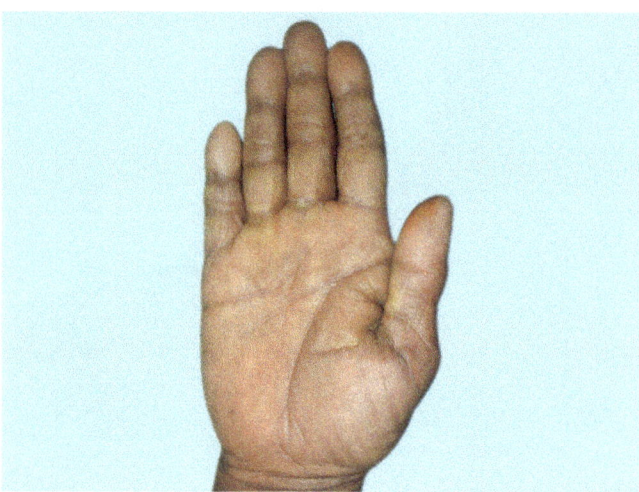

FIG. 27: Tinea manuum, chronic scaly hyperkeratosis involving the palmar as well as the dorsal aspect of the hand.

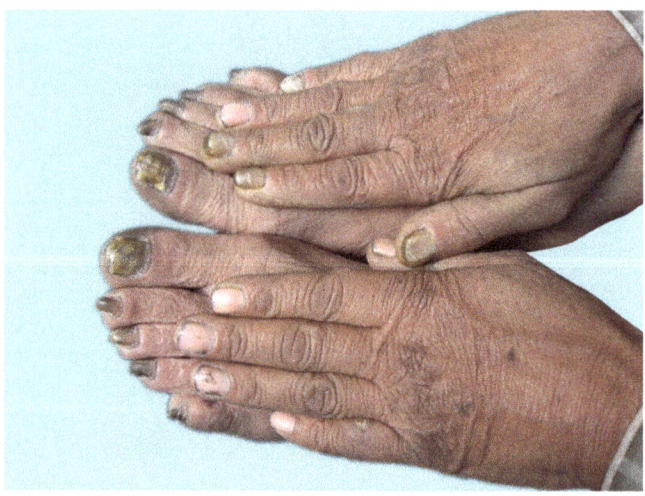

FIG. 28: One hand and two feet involvement in dermatophytosis.

Management Considerations for Tinea Pedis and Manuum

Mild interdigital involvement can usually be treated with topical azoles, allylamines, or tolnaftate. However, for chronic hyperkeratotic infection, oral antifungals are essential. A prolonged course of therapy is required.

Changes in the Pattern of Tinea Infections/Recalcitrant Dermatophytosis

The presentation and epidemiology of superficial dermatophytosis have rapidly changed during the last decade or so. In today's scenario, the following changes are being increasingly observed pertaining to superficial

| BOX 1 | Changes in the presentation of superficial dermatophytosis. |

- *Involvement of unusual locations*:
  ○ Rising incidence of tinea faciei
  ○ Tinea genitalis (males and females)
  ○ Superficial dermatophytosis of scalp skin
  ○ Tinea auricularis
  ○ Tinea labialis
  ○ Tinea ciliaris and tinea blepharitis
  ○ Tinea of vellus hair
  ○ Tinea involving immunocompromised districts
- *Changes in morphology*:
  ○ *Tinea pseudoimbricata*
  ○ Arcuate, dumb-bell-shaped tinea corporis
  ○ Large, bizarre-shaped, or geographic patches of tinea corporis
  ○ Double-edged tinea
  ○ Ill-defined and unclear borders
  ○ Eczematous tinea
  ○ Tinea mimicking other dermatoses
- *Changes in clinical behavior*:
  ○ Unusually extensive diseases with or without comorbidity
  ○ Multifocal disease at presentation
  ○ Erythrodermic disease at presentation
  ○ Rapid progression with involvement of large body areas
  ○ Absence of inflammation
  ○ Exaggerated inflammation (especially post initiation of therapy)
  ○ Poor or partial response to standard dosing of conventional topical and systemic antifungals
  ○ Persistent eczematous changes post-therapy
  ○ Involvement of multiple family members
  ○ Coexistent bacterial infections, e.g., furunculosis
  ○ Frequent relapses/quick relapses
  ○ Disabling itch (frequent nocturnal aggravation)
  ○ Persistent itch after resolution
- Signs of steroid abuse or irritant dermatitis
- *Changes in the impact of disease*:
  ○ High impact on quality-of-life indices
  ○ Higher cost of therapy
  ○ Longer duration of therapy (>6–8 weeks)
  ○ Higher chances of treatment failure
  ○ More family members/close contacts affected

dermatophytotic infections **(Box 1)**. These changes are also responsible for major challenges in their management.

Unusually Extensive Disease

Tinea infections were conventionally limited to a part of the body. It has now become common to see the involvement of multiple anatomic sites including axillae, groins, trunk, hands and feet, and nails in a single patient **(Figs. 29 to 31)**.

Occurrence in Infants and Young Children

The presentation with extensive tinea lesions in small children is seen more often now. This is generally seen when either parents or close family members are involved and there is the sharing of clothing **(Figs. 32 to 34)**. Even in children, the disease tends to be extensive and atypical.

Unusual Morphology (Tinea Incognito)

There is a higher incidence of difficult-to-recognize presentations and unusual morphologies. These include the following morphological presentations.
- *T. pseudoimbricata*: This clinically manifests as a "ring-inside a ring" or "waves or rings" of tinea. This

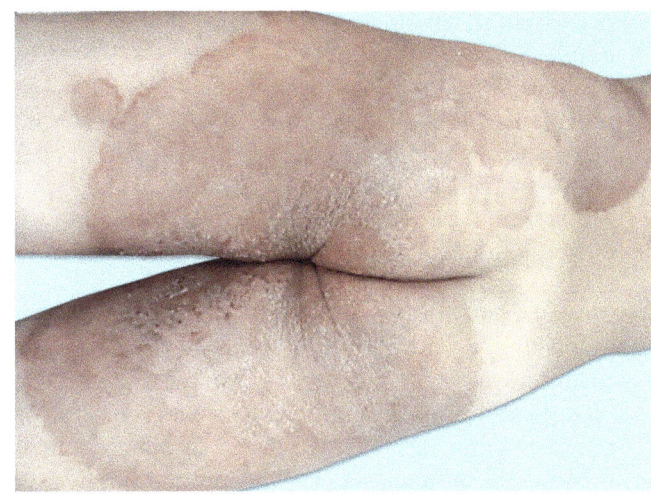

FIG. 31: Extensive tinea involving the trunk, buttocks, and legs (up to midthigh).

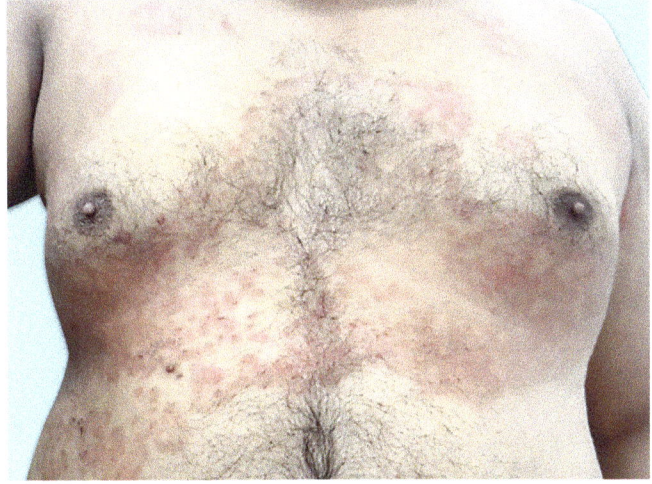

FIG. 29: Extensive tinea involving the trunk and extending to axillae as well.

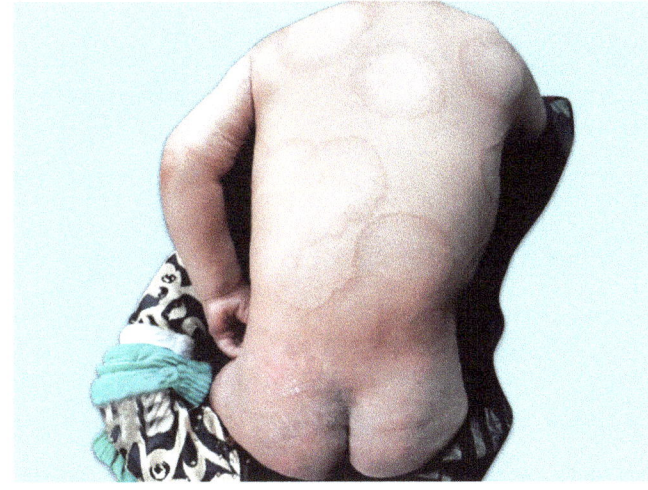

FIG. 32: Extensive tinea involving trunk in a 6-month-old infant.

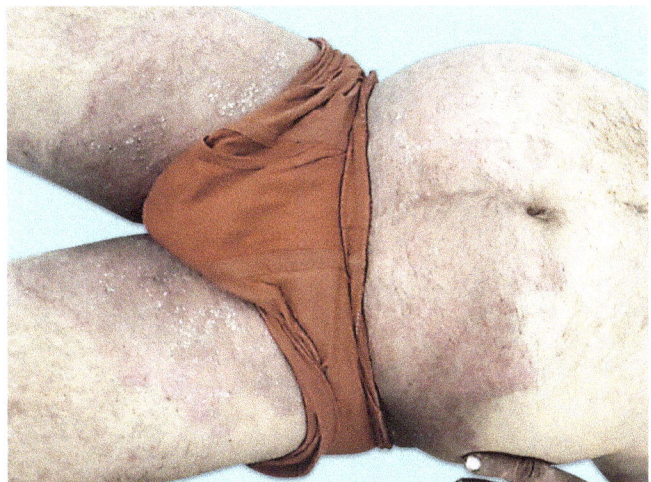

FIG. 30: Extensive tinea involving the lower abdomen up to the midthigh region. Both groins and genitalia were involved.

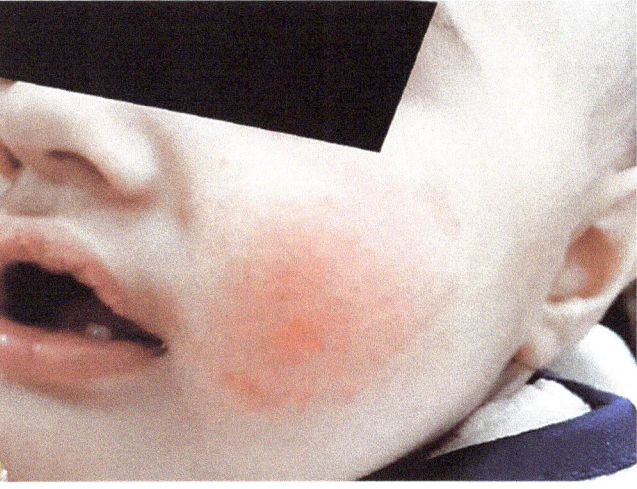

FIG. 33: Tinea faciei in a 3-month-old child.

presentation generally results from topical steroid application **(Figs. 35 to 37)**.

- *Pustular tinea*: Pustular presentation is generally seen in patients with tinea, who were on prolonged steroid use (systemic or topical) and have suddenly stopped it **(Figs. 38 and 39)**. This withdrawal is associated with a pustular flare with intense itching. Concomitant bacterial infection (furunculosis) may also be seen in some cases.
- *Tinea faciei*: This was a less commonly seen area of involvement. However, it is much more commonly seen now. This could be related to the irrational use of topical steroid preparations on the face and is common in the desire for fairer skin, for the treatment of melasma, or for any facial pigmentation **(Figs. 40 to 44)**. This form of tinea is generally accompanied by the

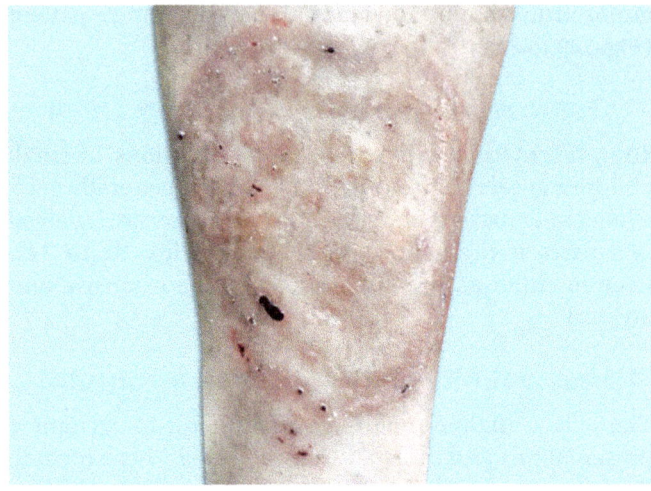

FIG. 36: *Tinea pseudoimbricata* involving the limbs.

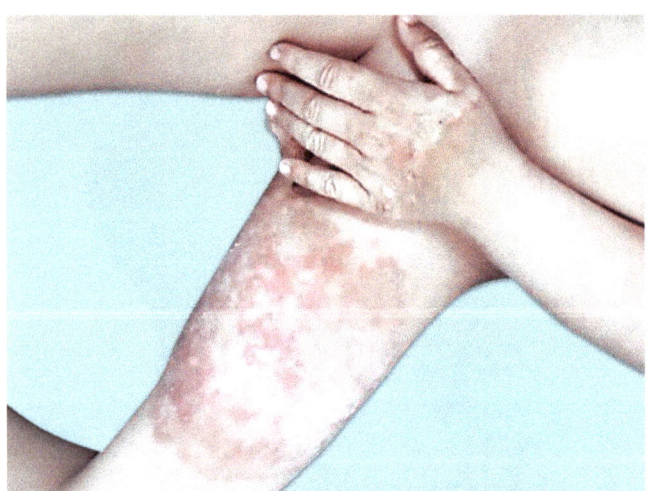

FIG. 34: Extensive tinea involving distinct areas of the body. There is involvement of the groin (tinea cruris) up to the midthigh) with limb extremity (tinea manuum) in a 2-year-old child.

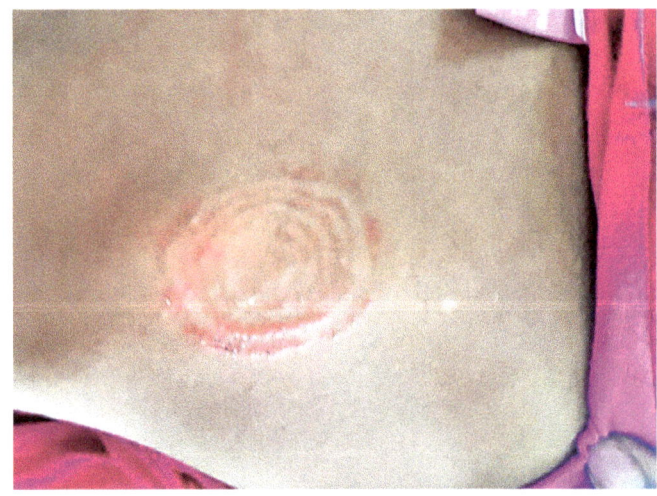

FIG. 37: *Tinea pseudoimbricata* in the groin area due to repeated steroid application.

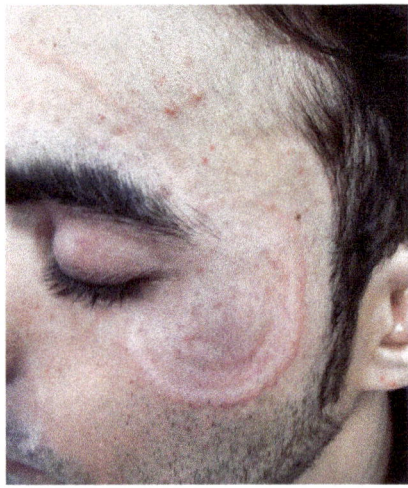

FIG. 35: *Tinea pseudoimbricata* involving the face.

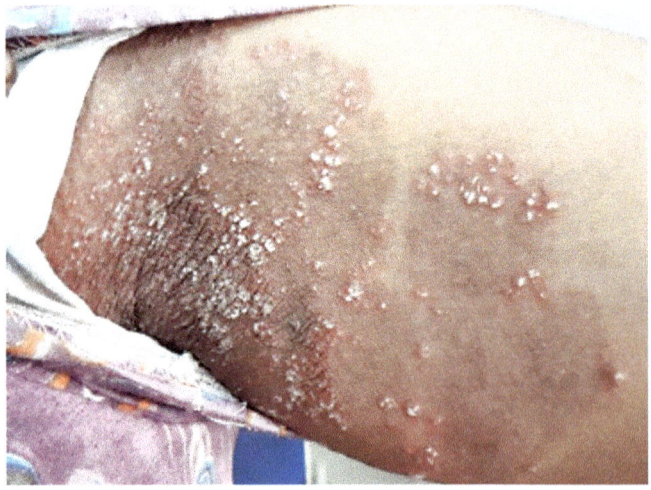

FIG. 38: Pustular tinea in a patient with prolonged steroid usage.

CHAPTER 3: Superficial Fungal Infections

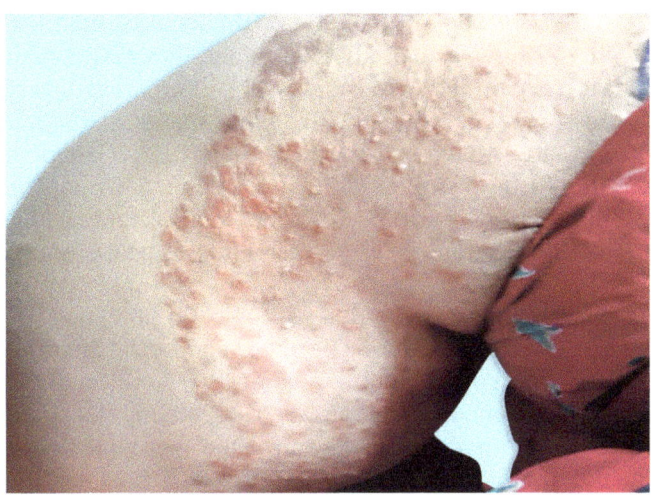

FIG. 39: Pustular and follicular inflammatory lesions in steroid modified tinea.

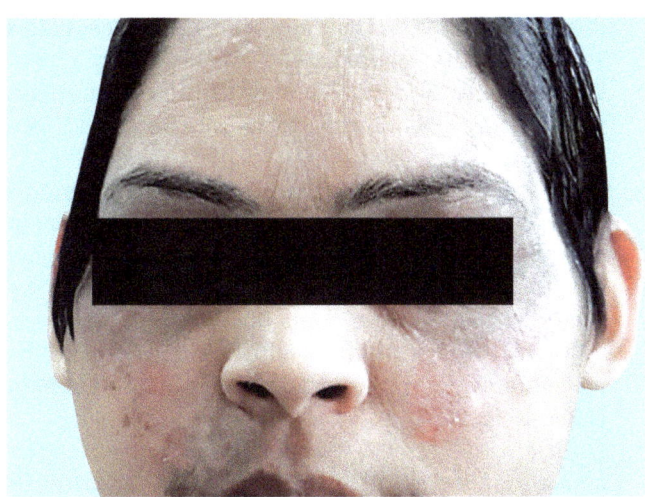

FIG. 42: Extensive tinea faciei involving almost the whole face, with indistinct margins.

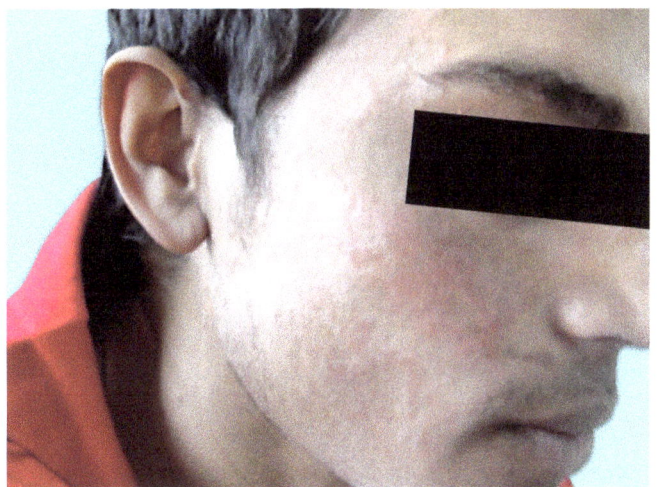

FIG. 40: Extensive *Tinea pseudoimbricata* involving the face.

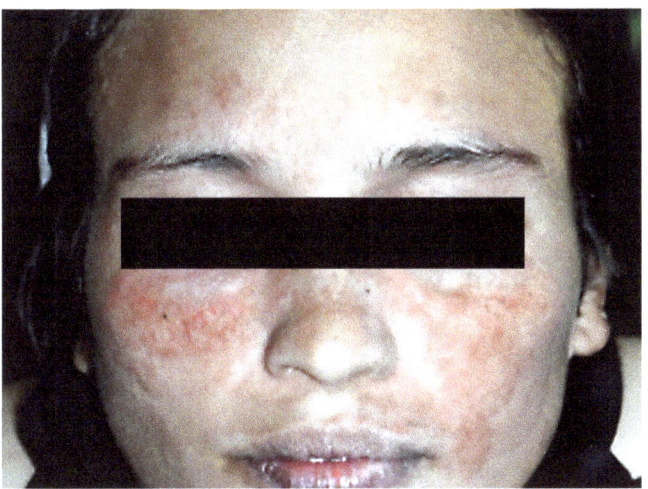

FIG. 43: Extensive bilaterally symmetrical tinea faciei with intense erythema, simulating a malar rash.

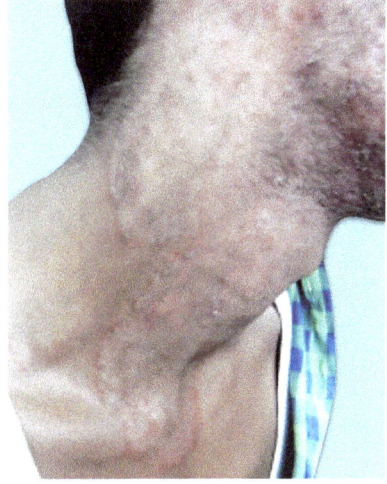

FIG. 41: Extensive tinea faciei extending up to the neck.

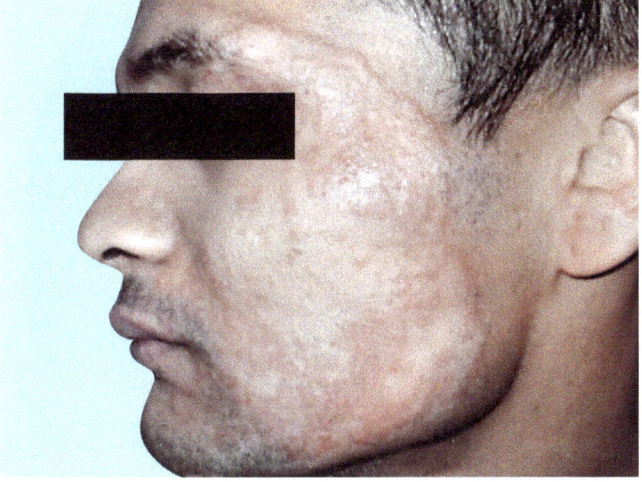

FIG. 44: Tinea faciei involving the whole central face, with extensive spread up to the sideburns and involvement of the eyebrow.

involvement of vellus hair in sideburns. It necessitates systemic antifungal drug use.
- *Tinea auricularis*: Involvement of the external ear, with a lesion extending up to the concha, is also seen now **(Fig. 45)**.
- *Tinea of the scalp*: This is also an emerging modification, where extensive involvement of the scalp skin, extending onto the adjacent skin of the forehead or the nape of the neck is seen. It tends to be noninflammatory. The extension of dermatophytosis to involve the terminal scalp hair even in adults necessitates prolonged systemic antifungal treatment **(Figs. 46 to 48)**.
- *Diffuse scaly tinea with ill-defined margins*: The conventional well-defined margins of tinea corporis tend to be very ill-defined in patients using steroids. The lesions also have diffuse scaling. They may appear very dry or very eczematous in certain areas. Every suspected scaly lesion with defined margins (whether or not well-defined) with or without central clearing, should be tested for fungal infection. This can be done with potassium hydroxide (KOH) scraping. This should be done before prescribing topical steroids **(Figs. 49 to 53)**.
- *Tinea of vellus hair*: This entity is being increasingly recognized, with more effective diagnostic techniques and closer examination. A clinical recognition of the involvement of vellus hair, even in seemingly localized tinea, has made us more aware of the need for systemic therapy in such cases. Tinea of vellus hair may be

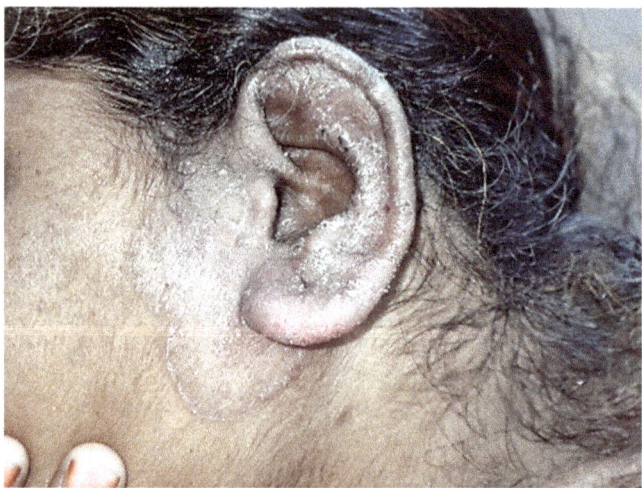

FIG. 45: Tine auricularis.

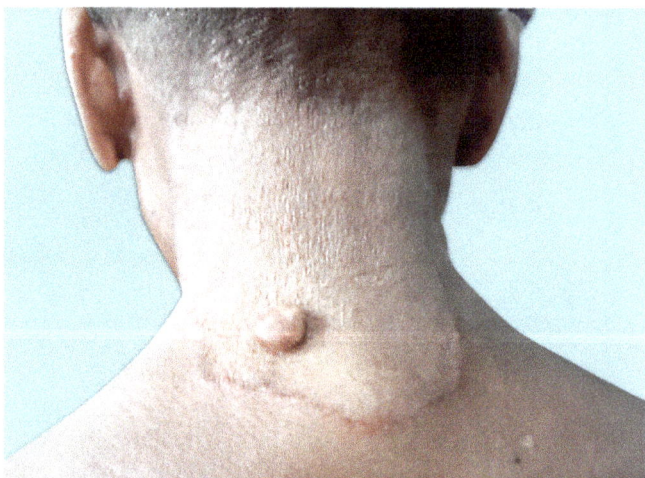

FIG. 47: Tinea of the posterior scalp with tinea corporis extending over the back of the neck.

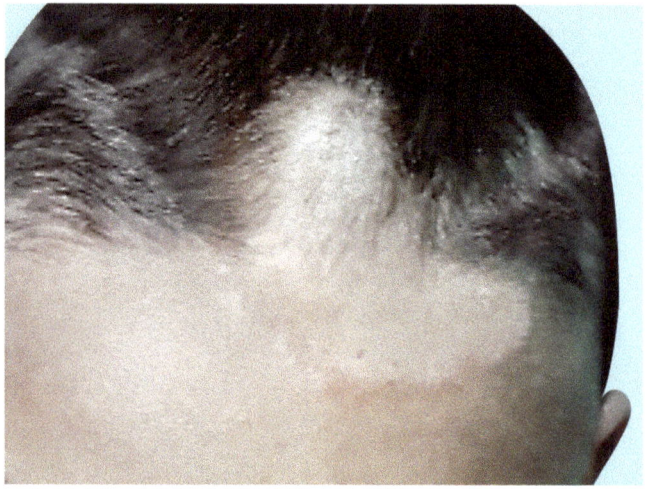

FIG. 46: Tinea of the scalp causing frontal hair loss. It extends on to the forehead skin.

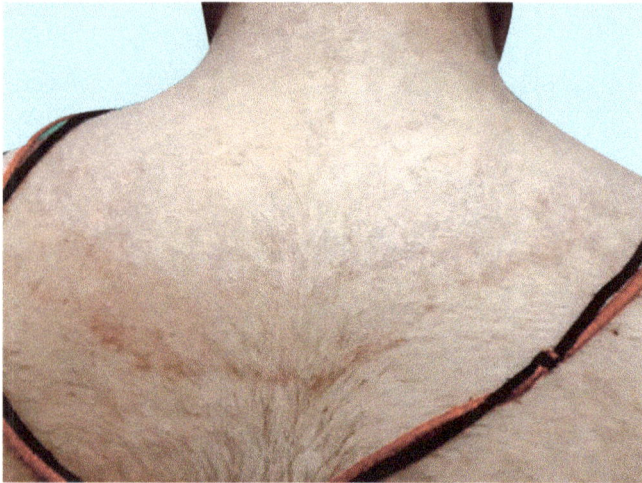

FIG. 48: Extensive involvement with tinea corporis that has contiguously extended to involve the scalp.

CHAPTER 3: Superficial Fungal Infections

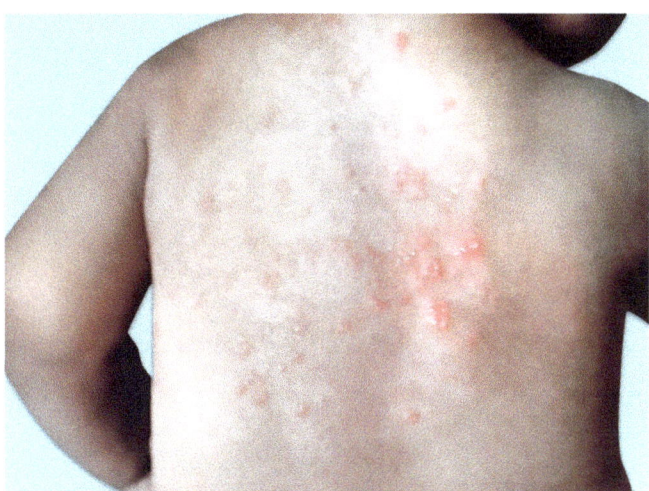

FIG. 49: Diffuse scaly tinea corporis in a young child. The lesion also has ill-defined margins. This presentation is commonly seen with steroid-modified tinea.

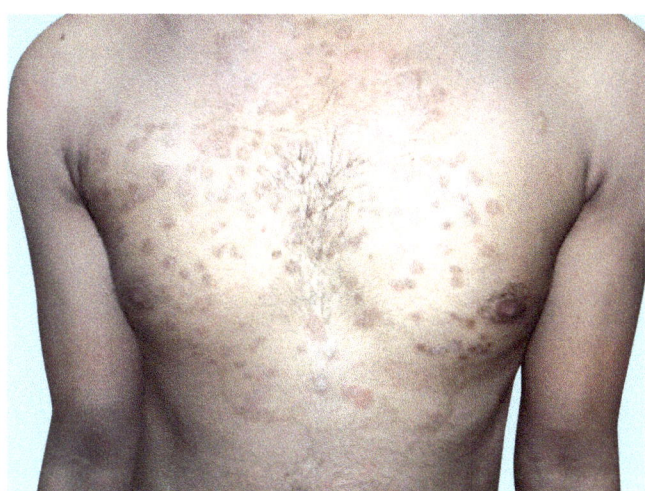

FIG. 52: Extensive truncal tinea corporis with numerous small lesions with very ill-defined margins.

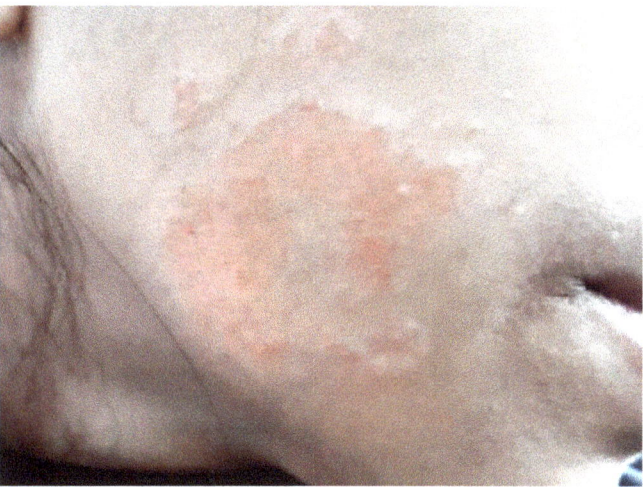

FIG. 50: Tinea faciei lesion with ill-defined margins. The erythema and scaling are secondary to topical steroid use.

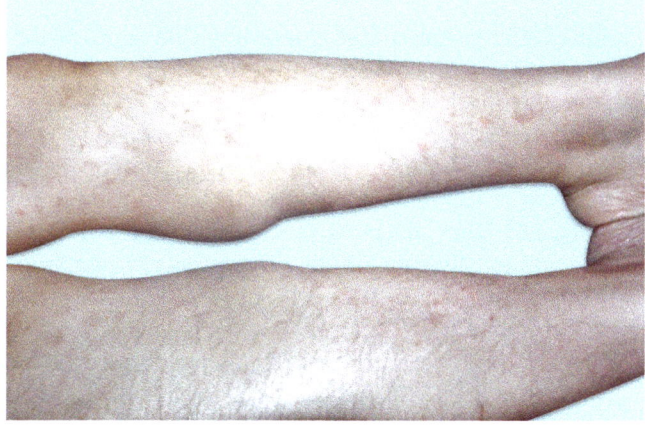

FIG. 53: Tinea corporis involving both legs with numerous, small, scaly lesions. The condition is highly steroid-modified.

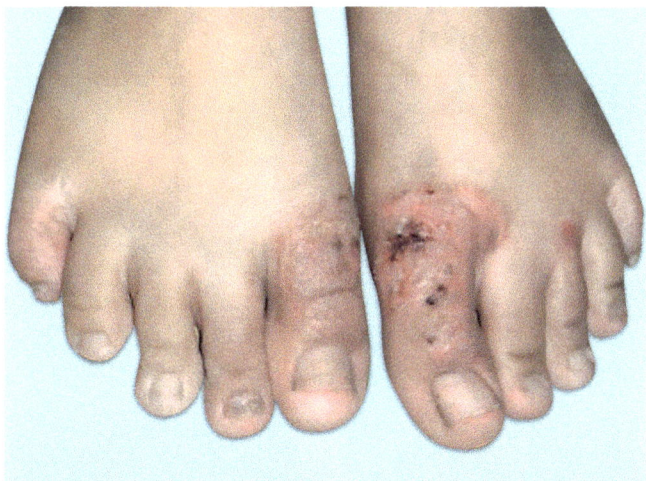

FIG. 51: Atypical symmetrical tinea pedis. The lesions appear very eczematous but have a defined margin.

responsible for relapse and poor treatment response in a large number of cases. It can be documented using a dermatoscope and KOH mount.
- *Tinea in immunocompromised districts*: An aberration in the immune control of a localized area of skin, affected by another disease process, is known as an immunocompromised district. There has been an increasing recognition of atypical tinea lesions appearing secondarily over such areas **(Fig. 54)**. These include areas such as amputation stumps, surgical incision sites, tattooed skin, and areas with resolved tinea lesions, apart from areas with topical steroid application. Immune-mediated dermatoses such as vitiligo and lichen planus are also known to develop preferentially at the sites of tinea corporis.

CHAPTER 3: Superficial Fungal Infections

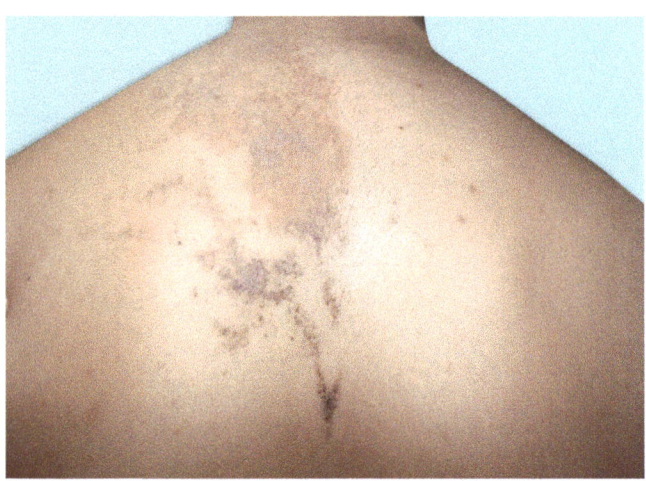

FIG. 54: Tinea corporis localizing to areas with segmental lichen planus on the back of a young male.

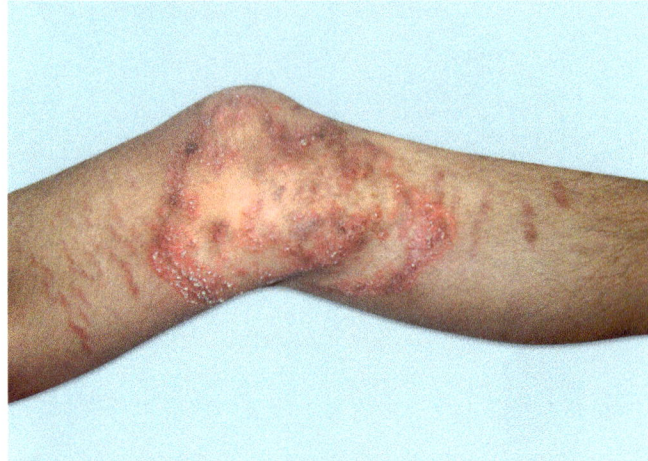

FIG. 55: Inflamed lesion of tinea corporis in a male with chronic steroid use as evidenced by extensive striae and erythema.

■ Signs of Corticosteroid or Irritant Use

Familiarity with signs and stigmata of steroid abuse as well as repeated use of irritants is important to recognize for the treating physician.

- Abuse of potent topical steroids is associated with striae and hypopigmentation. Striae mostly occur early with potent steroid-containing combinations **(Fig. 55)**. They are most pronounced in the flexures including axillae and thighs. The initial erythematous phase (striae rubra) is followed by whitish striae (striae alba).
- Occasional ulceration may be seen due to extreme thinning **(Figs. 56 and 57)**. These ulcers tend to become secondarily infected. Striae may assume a pseudoedematous appearance at times. Patients may deny continued usage; however, the depot effect of steroids ensures continued ulceration.
- *Red scrotum syndrome* (persistent scrotal erythema) is seen in some patients applying fixed-dose combinations containing topical steroids **(Fig. 57)**.
- *Lesional and perilesional hypopigmentation* develops within 3–4 weeks. It may be accompanied by atrophy and telangiectasia. It is also seen with intralesional steroid injections, especially in a linear pattern.
- Bacteria can concomitantly infect and complicate tinea lesions. This is due to local immunosuppression due to topical steroids.
- Signs of irritant dermatitis include erythema, brownish discoloration, scaling, and exfoliation. These may be seen over and around infected sites and are common to see due to the use of home remedies including crushed plant extracts or lotions, and over-the-counter preparations containing salicylic acid, sulfur, etc. Associated symptoms include burning, pain, and tenderness.

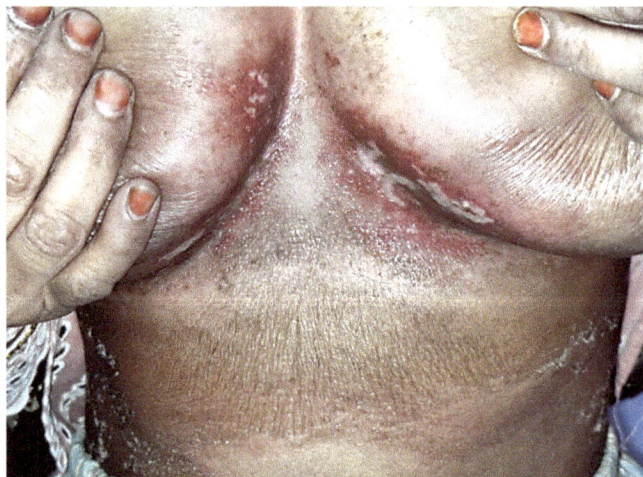

FIG. 56: An old lady with extensive tinea corporis, steroid induced striae, thinning of skin, ulceration of skin and secondary bacterial infection in the inframammary area.

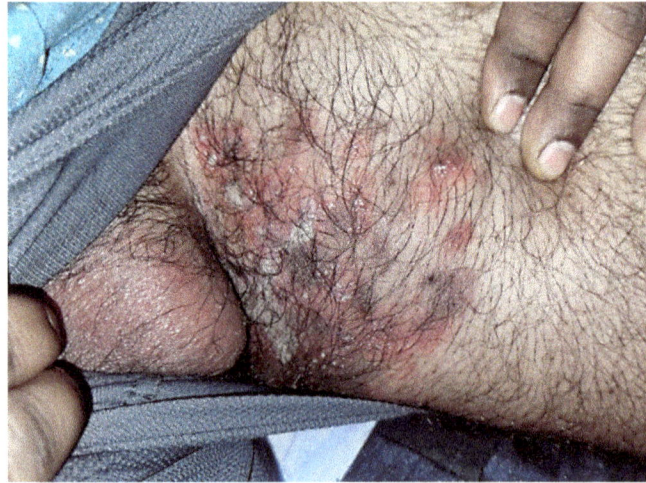

FIG. 57: Inflamed lesion of tinea cruris with secondary ulceration, infection, and red scrotal skin.

- Iatrogenic cushingoid syndrome may be seen in patients with extensive tinea and is suggestive of a possibility of systemic steroid intake over a long period of time. These include higher weight, truncal obesity, striking striae, acneiform eruption, hypertrichosis, and hirsutism.

Impact of Recalcitrant Dermatophytosis

The disease behaves like other chronic and recurrent disorders and has a significant bearing on the quality of life, emotions, and personal relationships of the patients. It may be responsible for feelings of hopelessness, shame, and anger, even suicidal ideation.

Also, the disease preferentially affects people from lower socioeconomic strata, and may often affect multiple family members. It also requires prolonged antifungal therapy. All this adds up to a significant financial burden. This in turn may contribute to poor compliance and consequently poor efficacy.

Management of Dermatophytosis

Investigations

- *Dermatoscopy*: It is an examination of skin and its appendages with a dermatoscope, an instrument with standard magnifying optics, and a transilluminating light source. It allows noninvasive, in vivo, subsurface visualization of various skin disorders. Dermatoscopy is the standard of care around the world and is now becoming increasingly popular and of diagnostic value, with many more indications being explored. It is a useful point-of-care test for tinea diagnosis. It offers several advantages as it enables rapid, non-invasive, and in vivo observation of fungal invasion. It can help identify suspect hair/nails for sampling. It can identify high-risk contacts as well as steroid-modified cases. The salient dermoscopic findings of superficial dermatophytosis are summarized in **Tables 3 to 5**.

TABLE 3: Dermoscopic findings in tinea capitis.	
Characteristic findings with a high predictive value but not seen in every case	Comma hairs (short hairs that bend and grow back toward the scalp, resembling a comma) **(Fig. 58)**
	Corkscrew hairs (short hairs that are coiled up like a corkscrew). Typical of *Trichophyton* infection and are seen less commonly in infection due to *Microsporum canis* **(Fig. 58)**
	Zigzag hairs (short hairs with several bends in them like a zigzag pattern)
	Barcode-like (Morse code-like) hairs **(Fig. 59)**
	Bent hairs **(Figs. 60 and 61)**
Common dermoscopic findings, but which are not diagnostic	Scale, follicular keratosis, and crusts **(Fig. 62)**
	Erythema
	Broken hairs and Black dots **(Fig. 63)**

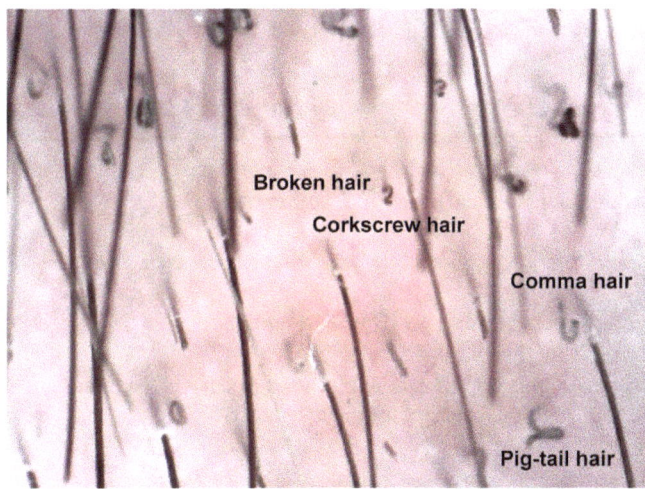

FIG. 58: Dermatoscopic image showing curved hair of various morphologies.

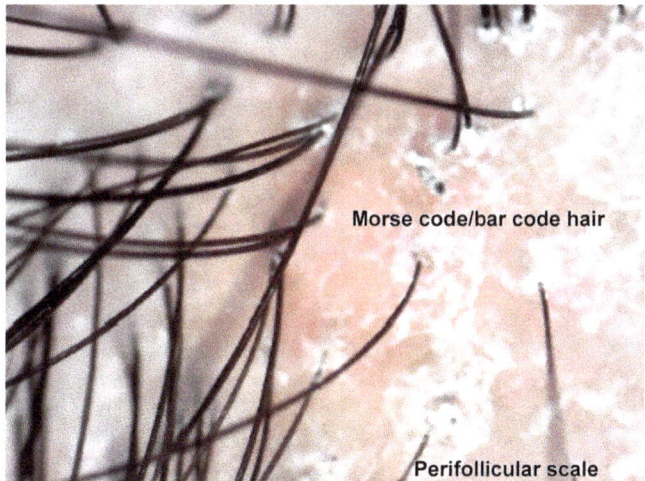

FIG. 59: Dermatoscopic image showing a single morse code hair.

CHAPTER 3: Superficial Fungal Infections

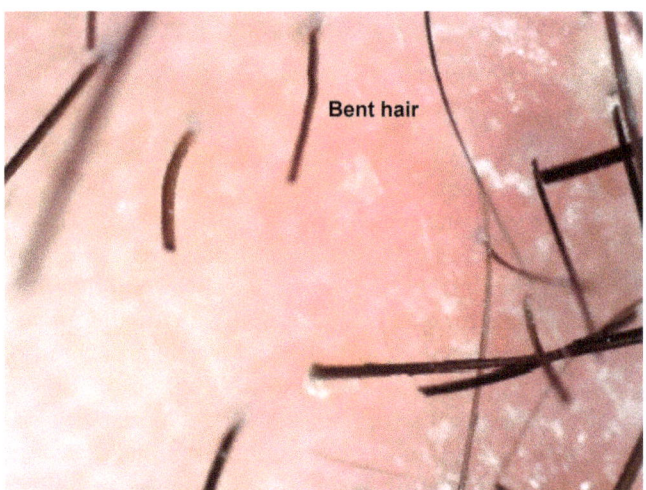

FIG. 60: Dermatoscopic image showing a bent hair.

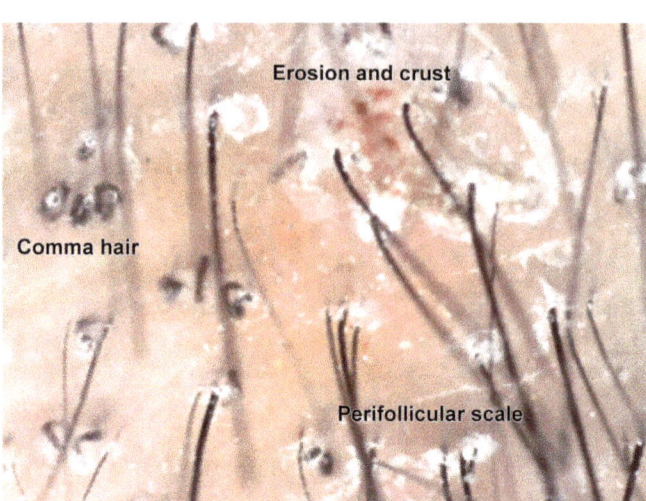

FIG. 62: Dermatoscopic image showing inflammatory changes with erosions, crusts along with other changes of tinea infection.

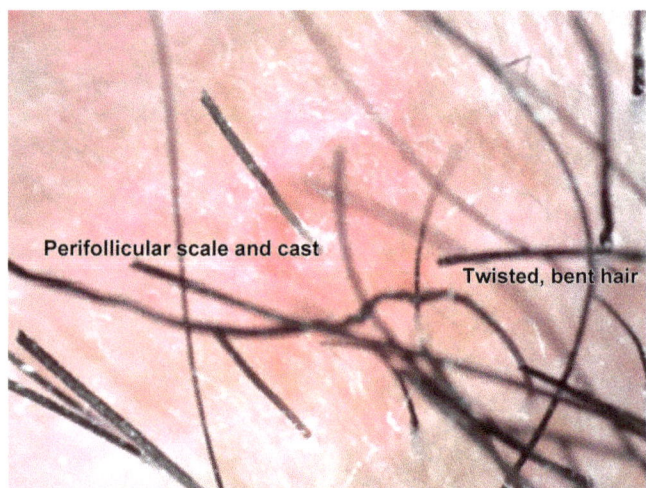

FIG. 61: Dermatoscopic image showing perifollicular scale along with twisted and bent hair.

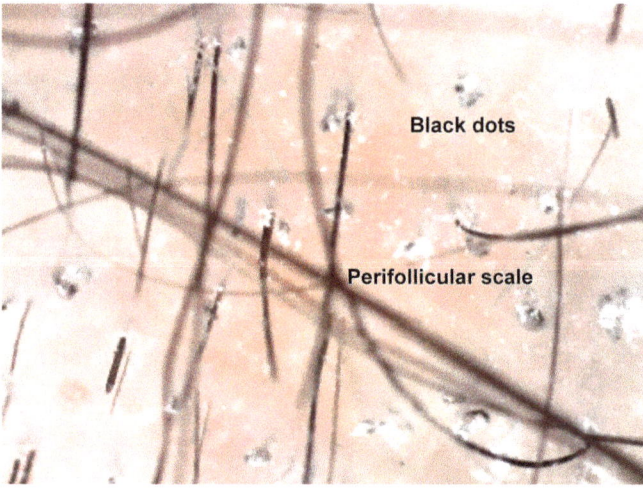

FIG. 63: Dermatoscopic image showing extensive perifollicular scaling along with black dots.

TABLE 4: Dermoscopic findings in onychomycosis	
Type of onychomycosis	**Onychoscopy features**
Distal lateral subungual onychomycosis	• Jagged edge of onycholysis with spikes (whitish longitudinal lines) on the proximal end of the onycholytic area **(Figs. 64 and 65)** • "Aurora Borealis" pattern—longitudinal striae of varying colors, white/yellow/brown/occasionally green within the onycholytic nail plate **(Fig. 66)** • Subungual "ruinous" appearance of the subungual hyperkeratosis **(Figs. 67A and B)** • Distal irregular termination—distal pulverization of the thickened nail plate • *Fungal melanonychia—multicolored pigmentation*: Yellow/brown/gray/black/red which is wider in the distal end (black reverse triangle) in association with thick subungual hyperkeratosis • Leukonychia—homogenous/or punctate • Superficial transverse striation—fine onychoschizia
Dermatophytoma	Round yellow-orange subungual area, connected by a thin band to the distal edge of the nail plate **(Fig. 68)**

Continued

CHAPTER 3: Superficial Fungal Infections

Continued

Type of onychomycosis	Onychoscopy features
Superficial white onychomycosis	• White, opaque, friable spots of scaling distributed irregularly along the nail **(Fig. 69)** • Application of interface media leads to the disappearance of scales • Grid pattern of scaling
Endonyx onychomycosis	• Onychoschizia • Absence of subungual hyperkeratosis or onycholysis • Application of interface media leads to the disappearance of scales • Milky white leukonychia **(Fig. 70)** • Dendritic pattern
Proximal subungual onychomycosis	• White discoloration below the nail plate in the lunula • Linear-edged white patch expanding distally

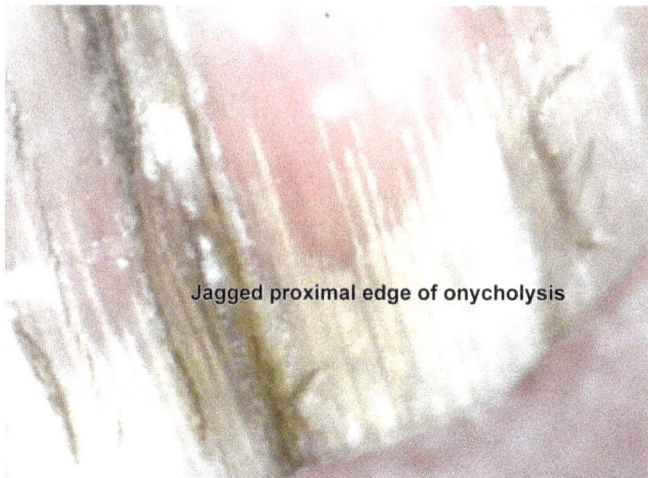

FIG. 64: Dermatoscopic image showing the proximal jagged edge of onycholysis in tinea unguium.

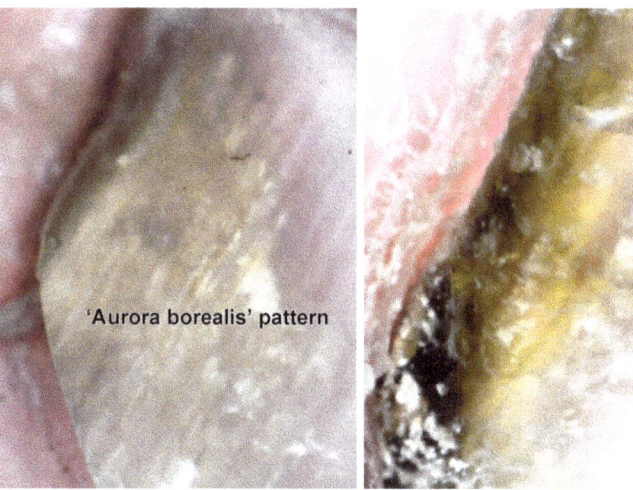

FIG. 66: Dermatoscopic image showing a spectrum of color changes through the nail plate, the so-called "Aurora Borealis pattern."

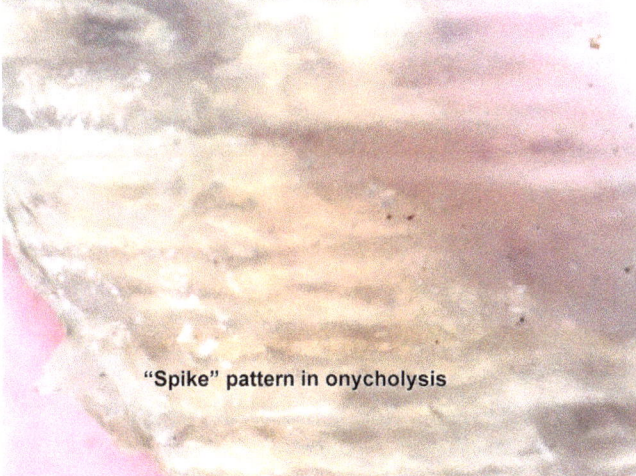

FIG. 65: Dermatoscopic image showing the presence of spikes within the onycholysed area.

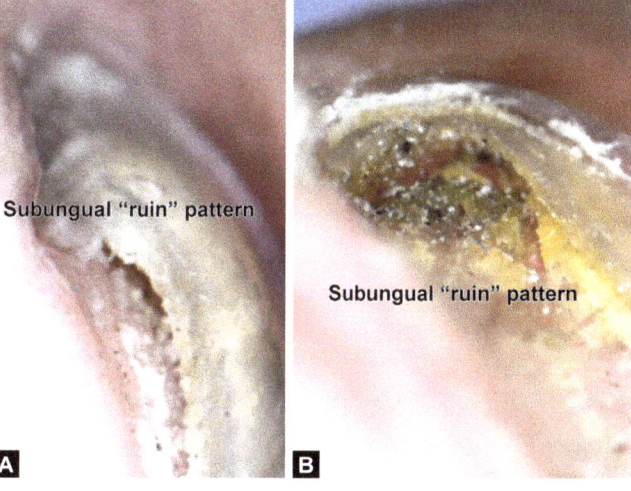

FIGS. 67A AND B: Dermatoscopic image of the distal edge showing subungual ruin appearance.

CHAPTER 3: Superficial Fungal Infections

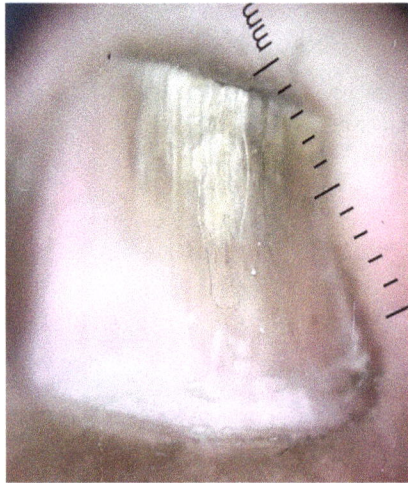

FIG 68: Dermatoscopic image of a case of dermatophytoma.

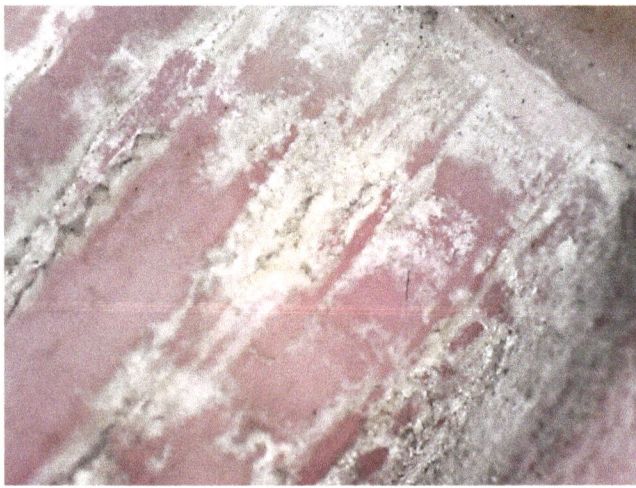

FIG. 69: Dermatoscopic image of a case of superficial white onychomycosis.

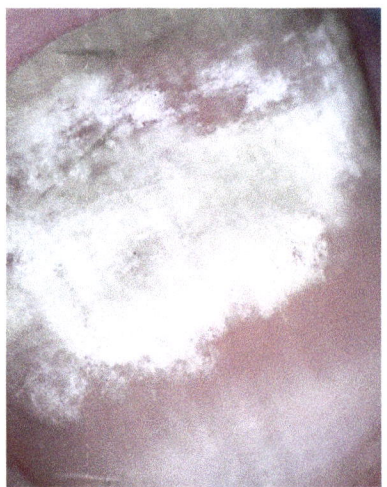

FIG. 70: Dermatoscopic image of a case of endonyx.

TABLE 5: Dermoscopic findings in dermatophytic skin infections.

Type of cutaneous fungal infection	Dermoscopic features
Tinea corporis	• Diffuse erythema (**Fig. 71**) • Whitish scales, especially peripherally (**Fig. 72**) • Follicular micropustules, especially peripherally (**Fig. 71**) • Brown spots surrounded by a white-yellowish halo • Wavy hair, broken hair, bent hair within the lesion (**Fig. 73**) • Morse code hairs of vellus hairs
Tinea cruris	• Features similar to tinea corporis • Morse code hair • Easily deformable hair • Transparent hair (**Fig. 74**)
Tinea mannum or pedis	• Whitish scales along the palmar and plantar creases • Brownish scales showing dried vesicles • Areas of intense erythema
Tinea incognito	• Morse code hairs • Damaged vellus hairs • Follicular micropustules • Concentric areas of erythema separated by scales • Easily deformable hairs that look transparent • Bent hair • Telangiectasia (**Fig. 75**)

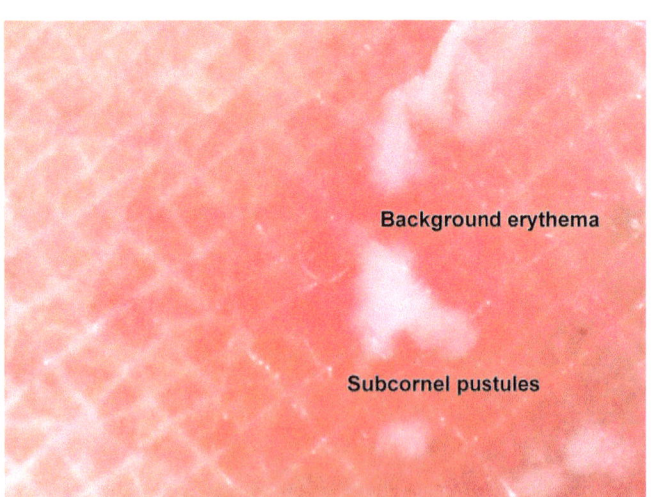

FIG. 71: Dermatoscopic image of extensive background erythema with superficial pustules in a steroid-modified tinea.

CHAPTER 3: Superficial Fungal Infections

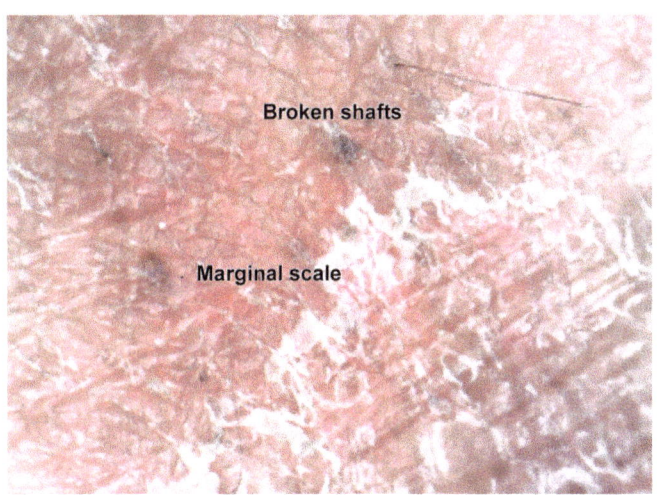

FIG. 72: Dermatoscopic image showing the marginal scale of tinea which was hardly visible on naked eye examination. Broken hair shafts as suggested by black dots, show extensive follicle involvement.

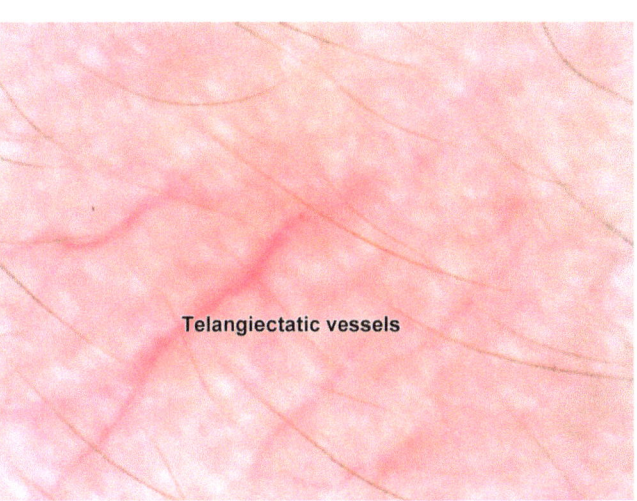

FIG. 75: Dermatoscopic image showing broad telangiectatic vessels due to prolonged steroid abuse.

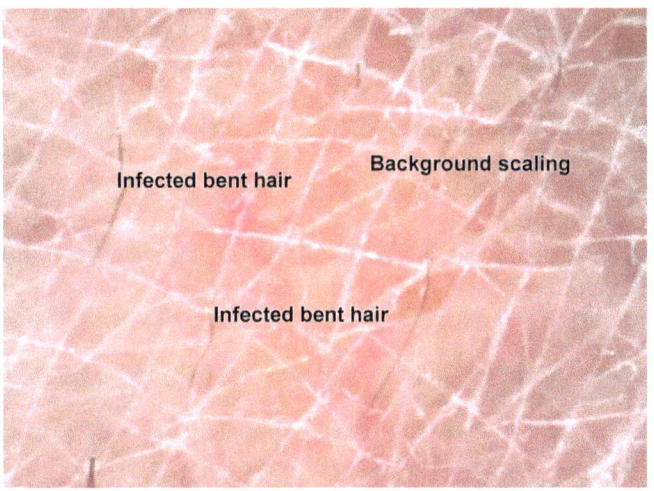

FIG. 73: Dermatoscopic image showing multiple bent hairs, possibly infected, with background scaling accentuated in skin creases.

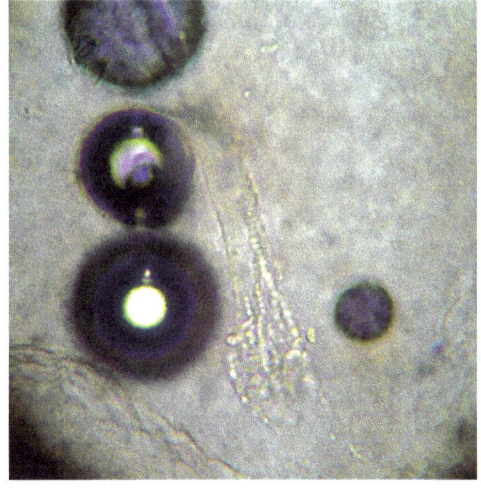

FIG. 76: Presence of dermatophyte septate hyphae under low power [potassium hydroxide (KOH) mount 400×].

- *Direct microscopy*: Dermatophytes can be seen as septate hyphae with an even diameter along their length **(Fig. 76)**. These can be demonstrated in superficial skin scrapings taken from the scaly part of the skin lesions. KOH 10% is used to mount these scrapings, so as to dissolve the keratin which helps in observing the characteristic hyphae. Direct microscopy of hair samples shows the presence of hyphae either inside the hair shaft (endothrix) or on the surface of the shaft (ectothrix infection). For nail samples, a higher strength of KOH or prolonged incubation may be needed to dissolve the thicker nail keratin before the characteristic hyphae can be visualized.
- *Fungal culture*: It is not done routinely. It is usually done in Sabouraud dextrose agar (SDA) (with chloramphenicol and cycloheximide) at 26–28°C,

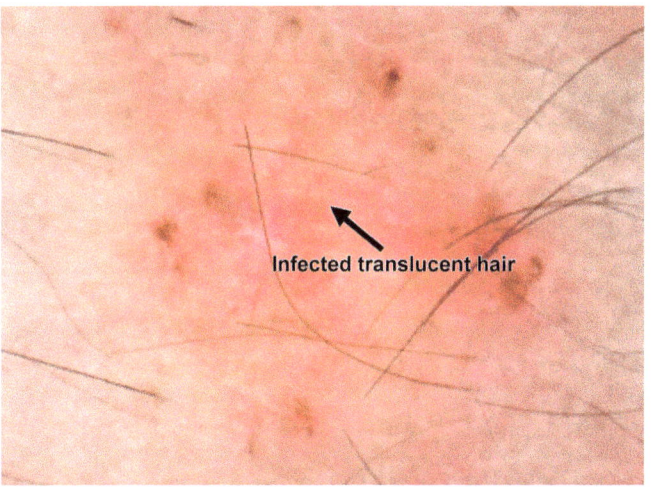

FIG. 74: Dermatoscopic image showing an infected translucent hair.

in which the dermatophytes grow readily. Cultures should be incubated for three weeks before reporting negative
- *Histopathology*: It is a useful investigation in cases of nail invasion especially when repeated direct microscopy and cultures are negative. In histopathological specimens' hyphae can be seen with periodic acid–Schiff (PAS) stain inside the lamellar structure of the nail plate, lying parallel to its surface **(Fig. 77)**. Histopathology cannot identify the species or differentiate between viable and nonviable organisms.

Treatment

- Although, similar antifungal agents (topical or systemic) are used for the treatment of most of these infections, the treatment regimen varies according to the site of involvement.
- The important systemic drugs available for use are summarized below **(Table 6)**.
- The commonly used topical antifungals are summarized in **Table 7**.
- The commonly used treatment regimens are summarized below **(Table 8)**.
- Additional treatment options are summarized in **Table 6**.

Nail Lacquers

Topical nail lacquers such as 8% ciclopirox and 5% amorolfine, can be used alone or in combination with

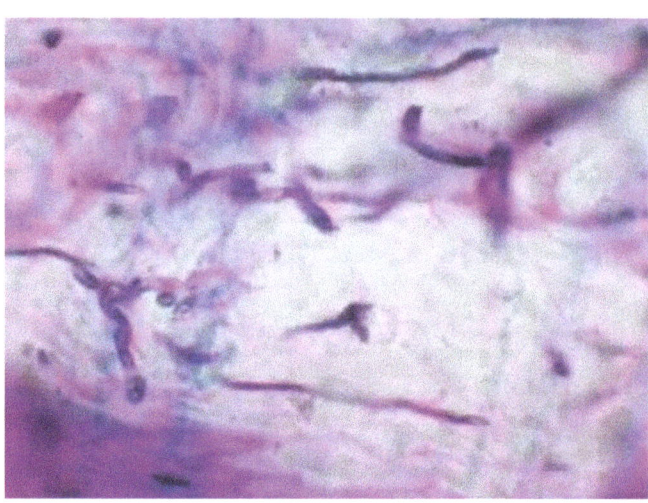

FIG. 77: Fungal invasion in the nail plate structure [periodic acid–Schiff (PAS)-stained nail plate biopsy 400×].

systemic antifungals. The common side effects of nail lacquer include transient periungual erythema or burning at the site of application and bluish or yellow-brown discoloration with the use of amorolfine which clears upon discontinuing treatment.

Device-based Therapies

Low cure rates and high relapse rates in onychomycosis even with highly efficacious antifungals have led to the development of newer treatment options to ensure drug penetration, drug persistence, mycological cure, and

TABLE 6: Systemic antifungals.			
Drug	Antifungal effect	Mechanism of action	Common reported side effects
Griseofulvin	Fungistatic	Inhibition of intracellular microtubules	Headache, nausea, exacerbation of systemic lupus erythematosus, and porphyria
Ketoconazole, fluconazole, and itraconazole	Fungistatic	Inhibition of ergosterol synthesis	Hepatitis (most common with ketoconazole), headache, and nausea
Terbinafine	Fungicidal	Inhibition of squalene epoxidase	Gastrointestinal disturbance, skin rash, pruritus, taste disturbance, and rarely hepatitis

TABLE 7: Topical antifungals.			
Drug	Formulation	Mechanism of action	Common reported side effects
Azoles including miconazole nitrate 2%, clotrimazole 1%, luliconazole 1%, sertaconazole nitrate 2%, etc.	Cream, lotion, and powder	Inhibition of ergosterol synthesis	Rare, itching, and burning
Allylamines (terbinafine)	Cream	Inhibition of squalene epoxidase	Rare, itching, burning, and rash
Tolnaftate	Cream	Inhibition of squalene epoxidase	Skin irritation-redness and burning
Ciclopirox	Shampoo and nail lacquer	Chelates polyvalent metal cations, such as Fe^{3+} and Al^{3+}	Skin irritation
Amorolfine	Cream and nail lacquer	Inhibits ergosterol synthesis in two steps: (1) The delta 14 reduction and (2) the delta 7–8 isomerization	Redness and itching

TABLE 8: Treatment regimens for common dermatophytosis.			
Indication	Drug	Dosage	Duration of therapy
Tinea unguium	Terbinafine	250 mg once a day	6 weeks for fingernails, 12 weeks for toenails
	Itraconazole	200 mg BID	1 week for each month for consecutive 2 months for fingernails and consecutive 3 months for toenails
	Fluconazole	150–300 mg/week	Around 9–12 months
Tinea corporis/cruris/faciei	Terbinafine	250 mg OD	2–4 weeks
	Itraconazole	100 mg OD	1–2 weeks
	Fluconazole	150 mg/week	2–4 weeks
Tinea capitis	Griseofulvin	5–25 mg/kg/day	6–8 weeks
	Terbinafine	5 mg/kg/day	4–6 weeks
Tinea pedis/tinea manuum	Terbinafine	250 mg OD	4–6 weeks
	Itraconazole	200 mg BID	2 weeks
Tinea barbae	Griseofulvin	1 g OD	4–6 weeks
	Terbinafine	250 mg OD	

Note: Most of the dermatophytosis requires much longer therapy now.
(BID: twice daily; OD: once daily)

effective prevention of relapse. These include device-related therapies; physical measures to enhance drug penetration through nails; and the development of synergistic combinations. There are two US FDA-approved laser systems—Pinpointe (NuvoLase Inc.) and Genesis Plus (Cutera Inc.), both approved to produce a temporary enhancement of clear nails in patients with onychomycosis. Potential phototherapy treatments for onychomycosis have been evaluated in podiatric literature. These include three light-based technologies: ultraviolet light therapy, near-infrared photoinactivation therapy, and photothermal ablative antisepsis, for use in OM.

Surgical Treatment
Surgical avulsion followed by topical therapies can be considered for single nail onychomycosis, not responsive to standard therapies or infection with nondermatophyte species; however, the results are not very encouraging.

Nondermatophytic Mold Onychomycosis

Nondermatophyte molds can cause nail infections, accounting for 1.5–6% of all onychomycosis. Causative organisms include *Scopulariopsis brevicaulis*, *Aspergillus*, *Fusarium*, *Onychocola canadensis*, and *Scytalidium*.

Clinical Features
- Features of nondermatophytic mold (NDM) onychomycosis are similar to dermatophyte onychomycosis, but there are subtle differences.

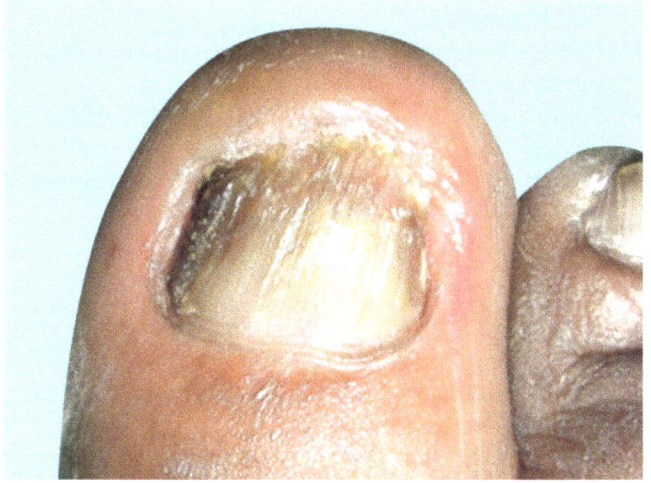

FIG. 78: Nondermatophytic mold (NDM) onychomycosis. Fungal culture showed growth of *Aspergillus fumigatus*. Note the lateral black discoloration.

- Various types of nail involvement can be seen in the form of distal and lateral subungual onychomycosis (DLSO) **(Fig. 78)**, proximal subungual onychomycosis (PSO), superficial white onychomycosis (SWO), and total dystrophic onychomycosis (TDO) **(Fig. 79)**.
- Other clinical clues are the presence of periungual inflammation **(Fig. 79)**, brown discoloration of the nail plate, and absence of concomitant skin involvement or tinea pedis.

Diagnosis
- These molds are ubiquitous; hence, their isolation in fungal cultures is not by itself considered a proof of

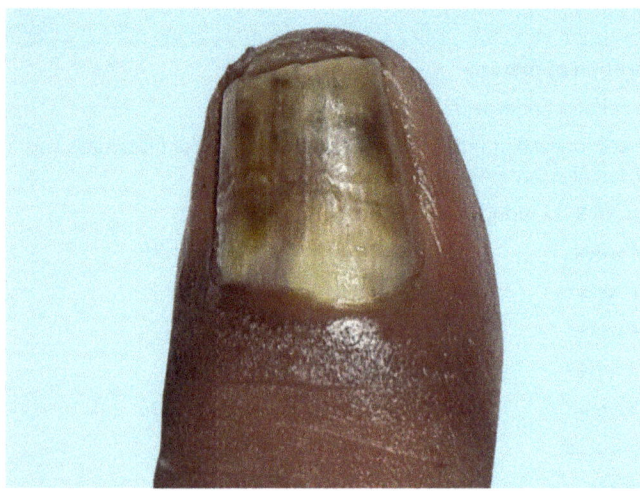

FIG. 79: Nondermatophyte mold (NDM) onychomycosis involving a single nail, showing significant periungual inflammation and swelling of the proximal nail fold.

causation. They are considered pathogenic only if nail abnormalities are consistent with a diagnosis of NDM onychomycosis.
- Positive direct microscopic examination shows hyphae in nail keratin.
- Failure to isolate dermatophyte species in fungal culture.
- Growth of more than five colonies of the same mold in at least two consecutive samples.

Treatment

- NDM's are often difficult to eradicate, so a combination of approaches is required.
- Newer antifungals, especially itraconazole have a broad-spectrum activity.
- *Aspergillus* infection responds well to systemic terbinafine or itraconazole. *Scopulariopsis* species can be treated with terbinafine; however, the duration of therapy may be prolonged.
- Treatment of other molds is often challenging and is best handled with a combination of oral, topical, and surgical methods.

Candidiasis or Candidosis

This is a range of superficial fungal infections of the skin, nails, and mucosae caused by yeasts belonging to the genus *Candida*. Causative organisms include approximately 200 species of *Candida* including *Candida albicans* (70–80% of infections), *Candida glabrata*, *Candida tropicalis*, *Candida krusei*, *Candida dubliniensis*, and *Candida parapsilosis*. The factors predisposing to candidal infections are outlined in **Box 2**.

BOX 2 | Factors predisposing to Candidiasis.

Endocrine factors:
- Diabetes
- Cushing's syndrome
- Pregnancy
- Addison's disease
- Hypothyroidism
- Hypoparathyroidism

Mechanical factors:
- Local occlusion and high moisture levels causing maceration
- Obesity
- Local tissue damage like burns, abrasions

Immunodeficiency:
- Acquired immunodeficiency syndrome (AIDS) and DiGeorge syndrome (defective T-lymphocyte function)
- Chronic granulomatous disease (defective macrophage function)
- Myeloperoxidase deficiency (defective neutrophil function)
- Severe combined immunodeficiency syndrome
- Malignancy, such as leukemia and lymphomas

Iatrogenic factors:
- Prolonged antibiotic use (disturbing the normal flora)
- Glucocorticoids
- Oral contraceptives
- Immunosuppressives

Acute Pseudomembranous Candidiasis or Oral Thrush

Clinical Features

- Oral candidiasis can present with various clinical patterns with acute pseudomembranous candidiasis being the most common form.
- It is characterized by a grayish-white semiadherent membrane in the buccal mucosa, tongue, palate, or gingiva **(Fig. 80)**.
- The base of these plaques is moist, red, and macerated.
- In immunosuppressed patients, lesions may extend into the pharynx and esophagus causing odynophagia.

Differential Diagnosis

- Oral lichen planus
- Herpetic infection
- Erythema multiforme
- Mucositis due to viral fever or chemotherapeutic agents

Angular Cheilitis (Perleche)

Clinical Features

- This is another common form of oral candidiasis.
- It presents as erythema, maceration, and fissuring at the oral commissures, usually bilaterally **(Fig. 81)**.

CHAPTER 3: Superficial Fungal Infections

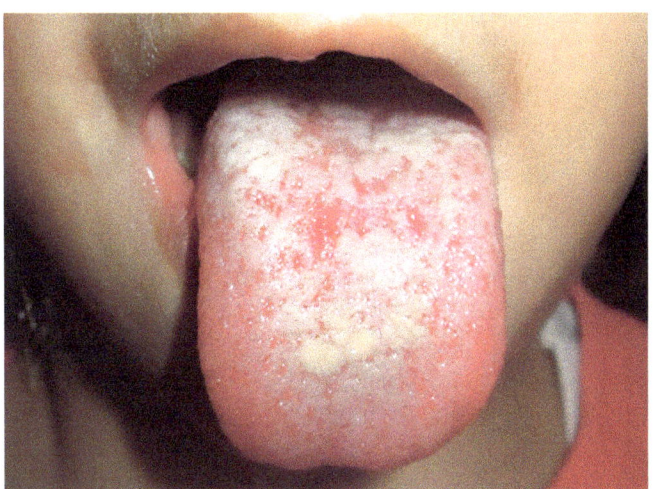

FIG. 80: Oral pseudomembranous candidiasis/thrush.

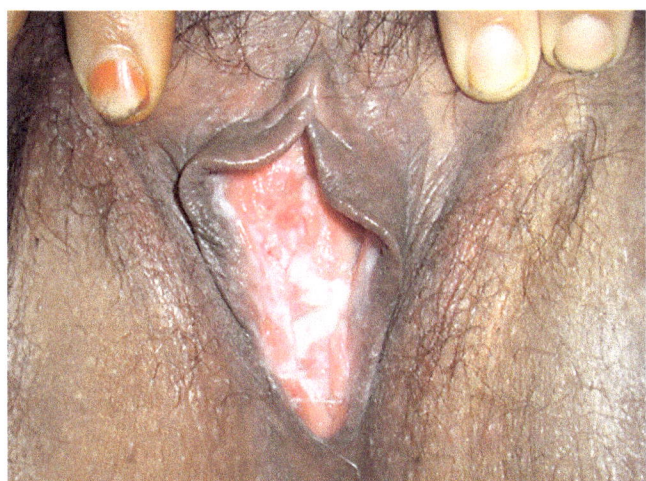

FIG. 82: Vulvovaginal candidiasis.

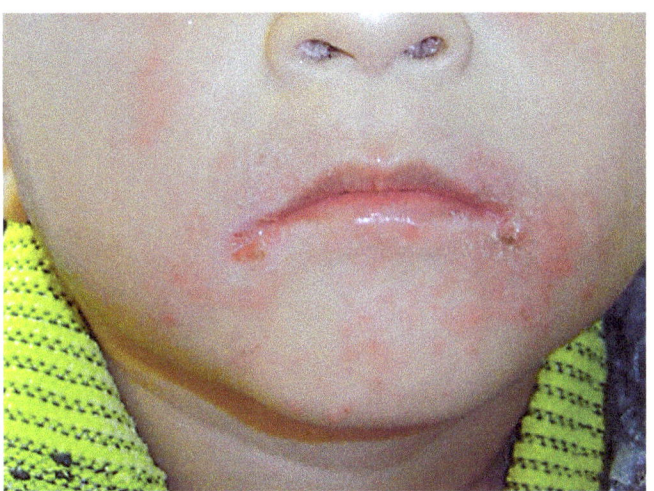

FIG. 81: Angular cheilitis in a young child.

- This condition can also be associated with the presence of coagulase-positive *Staphylococcus aureus* and gram-negative bacteria apart from *Candida* infection.
- As the etiology is multifactorial, management also needs to be multifactorial.
- The patient should be seen in totality, including the nutritional status.

Treatment
- General measures, such as maintenance of oral hygiene and removal of dentures at night.
- Topical Nystatin suspension (400,000–600,000 units) applied four times a day.
- Clotrimazole mouth paint applied five times a day for 10–14 days.
- For chronic and severe cases like hyperplastic or atrophic candidiasis, oral antifungals are needed, such as fluconazole (100-200 mg/day) and itraconazole (100-200 mg/day).

Vaginal and Vulvovaginal Candidiasis

It is a common infection seen in almost 75% of all women at least one time during their lifetime. Causative organisms include *C. albicans* (80–90% of cases) followed by *Candida glabrata*.

Clinical Features
- Severe itching, burning, and thick white creamy discharge per vaginum is characteristic **(Fig. 82)**.
- On per speculum examination, whitish plaques over the vaginal walls with erythema and edema can be seen.
- Recurrent candidal vulvovaginitis (four or more symptomatic episodes per year) may be seen in 5% of cases.
- The predisposing factors include pregnancy, diabetes mellitus, broad-spectrum antibiotic usage, immunosuppression, obesity, steroid use, and tightfitting synthetic undergarments.

Treatment
- Single 150 mg dose of fluconazole along with topical imidazoles (intravaginal pessaries or creams).
- For recurrent vulvovaginal candidiasis, a weekly fluconazole 150 mg tablet orally or clotrimazole 500 mg tablet intravaginally can be used effectively.

Candidal Balanitis and Balanoposthitis

Clinical Features
- It is common in uncircumcised sexually active males, accounting for 30–35% of cases of infective balanitis.
- It presents as tiny, fragile, papulopustules on the glans and prepuce.
- The lesions rupture to leave behind superficial erosions with a collarette of white scales **(Figs. 83 and 84)**.

CHAPTER 3: Superficial Fungal Infections

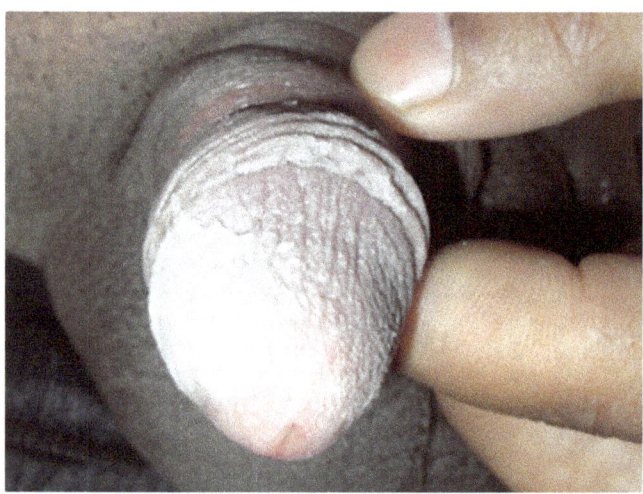

FIG. 83: Candidal balanoposthitis with characteristic white scale.

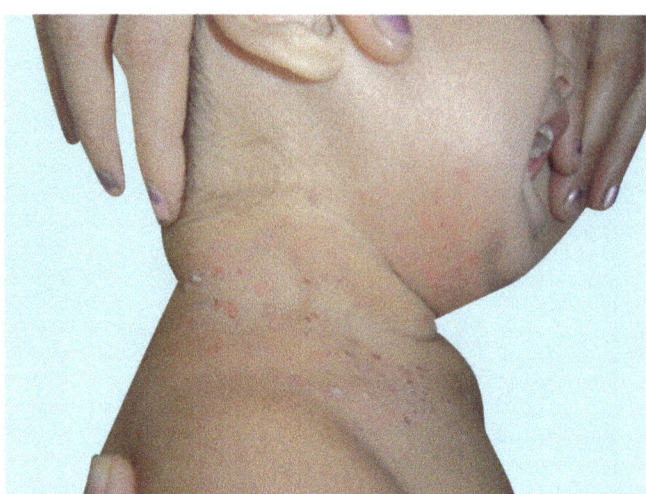

FIG. 85: Candidal intertrigo in an infant. The presence of satellite pustules is highly suggestive.

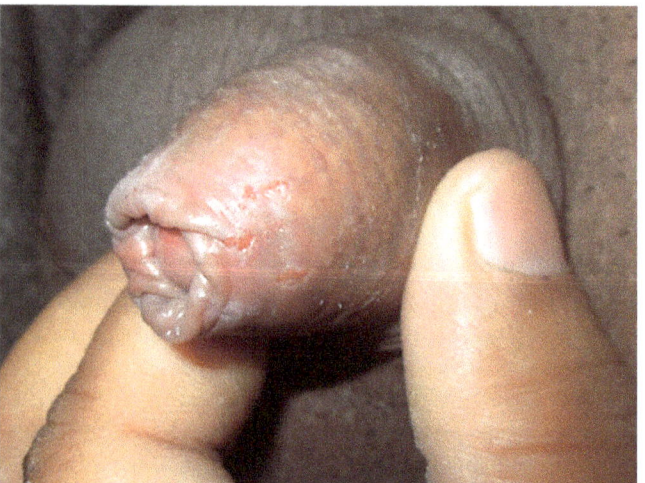

FIG. 84: Linear erosions over the glans, which is highly suggestive of candidal balanoposthitis (CBP).

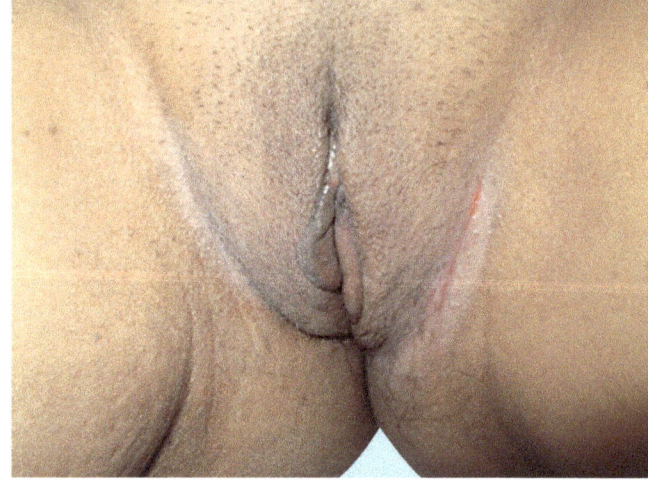

FIG. 86: Candidal intertrigo with moist, macerated intertriginous fissures.

- In immunosuppressed patients, there may be severe inflammatory changes of the glans, such as edema and ulceration.
- Small linear erosions are highly characteristic of this condition **(Fig. 84)**.

Candidal Intertrigo

This is the most common presentation of Candidiasis on glabrous skin.

Clinical Features

- It can present as pruritic, pink to red, moist areas, associated with satellite vesicopustules **(Fig. 85)**.
- Commonly involves the armpits, groins **(Fig. 86)**, intergluteal, interdigital, and submammary regions.
- The vesicopustules may rupture to leave behind a collarette of white scales. In severe cases, there may be fissure formation.

Differential Diagnosis

- Tinea cruris
- Erythrasma
- Bacterial intertrigo
- Flexural psoriasis
- Seborrheic dermatitis

Perianal Candidiasis

Clinical Features

- Candidal infection in the intergluteal and perianal area may present as pruritus ani.

- Characterized by redness, maceration, and oozing in the perianal region **(Fig. 87)**.
- Candidal superinfection on preexisting plaques of psoriasis or extramammary Paget's disease may also be present in this area.

Candidal Paronychia

Inflammation of the nail fold due to *Candida* is common in housewives and food handlers due to prolonged water contact. There is a significant role of bacterial coinfection and contact irritant dermatitis as well.

Clinical Features

- Early stages present with redness, swelling, and tenderness of the proximal nail fold.
- Later, there is a loss of cuticle and separation of the proximal nail fold from the nail plate **(Fig. 88)**.
- In chronic cases, the nail plate is thickened and brownish with Beau's lines, distal onycholysis, and extensive nail damage in long-standing cases.
- At this chronic stage, there is much fibrosis of the proximal nail fold. This impedes the penetration of topical and systemic therapy. Hence, this condition becomes all the more difficult to treat.

Candidal Onychomycosis

Clinical Features

- The most common presentation is DLSO with subungual hyperkeratosis in addition to paronychia **(Fig. 89)**.
- In a few cases, there is a presence of only erosions of lateral and distal nail plates along with paronychia.

Treatment

- Prolonged topical antifungal treatment is required for chronic paronychia, in addition to minimizing wet work.
- In proven cases of candidal onychomycosis, oral fluconazole, and itraconazole can be used successfully. Itraconazole as continuous or pulse regimen; and fluconazole as 50 mg/day or 300 mg/week to be continued for a minimum of 4 weeks for fingernail and 12 weeks for toenail onychomycosis.

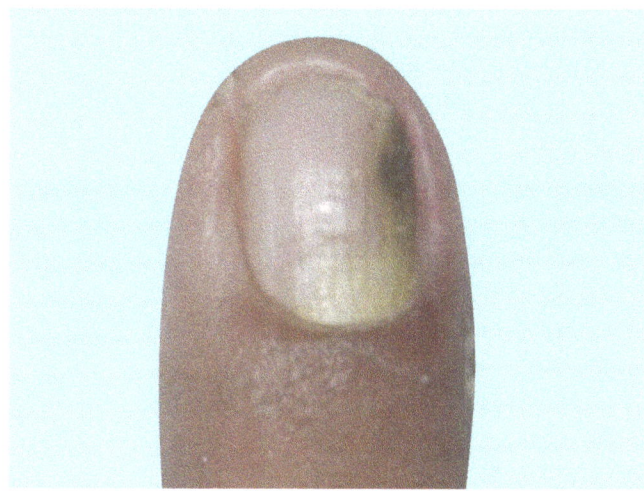

FIG. 88: Candidal onychomycosis with swelling and erythema of proximal and lateral nail fold. Note the absence of cuticles and secondary nail dystrophy.

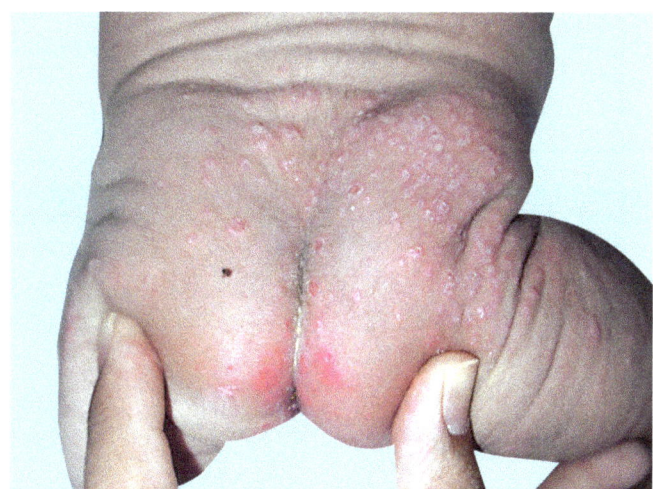

FIG. 87: Perianal candidiasis in an infant with characteristic satellite pustules.

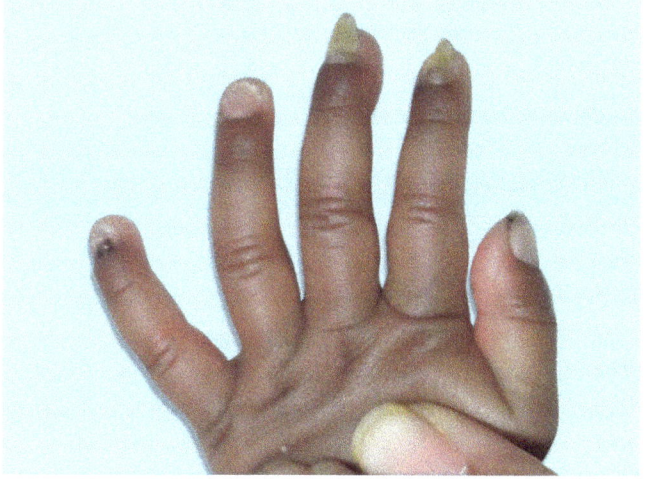

FIG. 89: Candidal onychomycosis in a young child.

Diaper Candidiasis or Candidal Diaper Dermatitis

Clinical Features
- There are red, moist macules with satellite pustules at the borders.
- In long-standing cases or with immunosuppression, there is the formation of brownish nodules on the buttocks, genitalia, upper thigh, and perineum. This is known as granuloma gluteale infantum **(Fig. 90)**.

Diagnosis
- The confirmation of the diagnosis is by demonstration of budding yeast cells (2–6 × 3–9 μm) **(Fig. 91)** with narrow bases accompanied by hyphae or pseudohyphae on light microscopy.
- *C. albicans* grows easily on cycloheximide-free SDA at 37°C; with whitish mucoid colonies appearing in 2–5 days. However, the plate should be incubated for one week before reporting it as negative.
- *Histopathology* shows subcorneal neutrophil accumulation. The yeast cells can be demonstrated in stratum corneum with PAS or methenamine silver stain.

Treatment
Apart from specific therapy for candidiasis, it is important to treat or alter the underlying predisposing factors such as diabetes mellitus, Addison's disease, Cushing's syndrome, and other causes of immunosuppression. Specific therapy includes:
- *Topical therapy* including topical polyene compound nystatin and topical imidazoles, such as miconazole nitrate 2% and clotrimazole 1%
- *Systemic therapy* including drugs such as fluconazole, and itraconazole which are summarized in **Table 9**. The major adverse effect of ketoconazole is hepatotoxicity.

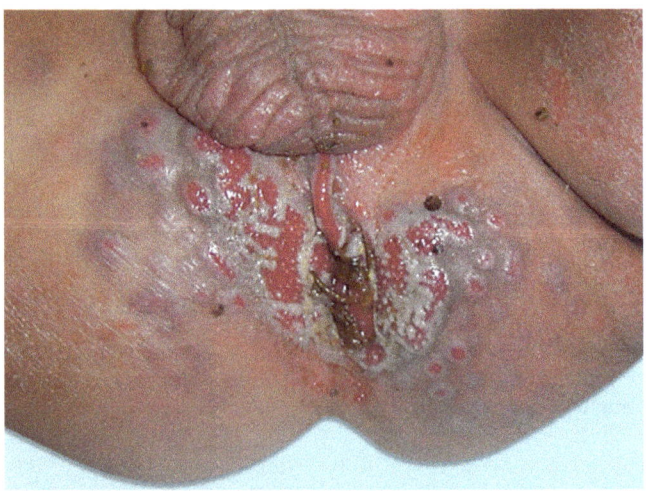

FIG. 90: Diaper involvement, granuloma gluteale infantum in a young child.

Note: Chronic occlusion caused by wet diapers creates an ideal condition for *Candida* infection with species from the patient's own gut flora.

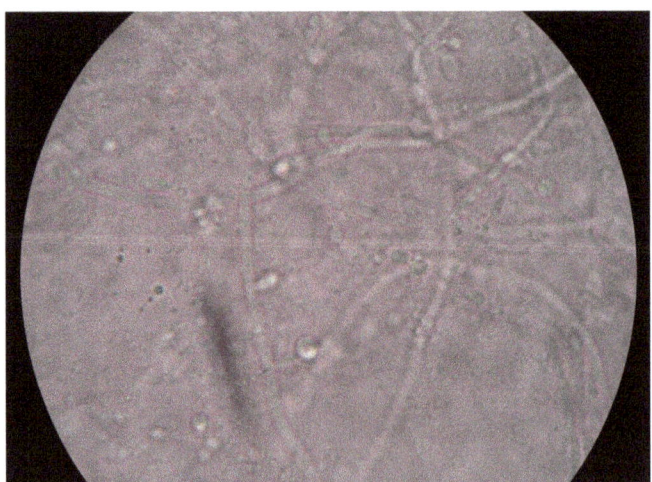

FIG. 91: *Candida* pseudohyphae and budding yeasts [potassium hydroxide (KOH) mount 400×].

TABLE 9: Oral treatment options for various clinical types of cutaneous candidiasis.

Indication	Drug	Dosage	Duration of therapy
Oropharyngeal candidiasis	Itraconazole	100 mg OD	7 days
	Fluconazole	100–200 mg OD	7 days
Vulvovaginal candidiasis	Itraconazole	600 mg stat	Single dose
	Fluconazole	150 mg stat	Single dose
Recurrent vulvovaginal candidiasis	Fluconazole	150 mg on 0, 3, and 7 days, then 150 mg/week for 6 months	–
Candidal onychomycosis	Itraconazole	200 mg BD for 7 days in a month (one cycle)	Two to three cycles
	Fluconazole	300 mg/week	4 weeks for fingernails and 12 weeks for toenails

(BD: twice daily; OD: once daily; stat: immediately)

Pityriasis Versicolor (Tinea Versicolor)

It is a chronic infection characterized by hypopigmented or hyperpigmented coalescing scaly macules over the trunk. Causative organisms are fungi of *Malassezia* species including lipophilic yeasts such as *Malassezia furfur, Malassezia pachydermatis, Malassezia sympodialis, Malassezia globosa*, etc. The yeast form of these organisms is a part of the resident flora of the skin, whereas the hyphal phase is implicated in producing skin lesions. It is more common in teenagers and young adults, more commonly seen in hot and humid climate

Clinical Features

- Hypopigmented **(Fig. 92)** or hyperpigmented coalescing macules **(Fig. 93)** with characteristic furfuraceous or fine branny scales are characteristic.

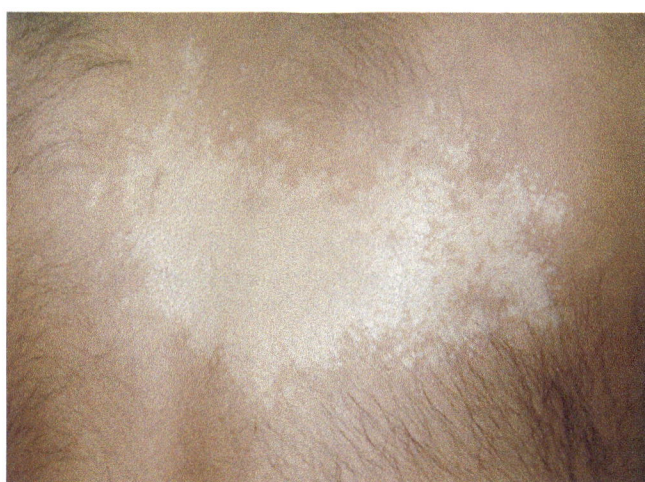

FIG. 92: Hypopigmented pityriasis versicolor. The lesions can be isolated or confluent. Mild scaling can be appreciated.

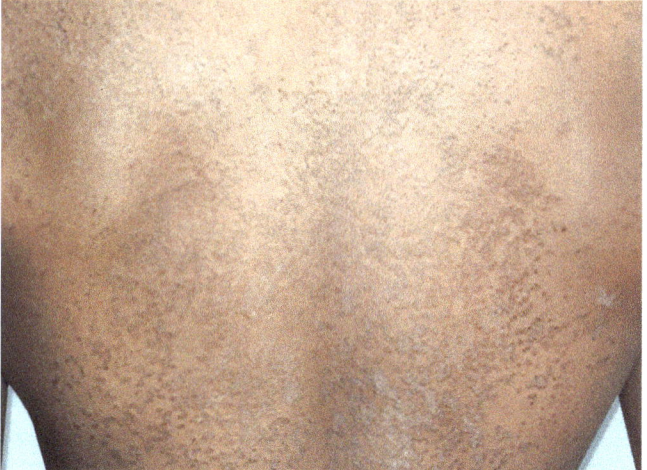

FIG. 93: Hyperpigmented pityriasis versicolor.

- The scale can be demonstrated on lightly scratching the skin (scratch sign).
- Sites of predilection are the sternal region, sides of the chest, upper arms, abdomen, back, neck, and intertriginous areas.
- The patients are usually asymptomatic.

Diagnosis

- Direct microscopic examination of lesional scrapings demonstrates fungus easily. A combination of mycelium (2–5 μm wide and 25 μm long) with spherical thick-walled yeasts (2–8 μm wide) commonly referred to as "spaghetti and meatballs" or "banana and grapes" appearance, confirms the diagnosis **(Fig. 94)**.
- Wood's lamp examination may show yellow fluorescence of involved skin.
- The organism can also be cultured in lipid-enriched media but this is rarely resorted to in clinical practice.

Differential Diagnosis

- Pityriasis alba
- Pityriasis rosea
- Seborrheic dermatitis
- Tinea infection
- Secondary syphilis (always rule out)
- Vitiligo
- Erythrasma
- Psoriasis
- Pityriasis rubra pilaris

Treatment

- Treatment options are summarized in **Table 10**.
- Patients must be counseled that hypopigmentation may take a further 2–3 months to resolve.

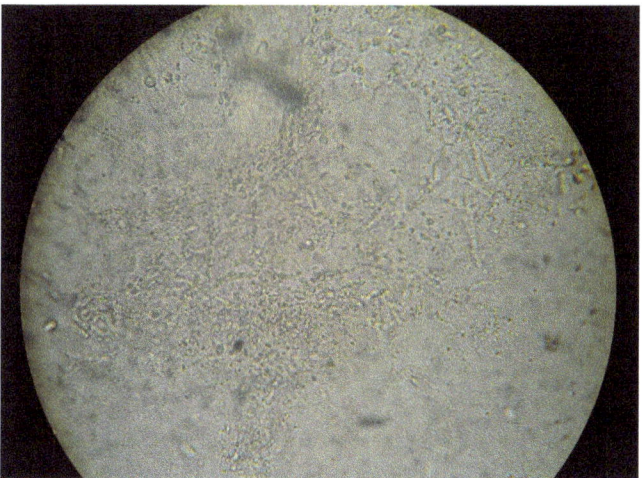

FIG. 94: Spaghetti and meatballs appearance [potassium hydroxide (KOH) mount 400×].

CHAPTER 3: Superficial Fungal Infections

TABLE 10: Treatment options for pityriasis versicolor.	
Topical	Systemic
Selenium sulfide 2.5% shampoo (left on for at least 10 minutes) for 14 days	Ketoconazole 400 mg stat or 200 mg daily for 7 days
Ketoconazole 2% shampoo (at least for 5 minutes) for 3 days	Itraconazole 200 mg daily for 7 days or 400 mg stat
Miconazole nitrate 2% cream BD for 3 weeks	Fluconazole 400 mg stat
(BD: twice daily; stat: immediately)	

- Relapses are very common. General measures such as wearing nonocclusive clothing and avoiding excessive sweating, help in reducing the risk of relapse.
- Oral antifungals in prophylactic doses can decrease the chances of relapse. Oral ketoconazole 400 mg or fluconazole 400 mg can be repeated at monthly intervals for the same.
- Similarly, topical antifungal shampoos or zinc pyrithione bars can also help.

Piedra or Trichomycosis Nodularis

It is a superficial fungal infection of the hair shaft more commonly seen in tropical countries with hot humid climates. White piedra is more common in temperate climates. Causative organisms are *Piedraia hortae* for black piedra and pathogenic species of *Trichosporon beigelii* for white piedra. Transmission of infection in close family members is common.

■ Clinical Features

- Black piedra is characterized by the presence of multiple, firmly adherent, dark, pinhead-sized, hard nodules on the hair of the scalp and less frequently on brows, lashes, or beard **(Fig. 95)**.
- White piedra presents with multiple, white, or beige colored soft, less adherent nodules. It is more common in beards, mustache, and pubic hair.
- In both forms, the patient may not be aware of the infection in the early stages. It is only when a large number of nodules have formed, then they are visible in wet hair.

■ Diagnosis

- The nodules can be seen adhering to the hair shaft **(Fig. 96)**. Upon removal and dissolution in KOH, the nodules of black piedra show brown septate hyphae along with chlamydoconidia. White piedra nodules demonstrate hyphae, arthroconidia, and budding cells under KOH examination.

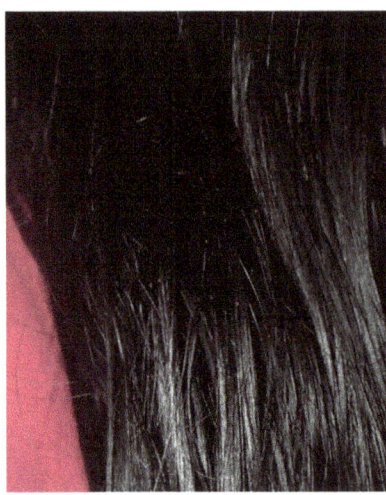

FIG. 95: Piedra in long hair. Note the barely visible dark brown concretions attached to the hair shaft along its length. The concretions can be made more visible by wetting the hair.

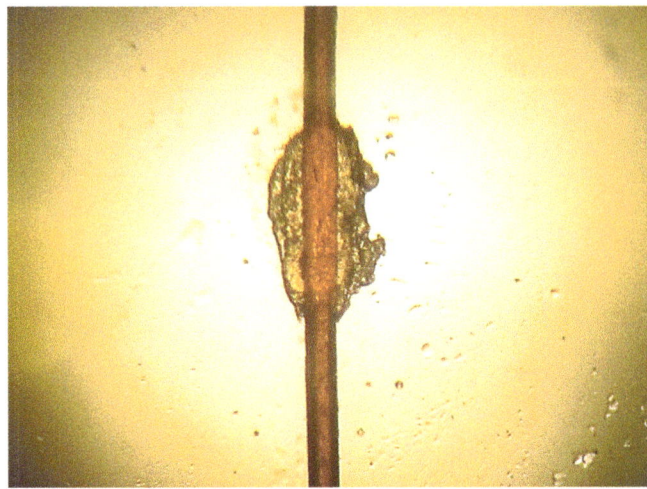

FIG. 96: Piedra nodules adherent to the hair shaft [potassium hydroxide (KOH) mount 100×].

- The fungus can be grown in SDA with cycloheximide to form black colonies. *Trichosporon* can be grown in SDA and is inhibited by cycloheximide.

Differential Diagnosis
- Nits
- Hair casts or peripilar casts

Treatment
- Cutting or shaving the infected hair shaft is a simple and curative treatment modality for both black and white piedra.
- Various topical and systemic antifungals have been reported to have low efficacy such as topical imidazoles, ciclopirox, selenium sulfide 2%, oral azoles, and oral terbinafine.

CHAPTER 4

Subcutaneous Mycoses

Introduction

Subcutaneous mycoses are fungal infections involving deeper skin, subcutaneous tissue, fascial planes, bones, or various organ systems. They have a protracted clinical course and significant morbidity. Key infections include sporotrichosis, chromoblastomycosis, pheohyphomycosis, mycetoma, subcutaneous zygomycosis (entomophthoromycosis and mucormycosis), and lobomycosis.

Cutaneous Sporotrichosis

- It is a chronic infection, caused by *Sporothrix schenckii*.
- Skin lesions develop at the site of traumatic inoculation.
- It occurs worldwide in warm and humid regions. In India, endemic areas are in the sub-Himalayan belt extending from Himachal Pradesh to Assam.
- *S. schenckii* is a dimorphic yeast, a complex of five important species including *Sporothrix albicans*, *Sporothrix brasiliensis*, *Sporothrix mexicana*, *Sporothrix globosa*, and *Sporothrix schenckii sensu stricto*.
- Occupations such as agriculture, gardening, foresting, nursery, and veterinary work are particularly at risk.
- The incubation period is an average of 3 weeks.

■ Clinical Features

- The primary lesion is a small, indurated, progressively enlarging papulonodule, at the inoculation site.
- It may ulcerate (sporotrichotic chancre) with or without transient satellite adenopathy.
- Various clinical variants are described including lymphocutaneous sporotrichosis, fixed cutaneous sporotrichosis, or extracutaneous/systemic disease.

Lymphocutaneous Sporotrichosis

- It is the classic form **(Fig. 1)** accounting for 70–80% of the cases. A string of nodules may appear along the draining lymphatics.
- Secondary lesions present as erythematous papules, nodules, or plaques with smooth or verrucous surfaces **(Fig. 2)**.
- Some may soften, ulcerate, and produce seropurulent discharge. They are mostly asymptomatic.

Fixed Cutaneous Sporotrichosis

- The infection remains confined to a single skin lesion at the inoculation site **(Fig. 3)**.
- Lesions may be noduloulcerative or crusted erythematous to verrucous plaques **(Fig. 4)**.
- Rarely, they may resemble keratoacanthoma, facial cellulitis, pyoderma gangrenosum, prurigo nodularis,

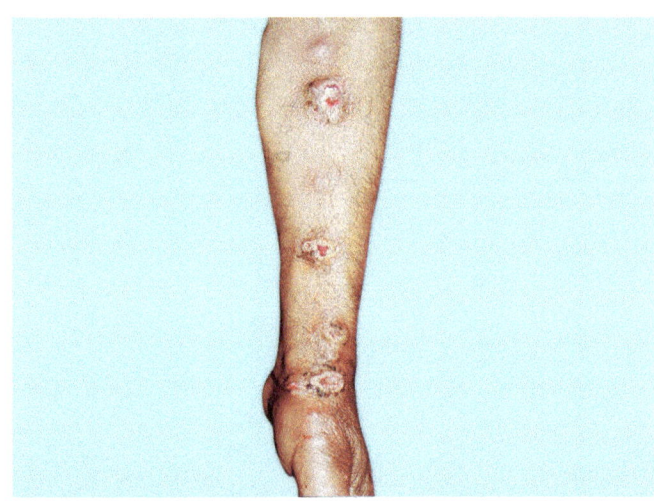

FIG. 1: Lymphocutaneous sporotrichosis involving the upper limb.

CHAPTER 4: Subcutaneous Mycoses

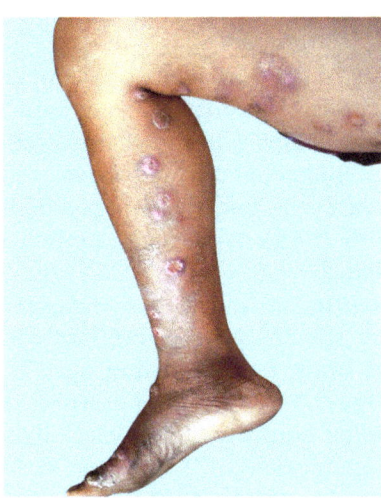

FIG. 2: In the lower limb, a string of noduloulcerative lesions appear along the lymphatics, proximal to the initial inoculation (injury) site.

soft tissue sarcoma, basal cell carcinoma, erysipeloid, or rosacea **(Figs. 5 to 7)**.
- This form is associated with higher host resistance and better therapeutic outcomes.

Multifocal or Disseminated Cutaneous Sporotrichosis

This refers to three or more lesions involving two different anatomical sites.

Extracutaneous Sporotrichosis
- Sporotrichosis may involve the osteoarticular, pulmonary, ocular, or central nervous system **(Fig. 8)**.
- It is a result of hematogenous spread in immunosuppressed patients.

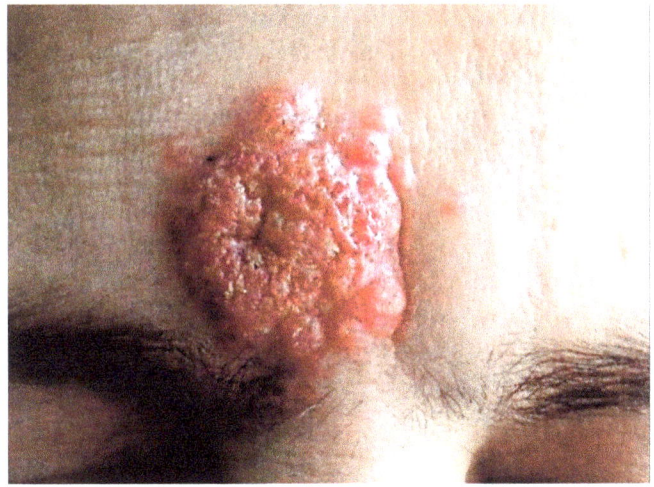

FIG. 3: Fixed cutaneous sporotrichosis. A large indurated granulomatous plaque over the forehead.

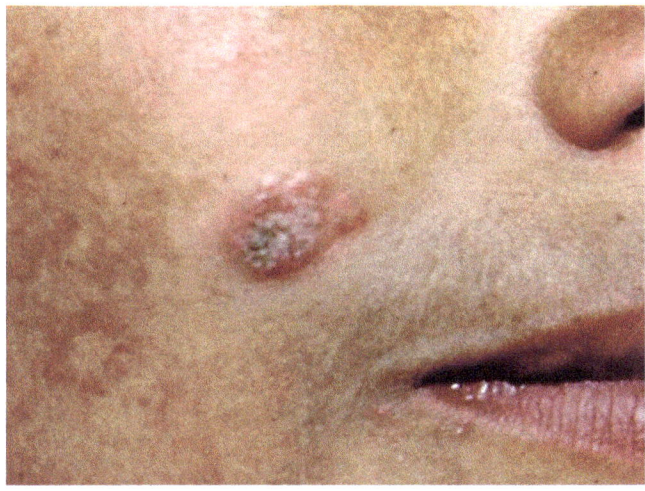

FIG. 5: Fixed cutaneous sporotrichosis over right cheek.

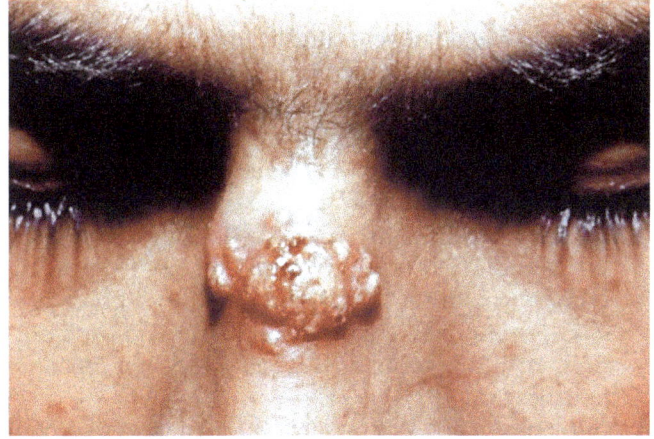

FIG. 4: Noduloulcerative lesion over the nasal bridge.

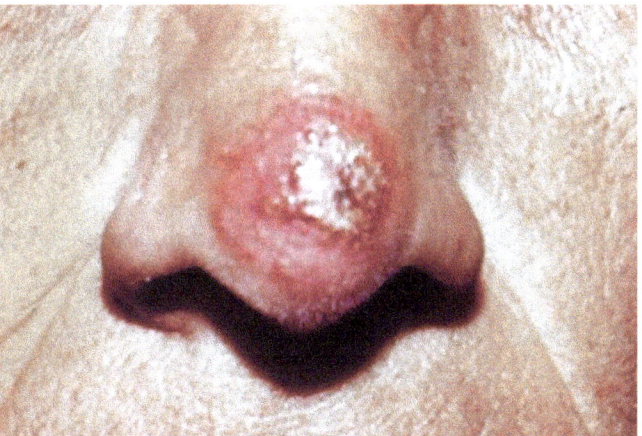

FIG. 6: Another lesion over the nose tip. The small papular lesions at the periphery of the primary lesion are suggestive of destabilization of the lesion and result from the trauma of surgery or manipulation of the lesion.

CHAPTER 4: Subcutaneous Mycoses

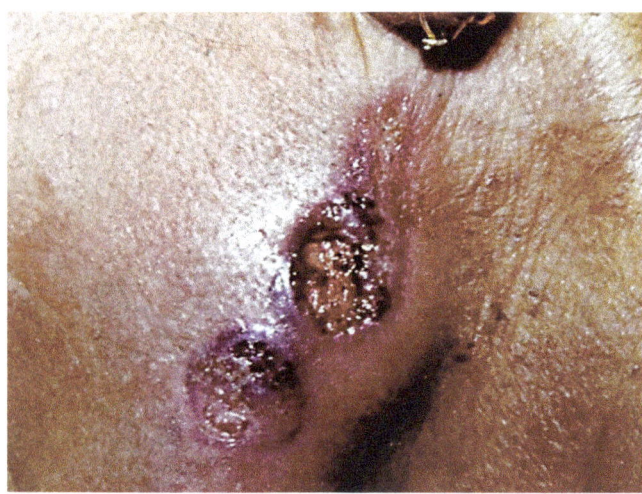

FIG. 7: Ulcerative variant of cutaneous sporotrichosis presenting as painless, nonhealing ulcers involving the left mandibular area.

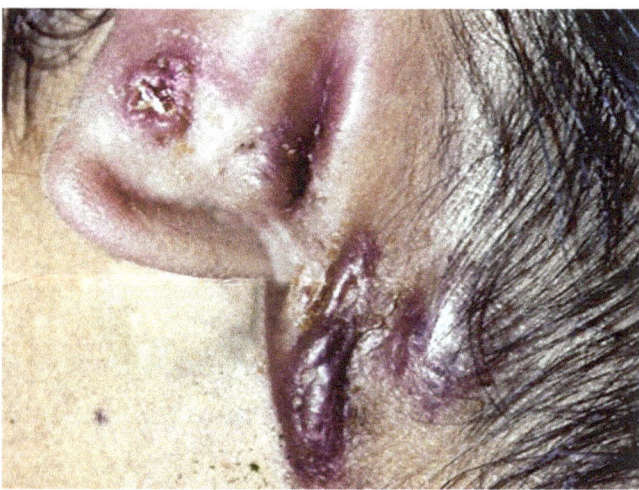

FIG. 8: Noduloulcerative lesions involving ear pinna and retro-auricular area as a result of inoculation with *Sporothrix schenckii* following ear prick.

- Manifestations include sinusitis, osteoarticular disease, meningitis, and endophthalmitis.
- Pulmonary disease is rare and may manifest as cough, low-grade fever, weight loss, mediastinal lymphadenopathy, or cavitation.
- Extracutaneous sporotrichosis has been reported as an emerging mycosis in human immunodeficiency virus (HIV) seropositive individuals in recent years.

Differential Diagnosis

- Cutaneous leishmaniasis
- Nocardiosis
- Chromoblastomycosis
- Paracoccidioidomycosis
- Atypical mycobacteriosis

Diagnosis

The diagnosis of sporotrichosis is often clinical, which needs to be confirmed with investigations including:

- *Direct microscopy*: Fine needle aspiration cytology may show epithelioid cell granulomas, asteroid bodies and/or yeast cells, and cigar-shaped bodies [periodic acid–Schiff (PAS) or Gomori methenamine silver (GMS) stains].
- *Fungal culture*: Culture of *S. schenckii* from pus or biopsy specimen on Sabouraud dextrose agar (SDA) or brain heart infusion agar is diagnostic. The fungus exhibits temperature dimorphism which helps confirm the species. It is a mold at room temperature (26°C) and yeast in tissues (37°C). Lactophenol cotton blue (LCB) mounts demonstrate delicate branching septate hyphae with slender, short, conidiophores, and surrounding pyriform conidia, in a flower-like arrangement. Individual thick-walled, dark brown conidia can also be seen attached directly to the hyphae in a dense sleeve-like pattern.
- *Biopsy and histopathology*: Histopathological features are usually nonspecific. Acute or chronic inflammation is seen with characteristic zonation. There may be chronic epithelioid cell granuloma with foreign-body or Langhans giant cells. There may also be nonspecific chronic granulomatous inflammatory cell infiltrate. Fixed cutaneous sporotrichosis shows central ulceration, and hyperkeratosis at the edge, along with acanthosis and epidermal hyperplasia. Neutrophilic abscesses may be seen. Asteroid bodies which are cigar-shaped (1–2 × 4–5 μm), oval to round, or single budding forms of the yeast, can be visualized in 40–85% of cases. These are extracellular, 15–35 μm in diameter, and localized within abscesses. Splendore–Hoeppli phenomenon, characterized by several fungal organisms enveloped by eosinophilic material radiating centrifugally in a sunburst fashion, can be seen in sporotrichosis. The nodules are organized into three concentric zones; (1) the central necrotic zone containing amorphous debris and polymorphonuclear leukocytes (zone of chronic suppuration), (2) the middle tuberculoid zone is composed of epithelioid cells, giant cells (predominantly Langhans' type) and (3) the outer zone comprising numerous plasma cells, lymphocytes and fibroblasts with prominent capillary hyperplasia and proliferation. In older lesions, this zonation may become indistinct.
- *Intradermal test*: It is performed by using sporotrichin or peptidorhamnomannan (PRM) antigens to detect delayed hypersensitivity.

CHAPTER 4: Subcutaneous Mycoses

Treatment

- Treatment schedules recommended by the Infectious Diseases Society of America are empirical **(Table 1)**.
- Fixed cutaneous sporotrichosis is associated with high host resistance and minimal lesions. It may subside spontaneously.
- Oral administration of a saturated solution of potassium iodide (SSKI) is a useful treatment for uncomplicated cutaneous sporotrichosis due to its low cost and consistent efficacy. The starting dose is five drops three times a day, increased daily by five drops to a maximum of 30-40 drops. Thrice a day till complete regression. The development of metallic taste signifies the threshold for maximum tolerable dose. The response is evident within 2 weeks with healing in 4-32 weeks. Adverse effects include flu-like syndrome, excessive lacrimation, gastrointestinal upset, parotid swelling, acneiform or papulopustular eruption, and inflammation. Rare side effects include hypothyroidism, hyperthyroidism, iododerma, cardiac irritability, pustular psoriasis, etc.
- Treatment should be continued for at least 4-6 weeks after completing clinical remission.

Chromoblastomycosis

- It is a chronic infection localized to the skin and subcutaneous tissue.
- It is caused by brown-walled, round, nonbudding, dematiaceous fungi (sclerotic or copper penny bodies).
- It needs to be differentiated from pheohyphomycosis (cutaneous and extracutaneous infections caused by dematiaceous fungi). Both these infections are actually a continuum of different tissue forms of the causal fungus under the umbrella term "chromomycosis."
- Chromoblastomycosis is reported worldwide, especially in tropical and subtropical regions. Sub-Himalayan, eastern, and western coastal areas in India report most cases. The black-pigmented dematiaceous fungi are saprophytes; they include *Fonsecaea pedrosoi* (most common), *Cladophialophora (Cladosporium) carrionii, Phialophora verrucosa, Fonsecaea compacta*, and occasionally *Rhinocladiella aquaspersa*.
- The usual mode of infection is inoculation following minor injury.

Clinical Features

- The initial lesion is a small, painless, papule at the site of inoculation on exposed body parts. It enlarges to form warty nodules or plaques **(Fig. 9)**.
- In long-standing cases, unilateral, multiple, nodular, tumoral, and hyperkeratotic verrucous plaques are common **(Fig. 10)**. These are seldom associated with pruritus or pain.
- Small hemorrhages are common within the lesions **(Fig. 11)**.
- Autoinoculation or lymphatic spread can lead to satellite lesions.
- Extracutaneous spread to lymph nodes, brain, ileocecal region, tonsils, tracheobronchial tree, etc., is rare.

TABLE 1: Treatment recommendations for sporotrichosis.

Clinical manifestations	Preferred treatment (dose)	Alternative treatment	Duration and remarks
Uncomplicated cutaneous sporotrichosis	Itraconazole (200 mg/day)	• Terbinafine (500 mg BID) • SSKI (increasing doses as detailed above) • Fluconazole (400–800 mg/day) • Local hyperthermia	Treat for 2–4 weeks after lesions have resolved
Osteoarticular sporotrichosis	Itraconazole (200 mg BID)	• Liposomal amphotericin B (3–5 mg/kg/day) • Deoxycholate amphotericin B (0.7–1 mg/kg/day) until resolution	Switch to itraconazole after resolution and treat for a total of 12 months
Pulmonary sporotrichosis	Liposomal amphotericin B (3–5 mg/kg/day) then itraconazole (200 mg BID)	Deoxycholate amphotericin B (0.7–1 mg/kg/day) until recovery then, itraconazole (200 mg BID)	Treat less severe disease with itraconazole. Treat for at least 12 months
Disseminated sporotrichosis	Liposomal amphotericin B (3–5 mg/kg/day), then itraconazole (200 mg BID)	Deoxycholate amphotericin B (0.7–1 mg/kg/day) until recovery, then itraconazole (200 mg BID)	Treat with amphotericin B until objective improvement, and for at least 12 months. Suppressive therapy with itraconazole is needed
Sporotrichosis in pregnant women	• Treat only severe sporotrichosis with liposomal amphotericin B (3–5 mg/kg/day) or deoxycholate amphotericin B (0.7–1 mg/kg/day) • Treat with local hyperthermia (~45°C) for uncomplicated cutaneous sporotrichosis		Preferably, defer treatment for uncomplicated cases

(BID: twice daily; SSKI: saturated solution of potassium iodide)

CHAPTER 4: Subcutaneous Mycoses

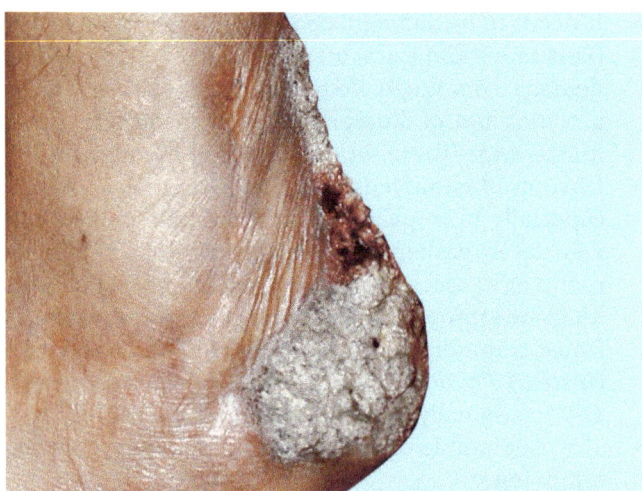

FIG. 9: Verrucous plaque over the heel is seen as a large, cauliflower-like lesion.

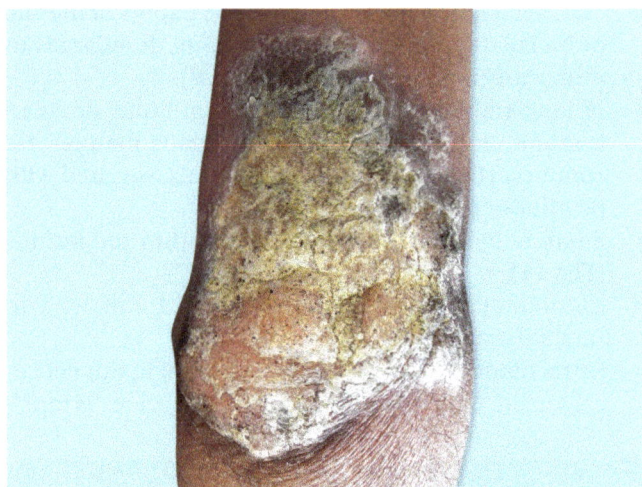

FIG. 10: Chromoblastomycosis seen as a large, hyperkeratotic, superficial, scaly, and verrucous plaque over the elbow.

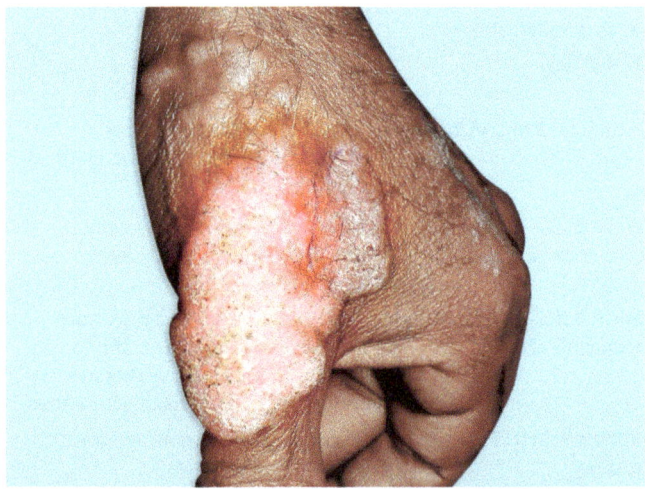

FIG. 11: Lesion of chromoblastomycosis over dorsal hand. The small, dark aggregates of clotted blood and fungal cells are characteristic and are likely to yield fungal cells in smears or histologic sections.

- For untreated cases, there is a risk of secondary complications such as recurrent infections, extracutaneous spread, malignant change, and risk of chronicity. Chronic lesions may develop squamous cell carcinoma.

Differential Diagnosis

- Tuberculosis verrucosa cutis
- Fixed cutaneous sporotrichosis
- Foreign body granuloma
- Lupus vulgaris
- Leprosy
- Cutaneous leishmaniasis
- Common warts
- Malignancy including squamous cell carcinoma and keratoacanthoma

Diagnosis

- *Direct microscopy*: Demonstration of characteristic small, round, thick-walled, brown-pigmented muriform cells, also known as the sclerotic bodies, is fairly diagnostic of chromoblastomycosis. These have longitudinal and transverse septae and are sized at 5–13 μm **(Fig. 12)**. These are evident in potassium hydroxide (KOH) mounts or hematoxylin and eosin-stained specimens of scrapings taken from the surface of lesions or tissue biopsies.
- *Histopathology*: Histological features include pseudoepitheliomatous epidermal hyperplasia, granulomatous inflammation with foreign body giant cells, and areas of microabscess formation. Fibrosis occurs in longstanding cases. The muriform cells (sclerotic or copper penny bodies) are often seen in deeper sections; whereas, hyphae and budding cells

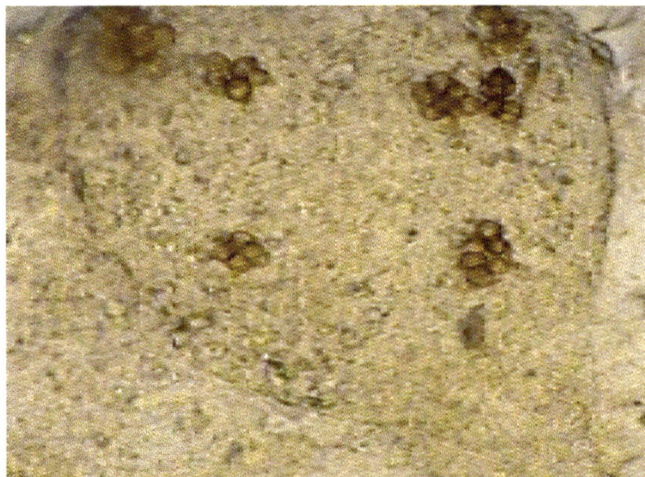

FIG. 12: Sclerotic bodies, as seen in potassium hydroxide (KOH) mounts. These are 5–13 μm, round, thick-walled, brown muriform cells, having longitudinal and transverse septa.

are present near the lesion surface. The presence of fungal cells or copper penny bodies, singly or in clusters, found within giant cells is diagnostic.
- *Fungal culture*: Culture can be attempted on SDA. Lesional biopsy, crust, or pus needs to be incubated at room temperature for at least 4 weeks. Culture is important for species differentiation.
- *Molecular diagnosis:* This is based on the identification or amplification of specific deoxyribonucleic acid (DNA) from ribosomal or internal transcribed spacer (ITS)-1 and ITS-2 regions of the recombinant DNA and the 5.8S sequence.

Treatment

- Treatment is difficult with a limited response to drugs, though spontaneous resolution is also rare. Infections caused by *F. pedrosoi* tend to be more resistant to therapy.
- Small lesions of shorter duration are best amenable to local destruction by surgical excision, cryotherapy, carbon dioxide (CO_2) laser, or local heat therapy.
- Topical heat therapy using chemical or electric pocket warmers at 42–46°C is an effective and safe option.
- For more extensive lesions, treatment with SSKI alone or in combination with other antifungal agents is widely used. These include itraconazole (200–400 mg/day) or terbinafine (500 mg/day) given over a period of 6–18 months or longer.
- The addition of 5-flucytosine (5-fluorocytosine) (50–150 mg/kg/day divided into four equal doses) may improve therapeutic outcomes. Using two or more treatment modalities yields better results.

Pheohyphomycosis

- This is a group of infections ranging from superficial to deep infections affecting skin and subcutis (subcutaneous pheohyphomycosis), viscera, central nervous system (cerebral pheohyphomycosis), or systemic involvement (disseminated pheohyphomycosis), commonly seen in patients with underlying immunodeficiency.
- These occur worldwide and, in all climates, without any racial or gender predilection.
- More than 100 different molds (generally saprophytes) belonging to 60 different genera have been implicated as etiological agents. These include the genera *Alternaria, Cladosporium, Phialophora, Curvularia, Exophiala, Fonsecaea, Wangiella*, and *Cladophialophora* as major pathogens.

Clinical Features

- Lesions are morphologically similar regardless of the implicated organism.
- The most typical presenting lesions are abscesses and cysts encapsulated in fibrous connective tissue, with no tendency to rupture.
- At times, papulonodules, verrucous or ulcerated plaques, nonhealing ulcers or sinuses, and scaly hyperkerototic lesions may be associated.
- Initial lesion is mostly asymptomatic or maybe a mildly painful subcutaneous nodule. This is followed by a slow increase to produce a painless cystic abscess **(Fig. 13)** which progresses to a verrucous plaque.
- Occasional manifestations include mycotic keratitis (contamination of corneal abrasion); pheomycotic "fungoma" (invasive paranasal sinus infection); cerebral pheohyphomycosis or disseminated infection in immunocompromised host **(Fig. 14)**.

Differential Diagnosis

- Cutaneous tuberculosis
- Cutaneous sporotrichosis
- Foreign body granuloma
- Abscesses and cystic lesions of varied etiology
- Chromoblastomycosis
- Mycetoma

Diagnosis

- *Direct microscopy*: The presence of brown, pigmented, septate hyphae with occasional branching, in KOH mounts from purulent discharge or skin scrapings is

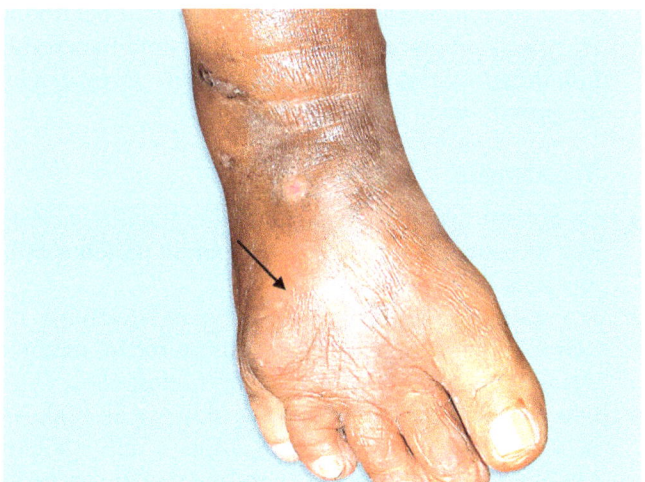

FIG. 13: Pheohyphomycosis presenting with diffuse induration involving the whole foot and ankle. There are painless encapsulated cystic abscesses containing purulent material with no tendency to rupture in a diabetic patient.

CHAPTER 4: Subcutaneous Mycoses

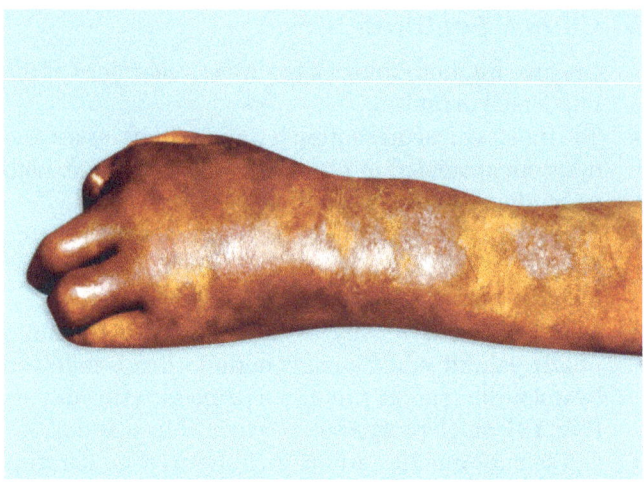

FIG. 14: Erythematous, indurated plaque over hand and forearm in an elderly diabetic. Diagnosis was established on the culture of *Cladosporium trichoides* from a skin biopsy. The patient later developed cerebral pheohyphomycosis.

highly suggestive. However, confirmation and species identification requires the recovery of organisms on suitable culture media.

- *Fungal culture*: Material obtained from surgical drainage, lesional biopsy, crusts, or pus is incubated at 30°C and 37°C for at least 4 weeks on SDA, malt extract agar, or potato dextrose agar. Depending upon the species, the colonies may be pigmented, gray, dark olive-gray, dark brown, or nearly black.
- *Histopathology*: The presence of brown-colored hyphae and yeast-like elements with giant cells against the background of granulomatous inflammatory reaction with a central neutrophilic abscess is pathognomonic. The cystic lesions are usually well-circumscribed, encapsulated granulomas with epithelioid histiocytic inflammatory reactions and giant cells. Fungal cells are prominent in the cyst wall lining.

Treatment

- Treatment options are limited. Therapeutic success can be expected in immunocompetent patients with localized disease.
- A combination of surgical excision, drainage or debridement, along with a maximum recommended dosage of antifungal drug is usually preferred.
- Oral itraconazole (200–400 mg/day, to as high as 800 mg/day, for 4–6 weeks) appears effective in pheohyphomycosis when combined with surgical excision.
- Amphotericin B (given intravenously at 0.5–1.0 mg/kg/day or intralesionally) has been used, with improved efficacy if combined with surgical excision.

- Voriconazole and posaconazole, have been found effective in disseminated or visceral infections both in humans and experimental animals.
- Combination therapy with different antifungal drugs provide the additional advantage of improved efficacy.

Mycetoma (Madura Foot, Maduromycosis, Maduramycosis)

- It refers to a chronic, localized, destructive infection of the skin, and/or subcutaneous tissue, fascia, muscle, and occasionally, the underlying bone and adjacent tissues.
- Classical triad including indurated tumor-like indolent swelling (tumefaction); sinuses; and presence of grains in the discharge or within the tissue, is highly characteristic for a mycetoma.
- The causative agents include gram-positive filamentous bacteria (actinomycetoma) or eukaryotic fungi (eumycetoma). Worldwide, actinomycetoma accounts for the majority of the cases, and approximately, 60% of these are due to *Nocardia brasiliensis*. The differences are summarized in **Table 2**.
- Mycetoma is most prevalent in latitudes 15–30° N (around the tropic of cancer). The disease is endemic in the Indian subcontinent. Actinomycotic mycetoma is common across India with the exception of northern regions (particularly Rajasthan), where eumycetoma occurs more frequently.
- Inoculation of causative agent usually follows a minor trauma, and the disease evolves slowly over a period of months to years. The incubation period varies from a few weeks to several years.
- Rural populations, aged 20–50 years, walking barefoot are particularly at risk.

Clinical Features

- The initial lesion is usually painless. It slowly progresses to a hard subcutaneous nodule usually involving exposed sites, especially the foot **(Fig. 15)**.
- It could develop on the back in individuals carrying soiled sacks **(Fig. 16)**.
- The slowly enlarging localized swelling progresses to form multiple nodules and sinuses, emitting purulent, seropurulent, or serosanguinous discharge mixed with grains of various colors. The presence of grains is a cardinal feature.
- Atypical sites could be buttocks, scalp, face, thigh, etc., **(Figs. 17 and 18)**.

CHAPTER 4: Subcutaneous Mycoses

TABLE 2: Comparative features of actinomycetoma and eumycetoma.

Features	Actinomycetoma	Eumycetoma
Etiological agents	Nocardia braziliensis (most common), Nocardia asteroides, Actinomadura madurae, Actinomadura pelletieri, Streptomyces somaliensis, and Nocardia caviae	Madurella grisea, Madurella mycetomatis, Leptosphaeria senegalensis, Curvularia geniculata, Pyrenochaeta romeroi, Phialophora jeanselmei, and Pseudallescheria boydii, Acremonium species, Fusarium species, Aspergillus nidulans, and Neotestudina rosati
Incubation period	Short incubation period with faster progression	Long incubation period with slower progression
Morphology of lesions	• Ill-defined indurated plaque that tends to merge with the surrounding skin • Sinuses are numerous with abundant discharge of pus and grains	• Well-defined, indurated encapsulated, plaque clearly delineated from surrounding skin • Sinuses are fewer with scanty discharge of pus and grains
Inflammation	Signs of inflammation are more pronounced at the sinus orifice	Signs of inflammation are less pronounced
Bone involvement	Bone involvement is early and severely destructive	Bone involvement is late and less destructive
Color of grains (causative agent)	White/yellow (*A. madurae, Nocardia asteroids,* and *Nocardia brasiliensis*), Red (*Actinomadura pelletieri*), yellow/brown (*S. somaliensis*)	Black-brown (*M. grisea, M. mycetomatis, Lepisanthes senegalensis, P. jeanselmei,* and *P. romeroi*), *C. geniculata,* white-yellow (*Acremonium* species, *P. boydii, A. nidulans,* and *N. rosati*)

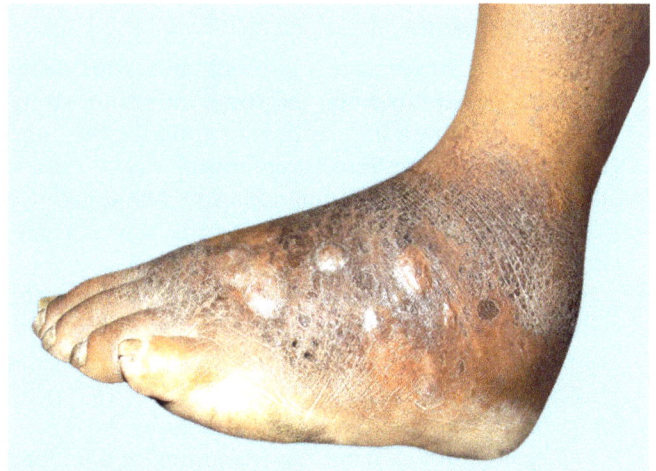

FIG. 15: Mycetoma foot. The most common presentation.

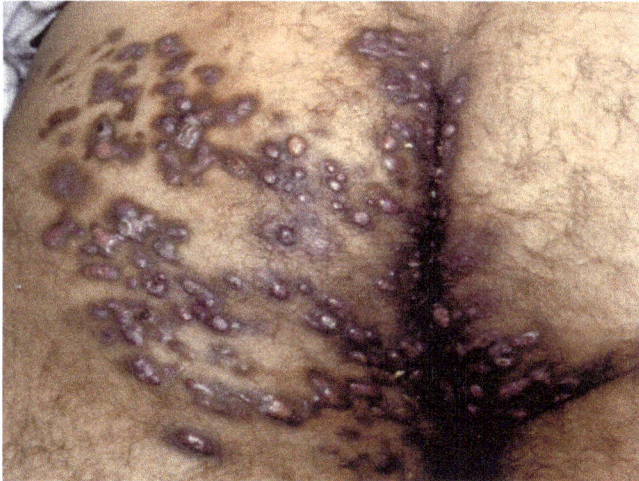

FIG. 17: Actinomycetoma over the gluteal area.

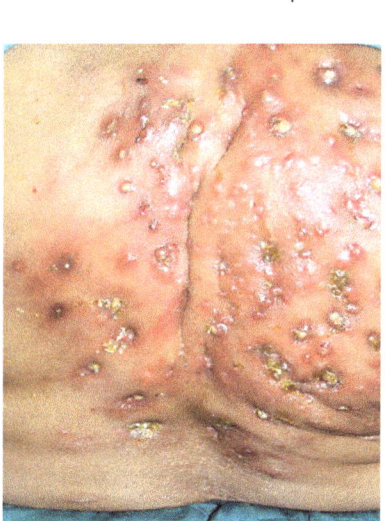

FIG. 16: Mycetoma over back. Note the multiple discharging sinuses.

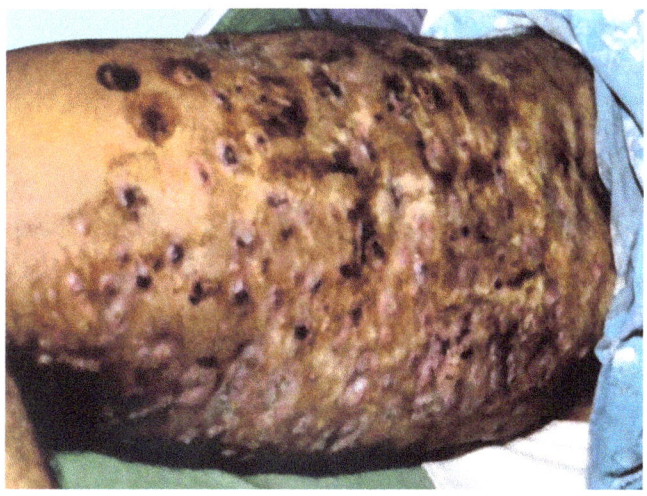

FIG. 18: Thigh involvement due to *Nocardia* species.

Complications

These include progressive deformity and disability, fungal osteomyelitis, secondary bacterial infections, destructive lesions, and pulmonary dissemination.

Differential Diagnosis

- Granulomatous cutaneous leishmaniasis
- Scrofuloderma
- Syphilis and yaws
- Osteomyelitis of pyogenic or tubercular origin
- Benign soft tissue tumors or carcinomas
- Actinomycosis
- Botryomycosis

Diagnosis

The investigations are directed at the identification of causative organisms and the extent of tissue involvement for deciding the mode of therapy.

- *Radiological investigations*: This helps assess disease extent and bony involvement. Soft tissue swelling, widening of intermetatarsal spaces, periosteal reaction, and osteolytic or osteosclerotic bony changes may be seen.
- *Direct microscopy*: Granules are aggregates of microcolonies of causative organisms that can be identified by gross and microscopic examination. They are preferably obtained from deeper tissue by direct extraction or fine-needle aspiration. Actinomycotic grains contain very fine filaments (<1 μm in diameter); whereas, fungal grains have short and broad hyphae (2–4 μm in diameter).
- *Culture*: This can be done on blood agar (for actinomycetes), on egg-containing media (for aerobic actinomycetes), or on SDA (for fungal species). Colonies are seen to grow in 7–10 days at 35–37°C.
- *Histopathology*: A focal pseudoepitheliomatous hyperplasia, with an acute or chronic granulomatous inflammatory infiltrate of neutrophils, lymphocytes, histiocytes, plasma cells, epithelioid cells, and Langhans giant cells is seen. It surrounds the granules in a sunray pattern (Splendore-Hoeppli phenomenon). The presence of grains of the causative organism in the tissue sections is confirmatory.
- *Serodiagnosis*: Techniques used are immunodiffusion or enzyme-linked immunosorbent assay (ELISA) based tests to detect antibodies against *N. brasiliensis*; however, serological responses are less reliable and not available for commercial use.

Treatment

Eumycetoma

- Generally, not amenable to antifungal drugs alone, needs additional surgical intervention including debulking or amputation. Indications include well-encapsulated, localized superficial lesions and failure of chemotherapy.
- Criteria for cure are clinical resolution, healing of sinuses, and absence of grains OR three consecutive negative findings of ELISA tests 1 month apart.
- Useful drugs include ketoconazole, voriconazole, and itraconazole. The duration of the treatment remains uncertain, and relapses are frequent.
- Itraconazole is preferred for its better efficacy and tolerability.
- Fluconazole is not effective and griseofulvin, amphotericin B, and terbinafine have shown limited or poor response.

Actinomycetoma

- Medical treatment is usually effective with drugs including cotrimoxazole, dapsone, amikacin, streptomycin, rifampicin, isoniazid, sulfadiazine, and sulfadoxine, prescribed in combinations to ensure better therapeutic outcomes and avoid resistance.
- Treatment must be continued until cure (usually more than a year).
- Other drugs used include amphotericin B, gentamicin, coamoxiclav, tetracyclines/doxycycline, linezolid, rifampicin, imipenem, ciprofloxacin, and linezolid (against *N. brasiliensis*).
- A few useful therapeutic regimens include:
  - Dapsone, 100–200 mg/day (6 months), maintained at 50 mg/day (1–2 years).
  - Combination of dapsone (100 mg/day), cotrimoxazole twice a day with streptomycin (1 g intramuscularly daily) for 1–2 months, with the first two drugs continued till clinical cure. Gentamicin may be equally efficacious.
  - *Welsh regimen (1987)*: Intensive phase is composed of 1–3 cycles, with each cycle composed of Injection amikacin 15 mg/kg/IV (2 divided doses) with cotrimoxazole tablets for 21 days. The cycles are administered at intervals of 15 days with the intervening period of maintenance phase (continuing co-trimoxazole).
  - *Ramam (two-step) regimen (2000)*: Intensive phase with crystalline penicillin 1 MU IV QID with gentamicin 80 mg IV BD and cotrimoxazole BD for

5-7 weeks. Maintenance phase of cotrimoxazole BD and amoxicillin 500 mg TDS for 2-5 months or complete clearance.
- *Modified two-step regimen (2007)*: Intensive phase with gentamicin 80 mg IV BD with cotrimoxazole BD for 4 weeks. Maintenance phase with doxycycline 100 mg BD with cotrimoxazole BD for 5-6 months or complete clearance.
- *Modified welsh regimen (2008)*: Intensive phase is composed of 1-3 cycles, with each cycle consisting of injection amikacin 15 mg/kg/IV (2 divided doses) with cotrimoxazole and rifampicin 10 mg/kg/day for 21 days. The cycles are administered at intervals of 15 days. Maintenance phase consists of continuing cotrimoxazole and rifampicin for 3 months.

CHAPTER 5

Deep Fungal Infections

Introduction

Deep fungal skin infections are chronic diseases caused by fungi resulting in systemic mycoses. These are acquired mostly by inhalation and affect internal organs due to subsequent hematogenous dissemination **(Fig. 1)**.

Systemic mycoses can be divided into two groups:
1. *Endemic mycoses*: These have a specific geographic niche due to the typical climatic conditions, flora, or fauna. They affect healthy people living in that area and are mostly asymptomatic. Examples include histoplasmosis, blastomycosis, coccidioidomycosis, paracoccidioidomycosis, and penicilliosis. These are now gaining worldwide importance as opportunistic infections with an increased incidence seen in human

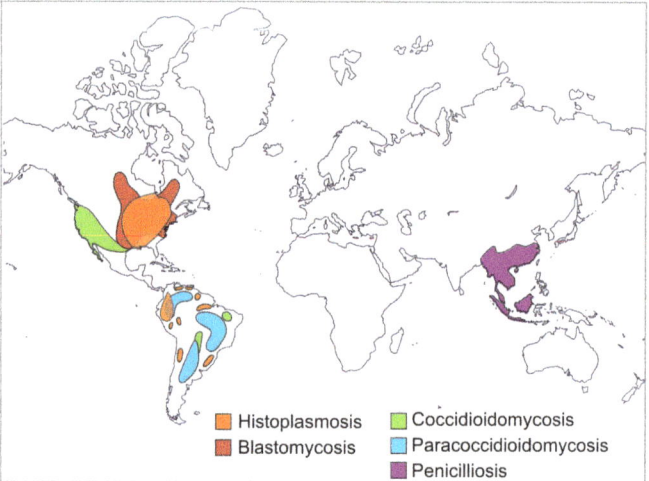

FIG. 2: Endemic areas of the various systemic mycoses.

immunodeficiency virus (HIV) infection cases. The endemic areas for the various systemic mycoses are outlined in **Figure 2**.
2. *Opportunistic mycoses*: These are seen in patients with immunosuppression including primary immunodeficiencies, HIV-AIDS (acquired immune deficiency syndrome), cytotoxic drugs, and chronic debilitating conditions. They do not have a specific geographic predilection. Examples include aspergillosis, fusariosis, disseminated candidiasis, and mucormycosis.

Histoplasmosis (Darling's Disease)

- It is a common granulomatous fungal disease of worldwide distribution, with the endemic area being the American continent.
- It is caused by *Histoplasma capsulatum*, which is a primary pathogen of the respiratory system. There are two varieties: (1) *H. capsulatum var. capsulatum*,

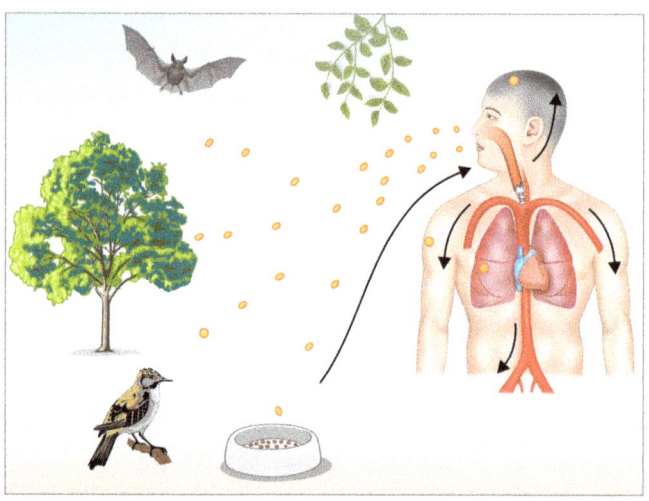

FIG. 1: Pathogenesis of systemic mycoses. The infections are usually acquired via inhalation from environmental sources such as soil, vegetation, bird or bat droppings, and laboratory sources. The organism forms a primary pulmonary focus. Hematogenous dissemination occurs to other organs in the setting of immunosuppression.

(2–5 μm causing classic histoplasmosis) and (2) *var duboisii* (10–15 μm causing African histoplasmosis).
- Infection is acquired by inhalation of microconidia, which generates a primary infection complex on reaching the alveoli, similar to tuberculosis. Hematogenous spread commonly occurs in immunocompromised patients, especially in HIV/acquired immune deficiency syndrome (AIDS).
- The natural habitat of the fungus is soil and detritus, especially enriched with bird and bat droppings.
- The incubation period varies from 3 days to 5 months, with an average of 10 days.
- Occupations such as miners, farmers, archaeologists, and builders are at greater risk.

Clinical Features

- In endemic areas, the disease is asymptomatic in 95% of infected individuals. However, in immunosuppressed patients, it becomes symptomatic.
- Pulmonary involvement is the most common mode of presentation; it could be acute pulmonary, chronic cavitatory, or disseminated infection.

Mucocutaneous manifestations are varied:
- Direct skin inoculation (exceedingly rare) can present as a painless ulcer with regional adenopathy. It usually resolves spontaneously over weeks to months.
- Secondary cutaneous involvement occurs due to hematogenous dissemination. Lesions are reported in a quarter of HIV-infected patients. It can present as papules, crusted plaques, pustules, nodules, mucosal ulcers, erosions, or lesions resembling molluscum contagiosum **(Figs. 3 and 4)** or acneiform eruptions. Less commonly reported presentations include purpuric lesions, localized and generalized dermatitis, vegetating lesions, rosacea-like eruption, keratotic papules with transepidermal elimination, erythroderma, pyoderma gangrenosum, panniculitis, diffuse hyperpigmentation, abscesses, and cellulitis.

Diagnosis

Diagnosis needs to be confirmed from the tissue specimens. Specimen collection depends on the organ affected and the extent of dissemination.
- *Direct microscopy*: Direct microscopy of a peripheral blood smear, buffy coat, bronchial brushings, bone marrow aspirate, etc., can be done. Staining with silver methenamine or Giemsa on blood smears or a buffy coat usually shows intracellular yeasts with characteristic budding **(Fig. 5)**.

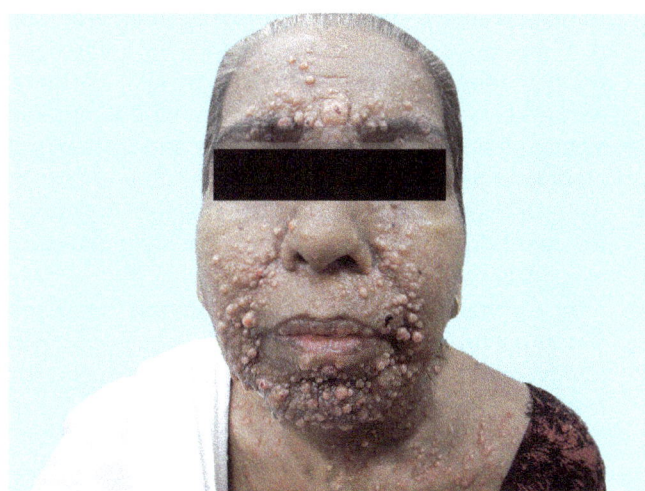

FIG. 4: Disseminated histoplasmosis in a human immunodeficiency virus (HIV)-positive woman.

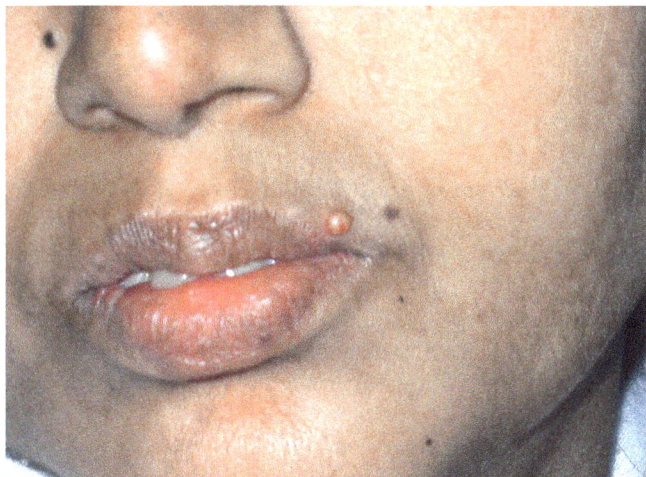

FIG. 3: Molluscum contagiosum-like lesion of cutaneous histoplasmosis in a human immunodeficiency virus (HIV)-positive woman.

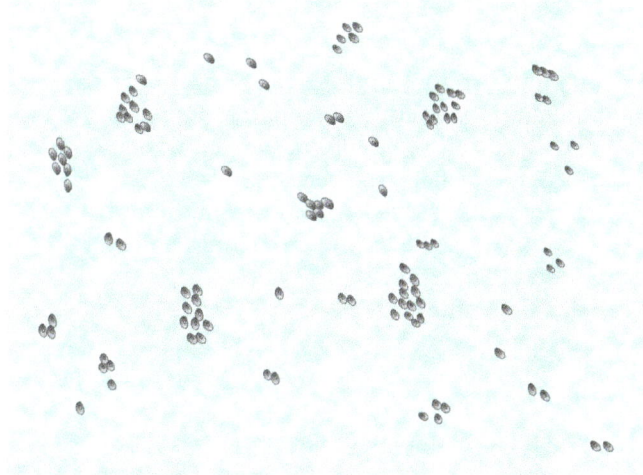

FIG. 5: Diagram showing staining with silver methenamine. Intracellular yeasts with characteristic budding is seen, with mother cell forming daughter yeast cells.

- *Histopathology*: Samples from the affected end organ, viz., lung tissue, skin, lymphatic tissue, liver, and spleen can show the fungus. These show the presence of granulomas, with or without caseous necrosis, and lymphohistiocytic infiltrates. Special stains such as periodic acid–Schiff (PAS), silver methenamine, and Grocott-Gömöri's stains are used to visualize the organism seen as yeast forms within or outside macrophages.
- *Fungal culture*: Although, fungal culture is the gold standard for diagnosis, the incubation time is very long (3–6 weeks).
- *Serology*: Immunodiffusion or complement fixation test (CFT) can be used for the diagnosis of histoplasmosis. Immunodiffusion is less sensitive but more specific as compared to CFT. Enzyme-linked immunosorbent assay (ELISA) increases the proportion of positive results to up to 75% of cases. Immune response is weak in an immunocompromised patient; thus, it may be negative in 60% of HIV patients. Serology is important in patients where clinical suspicion is high, and where culture and histological analysis is not possible or negative.
- *Antigen detection*: It is a sensitive diagnostic method for disseminated disease which helps early detection even by 24–48 hours.
- *Skin testing*: The histoplasmin skin test has been found useful in estimating the extent of population involvement; however, it is not reliable as a diagnostic test.

Treatment

- A rapid initiation of treatment is indicated due to a high risk of mortality with disseminated disease.
- An initial induction phase is needed to produce remission, followed by a suppressive maintenance phase to prevent relapses.
- Amphotericin B is the therapeutic agent of choice for induction. Conventional amphotericin B (0.7–1 mg/kg daily for 12 weeks) or liposomal formulation (dose of 3–5 mg/kg daily) can be used.
- Itraconazole is used in mild-to-moderate disease. A loading dose of 200 mg three times daily for 3 days is followed by maintenance with 200 mg, once or twice daily, depending on the severity of the infection. The drug may have to be continued life-long.
- Fluconazole (800 mg daily) has limited therapeutic efficacy. Newer azoles such as voriconazole and posaconazole have unclear role.

Blastomycosis

- It is primarily a respiratory mycoses caused by *Blastomyces dermatitidis*.
- The infection is mostly limited to North America, seemingly exclusive to the midwestern United States.
- It commonly affects male adults in the fourth decade of life.
- Predisposing factors include low socioeconomic status or concomitant diseases such as diabetes and HIV.

Clinical Features

- Primary pulmonary blastomycosis presents with cough, weight loss, chest pain, fever, and hemoptysis.
- Extrapulmonary blastomycosis is characterized by varying manifestations, with cutaneous involvement being the most frequent.
- Cutaneous features include papules or pustules with regional adenopathy, which undergo spontaneous resolution over weeks to months.
- Other lesions described include warty plaques, chronic ulcers, fistulae, panniculitis, and subcutaneous abscesses, often simulating cutaneous malignancy.
- Bone and joint involvement (osteomyelitis or septic arthritis); involvement of prostate, epididymis, fallopian tubes, and ovaries; central nervous system (CNS) involvement (meningitis, cerebral abscess, or granuloma formation) can occur.

Diagnosis

- *Direct microscopy*: Skin scraping, purulent material, bronchoalveolar lavage, sputum, urine, or cerebrospinal fluid (CSF) can reveal characteristic thick-walled, single-budding yeasts, of size 8–14 μm with a broad base **(Fig. 6)**.
- *Histopathology*: Tissue samples show a mixed inflammatory infiltrate with predominant polymorphonuclear cells. Noncaseating granulomas containing histiocytes and giant multinucleated cells can be seen. Special mycological stains such as Grocott-Gömöri and PAS, allow observation of single budding yeasts.
- *Fungal culture*: At 25–30°C, colonies appear in two weeks, initially as whitish, smooth colonies, which turn into gray-brown, hairy colonies. Microscopically, fine mycelium and piriform conidia are seen.
- *Serology*: Antibody testing has low sensitivity and specificity, however, antigen detection in body fluids is useful (sensitivity > 90%).

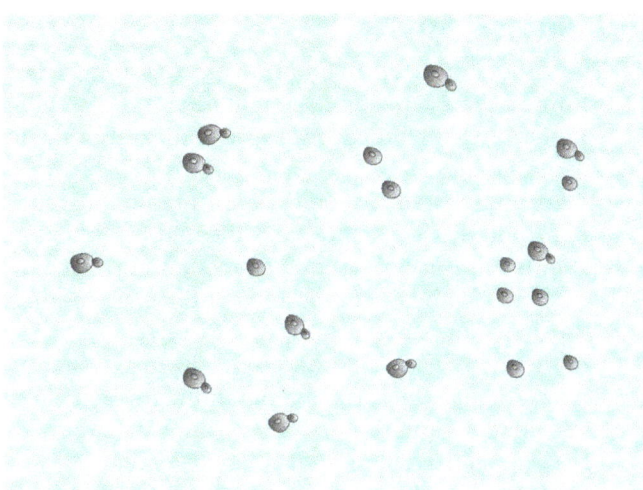

FIG. 6: Diagram showing thick-walled, single-budding yeasts of size 8–14 μm with a broad base, as seen on the Gomori methenamine silver stain.

Treatment

- For primary pulmonary form with mild symptoms, oral itraconazole, 200 mg twice daily for 4–6 months is the treatment of choice. Oral posaconazole, fluconazole, and voriconazole can also be tried
- For severe pulmonary blastomycosis or disseminated disease, intravenous (IV) amphotericin B deoxycholate (0.7–1 mg/kg alternate days) is indicated. Liposomal formulations (3–5 mg/kg) have also been used.

Coccidioidomycosis (San Joaquin Valley Fever)

- It is a pulmonary and extrapulmonary systemic disease caused by dimorphic fungus *Coccidioides immitis*.
- It is predominant in the arid zones of the American continent (Southwestern United States, Mexico, Central and South America).
- The infection is transmitted by inhalation of arthroconidia. Transmission by direct inoculation is rare.

Clinical Features

- It could be a primary pulmonary infection, chronic pulmonary infection, or disseminated disease. About 60% of infected individuals are asymptomatic.
- In symptomatic patients, flu-like syndrome with myalgia and fatigue are frequent with patients recovering in 2–3 weeks. Respiratory signs and symptoms include fever, cough, hemoptysis, miliary lesions, pneumonia, hilar adenopathy, and pleural effusion.
- Disseminated disease is seen with immunosuppression with skin being one of the most common organs affected. Others include lymph nodes, spleen, liver, kidneys, bone, joints, and CNS.
- Cutaneous lesions vary from papules, nodules, gummas, acneiform pustular lesions, ulcerated and verrucous plaques, scars, abscesses, and fistulae.
- Other manifestations include erythema nodosum, erythema multiforme, and Sweet's syndrome. Primary chancriform cutaneous coccidioidomycosis is a rare form caused by direct inoculation.

Diagnosis

Specimens for evaluation include sputum, bronchoalveolar lavage, transtracheal aspirate, pleural fluid, lung tissue, skin and bone biopsy, pus from abscesses, joint fluid, CSF, etc.

- *Direct microscopy*: Thick-walled mature spherules (80 μm) containing endospores, can be identified by hematoxylin and eosin **(Fig. 7)**. They do not take up Gram's stain but may be visualized with potassium hydroxide (KOH), Lugol's, or calcofluor white preparations.
- *Histopathology*: Coccidioidal granuloma is characterized by abundant polymorphonuclear leukocytes, eosinophils, lymphocytes, epithelioid cells, multinucleated giant cells, along with areas of necrotic tissue, and fibrosis. Double-walled spherules with endospores (varying from 10 to 80 μm) can be identified.
- *Fungal culture*: It can be done on brain heart infusion agar, potato-dextrose agar, and Sabouraud's dextrose

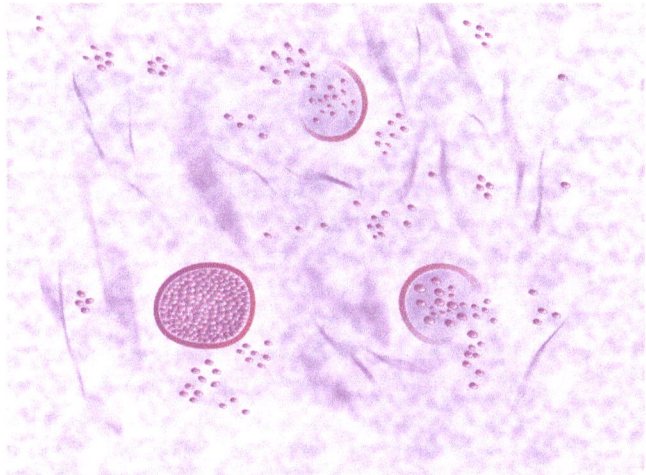

FIG. 7: Diagram showing thick-walled mature spherules of *Coccidioides*, measuring up to 80 μm in diameter. These contain endospores and can be identified by hematoxylin and eosin stain.

agar. After approximately 2–3 weeks of incubation at 28–30°C, a white, cottony mold grows resembling angel hair. Microcultures reveal arthrospores and barrel-shaped hyphae.
- *Serology*: Immunoglobulin M (IgM) antibodies can be detected between the first and third week of the disease, while immunoglobulin G (IgG) antibodies show up between weeks 2 and 28. The laboratory techniques used are enzyme immunoassays, immunodiffusion, and CFT. Levels are related to disease activity and response to treatment.
- *Molecular methods*: These include AccuProbe assays (a type of nucleic acid hybridization test) and conventional nested polymerase chain reaction (PCR).
- *Coccidioidin or spherulin skin tests*: A positive reaction is when the erythema and induration exceed 5 mm after intradermal injection of antigen.

Treatment

- *Severe, disseminated disease*: Amphotericin B deoxycholate (0.3–1.5 mg/kg IV daily); amphotericin B colloidal dispersion; and liposomal amphotericin B can be given for 1–4 months.
- *Mild disease*: The same regimen can be administered three times per week.
- *Extrapulmonary or severe disease*: Therapy may be prolonged; lasting 6 months to 1 year after the disease has become inactive.
  - Fluconazole (200–400 mg daily) and itraconazole (400 mg daily) are common alternatives.
  - Posaconazole (800 mg daily in divided doses given for 1–2 years) and voriconazole (3–4 mg/kg body weight IV or 200–300 mg orally daily) can also be used.

Paracoccidioidomycosis (South American Blastomycosis)

- It is a systemic disease caused by *Paracoccidioides brasiliensis*, acquired mainly by inhalation leading to respiratory symptoms.
- It is endemic in Southern Mexico, parts of Central America, and South America.
- The natural habitat of *P. brasiliensisis* is the soil and it infects the host through the respiratory tract, leading to the formation of a primary pulmonary complex with the persistence of viable fungi, also called latent focus. Transitory hematogenous dissemination resulting with extrapulmonary latent foci also occurs, simultaneously.
- Comorbidities such as alcoholism, malnutrition, and immunosuppression predispose to dissemination.

Clinical Features

- The association with immunosuppression is less common than expected. The majority of the patients suffer from subclinical infection and are clinically asymptomatic.
- When manifested, it could be an acute, subacute, or chronic disease. Lungs are affected in almost all patients with dry or productive cough and dyspnea associated with reticulonodular infiltrates on chest X-ray in the upper two-thirds of the lungs.
- Cutaneous lesions may originate from contiguous lesions, hematogenous dissemination, or rarely, from direct inoculation
- Face is the most common site of involvement.
- Classical oral/mucosal presentation is a superficial ulcer with a granular appearance and hemorrhagic points (mulberry-like stomatitis). Lip involvement may be seen as macrocheilia.
- Other morphologic types include papular, acneiform, verrucous lesions, fistulae, and abscesses. Lymph nodes, liver, and spleen are the classic sites affected in acute and sub-acute forms of the disease.

Diagnosis

- *Direct microscopy*: The gold standard for diagnosis is the identification of *P. brasiliensis* in 10% KOH tissue mounts. It is seen as round yeasts with characteristic multiple budding, with the parent cell being surrounded by multiple small buds. This is known as the "Captain's wheel" appearance **(Figs. 8A and B)**.
- *Histopathology*: Both hematoxylin and eosin (H&E) and special stains (silver methenamine or PAS) are required. A mixed granulomatous response with fibrosis and yeasts with a characteristic budding pattern is seen, respectively.
- *Fungal culture*: This can be done in Sabouraud's agar or brain heart infusion agar at 37°C but has low sensitivity.
- *Serology*: It is a useful tool for evaluating treatment response and disease recurrence. Immunodiffusion has sensitivity > 80% and specificity > 90%. CFT test can also be done. Antibody to a 43 kDa antigen can be assayed via immunoblot and this has high specificity.

Treatment

- Itraconazole (200 mg daily for 6–9 months for mild disease and 12–18 months for moderate disease) is considered the best treatment option.
- Sulfamethoxazole-trimethoprim (2,400 mg plus 480 mg daily for 12 months for mild cases and 24 months for moderate infection) can be used.

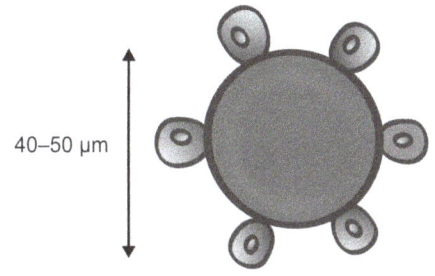

FIGS. 8A AND B: Diagram of Gomori methenamine silver stained specimen with round yeasts with characteristic multiple budding. The parent cell surrounded by multiple small buds is referred to as the "Captain's wheel"-like appearance.

- For severe cases, amphotericin B (0.75 mg/kg daily with a cumulative dose of 30 mg/kg) is the drug of choice.
- Voriconazole can also be used.

Cryptococcosis

- It is a pulmonary or disseminated infection acquired by inhalation of soil contaminated with *Cryptococcus neoformans* or *Cryptococcus gattii* (encapsulated yeasts), with a universal geographic distribution.
- The infection became commoner with the advent of the AIDS pandemic as the unique capsule allows the fungus to evade innate immunity, by preventing effective phagocytosis by host cells. Other virulence factors like the ability to grow at 37°C, melanin production, and the production of enzymes such as proteases, ureases, and phospholipase B, facilitate tissue invasion.
- Infection occurs by inhalation of spores.
- Symptoms are those of pneumonia, meningitis, or involvement of skin, bones, or viscera.
- CNS is the most common organ system affected.

- It mostly runs a benign course and resolves spontaneously; however, severe disease occurs in immunosuppressed hosts such as AIDS, primary immunodeficiency syndromes, pregnancy, organ transplantation, lymphoma treated with cytotoxic drugs, or high-dose corticosteroid therapy.

Clinical Features

- *Disseminated cryptococcosis*: A severe infection with multiorgan involvement in severely immunosuppressed HIV-positive patients [clusters of differentiation 4 (CD4) count < 100/µL].
- *Pulmonary cryptococcosis*: It presents as weight loss, prolonged fever, anorexia, fatigue, productive cough, dyspnea, chest pain, and hemoptysis.
- *CNS cryptococcosis*: It presents as subacute or chronic meningoencephalitis, or as a space-occupying lesion in the brain. The onset is insidious, with headache, behavioral changes, fatigue, drowsiness, blurred vision, etc.
- *Ocular cryptococcosis*: It accompanies CNS disease, the most common sign being papilledema (intracranial hypertension), followed by partial or total loss of vision and oculomotor nerve paralysis.
- *Cutaneous cryptococcosis*: Skin lesions can appear as a tubercle, nodule, or abscess at the site of penetration and with satellite lymphangitis and adenopathy. The initial lesion is a painless papule that softens and ulcerates giving rise to molluscum contagiosum-like lesions. Vegetating, crusted plaques **(Fig. 9)**, and vasculitic lesions may also be seen. HIV-positive patients undergoing highly active antiretroviral therapy (HAART) may develop immune reconstitution

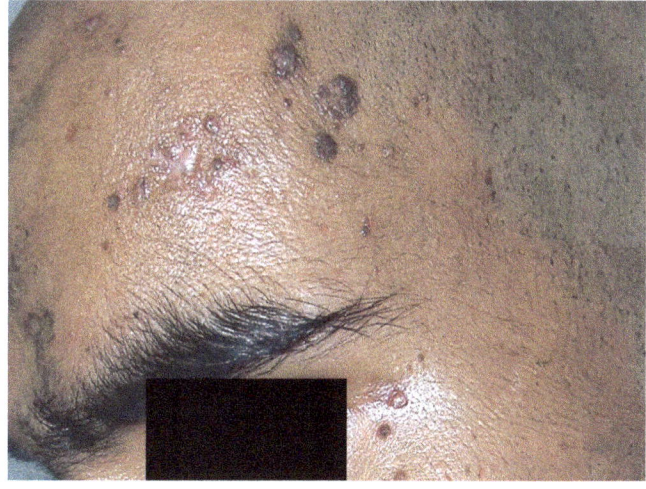

FIG. 9: Hyperpigmented papules and plaques of cutaneous cryptococcosis over the forehead in a young human immunodeficiency virus (HIV)-positive male.

inflammatory syndrome (IRIS). Scrofuloderma-like lesions can occur.
- *Urogenital cryptococcosis*: It is frequent but asymptomatic.
- Bone lesions are reported to occur but are relatively rare.

Diagnosis

The specimens used for diagnosis are CSF, pleural fluid, lymph, and specimens from lymph nodes, skin, lung, bone marrow, urine, and blood.
- *Direct microscopy*: Evaluation of CSF, blood, urine, or bone marrow aspirates with India ink or phase contrast microscopy shows *Cryptococcus* species. It is identified as a spherical or oval fungal element with a double-contoured cell wall, varying from 5 to 12 μm with a single bud through a narrow neck **(Fig. 10)**.
- *Histopathology*: *Cryptococcal* cells can be seen with a double-walled capsule. Special stains for selective staining include Mayer's mucicarmine (red) and alcian blue (blue). In immunocompetent hosts, compact epithelioid cell granulomas, with histiocytes, giant cells, and lymphocytes are seen with small spores (2–4 μm) and are few in number. In immunosuppressed, numerous spores (4–12 μm) with very little inflammatory tissue reaction are seen **(Fig. 11)**.
- *Fungal culture*: It is attempted on honey-agar media, Sabouraud's dextrose agar, or brain heart infusion agar. Pathogenic cryptococcal strains grow at 37°C, producing brown colonies in Staib medium (production of melanin).
- *Serology*: It lacks specificity; however, blood or CSF cryptococcal antigen detection by latex particle agglutination has high sensitivity and specificity, and titers correlate with the severity of infection. Antigen capsular detection can also be done by ELISA.
- *Molecular techniques*: These include ribosomal ribonucleic acid (rRNA) or conventional PCR to detect the fungus. Other investigations are based on organ involvement.

Treatment

- Mild/localized cryptococcosis without CNS involvement can be treated with oral fluconazole (400 mg daily for 6–12 months) or itraconazole (same dose and duration)
- CNS cryptococcosis with HIV-AIDS is treated with a combination of amphotericin B deoxycholate (0.7 mg/kg/day) and 5-fluorocytosine (or flucytosine) orally (25 mg/kg/day every 6 hours) for 3 weeks,

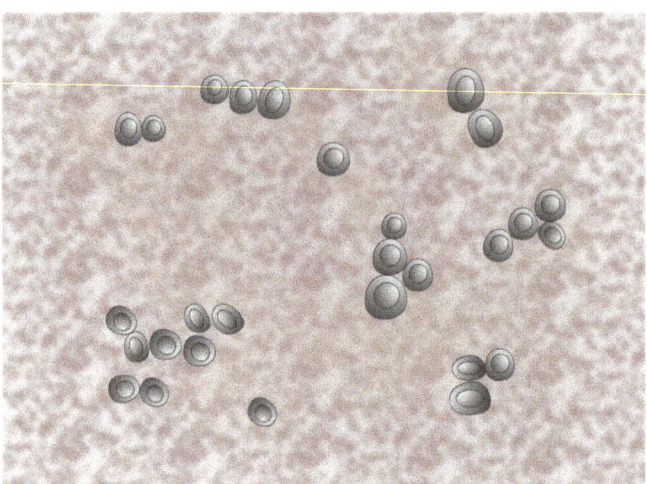

FIG. 10: Diagram showing *Cryptococcus* species as spherical or oval, 5–12 μm large, double contoured cells with a cell wall which stains negatively with India ink.

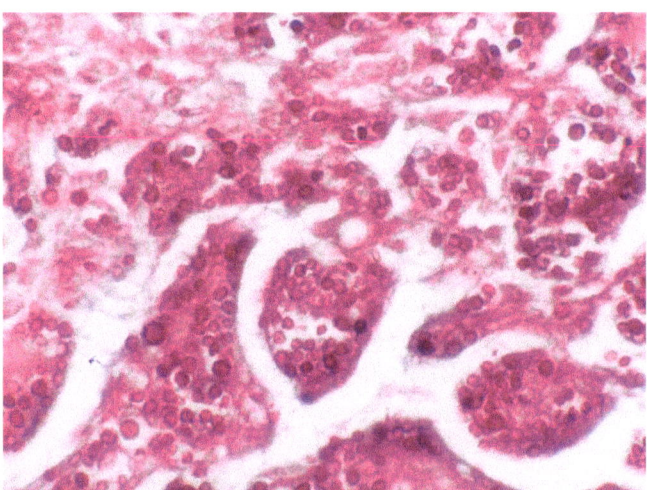

FIG. 11: Numerous cryptococcal spores in a tissue section.

followed by fluconazole (400–800 mg daily) for 6–8 weeks. For intracranial hypertension, mannitol and corticosteroids may not be very useful and it may require repeated lumbar puncture.
- In HIV-negative, the duration of treatment is 6 weeks.
- Other drugs include second generation triazoles, voriconazole, and posaconazole.

Talaromycosis (Penicilliosis)

- Talaromycosis (formerly penicilliosis) is caused by the thermally dimorphic fungus *Talaromyces marneffei* and is one of the AIDS-defining illnesses in South and Southeast Asia, South China, and north-east India.

- Multiorgan system involvement including cutaneous spread is common with clinical disease being more frequent in men.
- The infection is acquired by inhalation or through abrasions. After penetration, the fungal elements are phagocytosed by alveolar macrophages and undergo intracellular multiplication, followed by hematogenous spread.
- The infection carries a high mortality rate if left untreated.

Clinical Features

- It presents as a systemic disease in immunocompromised individuals, characterized by fever, weight loss, lymphadenopathy, hepatosplenomegaly, respiratory signs, skin lesions, and bony lesions.
- Varied skin lesions including papules with central necrosis, molluscoid lesions, nodules, gummas, and subcutaneous cold abscesses, more commonly on the face and neck. Mucosal ulcers or papules can be seen.
- In immunocompetent individuals, smooth papules may be seen.

Diagnosis

Specimens used are biopsy from skin lesions and reticuloendothelial system (lymph nodes, spleen, and liver), blood or sputum.
- *Fungal culture*: It is done on Sabouraud's dextrose agar, producing folded and velvety colonies at 27°C with a characteristic diffusion of red pigment around the colonies.
- *Histopathology*: Tissue biopsy shows intracellular parasites inside large macrophages. The appearance is similar to *H. capsulatum* but it reproduces by the formation of a septum in its middle **(Fig. 12)**.

- *Serology*: Immunofluorescence with monoclonal antibodies, as well as deoxyribonucleic acid (DNA) hybridization techniques, has been successfully used for diagnosis.

Treatment

- The fungus is sensitive to drugs such as amphotericin B, itraconazole, miconazole, and voriconazole. Variable sensitivity to 5-fluorocytosine and fluconazole is seen.
- For severe infections, the use of IV amphotericin B is recommended (0.6 mg/kg/day) for 2 weeks followed by oral itraconazole (200 mg BD) for 10 weeks.
- Milder infections can be treated with itraconazole, only.

Aspergillosis

- It is a systemic infection caused by *Aspergillus* species. which is a widespread fungus, found in soil, air, plants, and decomposing organic matter. *Aspergillus fumigatus* followed by *Aspergillus flavus*, *Aspergillus niger*, and *Aspergillus terreus* are the most common species causing aspergillosis.
- Risk factors for invasive aspergillosis include prolonged neutropenia, chronic graft versus host disease, bone marrow transplantation, and nosocomial spread.

Clinical Features

- Unremitting fever, unresponsive to broad-spectrum antibiotics is mostly seen.
- The most common invasion seen is invasive sinopulmonary aspergillosis (ISPA) characterized by sinus or chest pain, hemoptysis, and cough.
- Brain involvement (10% of patients) heralds a poor prognosis.
- Skin involvement occurs in the form of eschar, ulcer, and cellulitis. Plaques studded with pustules, nodules, abscesses, and folliculitis can also occur. Skin lesions are larger (2–3 cm) and fewer in number as compared to other opportunistic fungal infections.
- Eye involvement can be present as corneal ulcers **(Fig. 13)**.

Diagnosis

- *Galactomannan and serum (1-3)-β-D-glucan*: For early detection.
- *Sputum or bronchoalveolar lavage*: Isolation of fungus.
- *Chest X-ray*: Nodules, halo sign, consolidation, and cavitation.
- *Skin biopsy*: Skin biopsy for histology and culture.

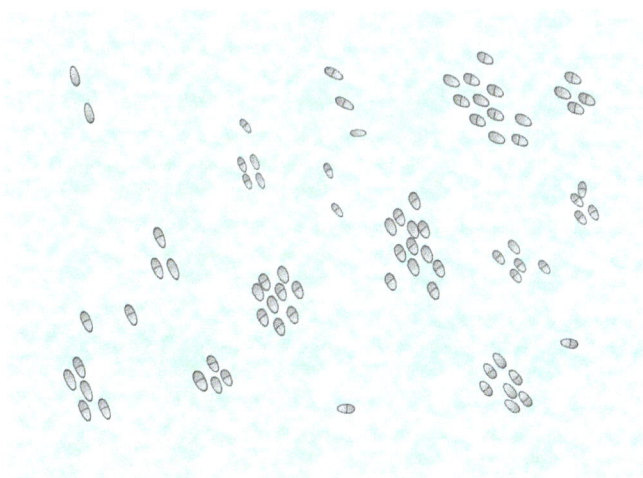

FIG. 12: Diagram showing *Talaromyces marneffei* reproducing by septum formation.

CHAPTER 5: Deep Fungal Infections

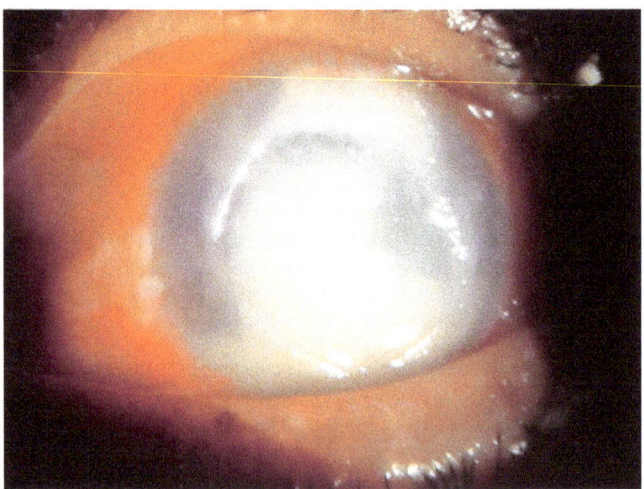

FIG. 13: Corneal ulcer due to *Aspergillus* species.

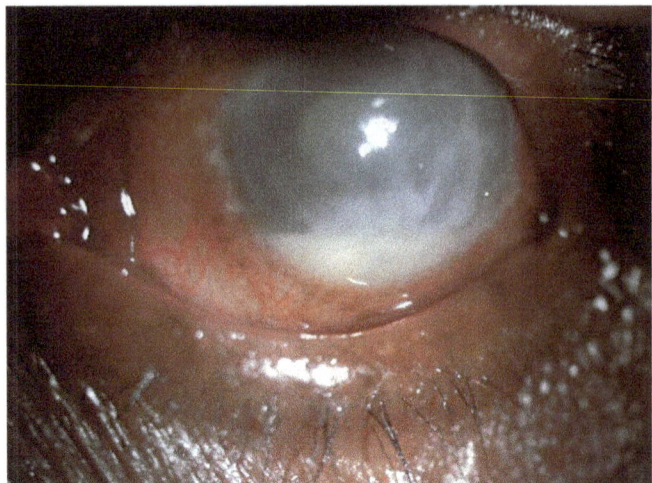

FIG. 14: Candidemia with endophthalmitis and hypopyon in a diabetic patient.

Treatment

- Voriconazole is the preferred agent for ISPA and disseminated aspergillosis.
- Liposomal amphotericin B, itraconazole and posaconazole are alternatives.
- Echinocandins (caspofungin, micafungin, and anidulafungin) are also active against *Aspergillus* species.
- Secondary prophylaxis is warranted post-recovery.

Systemic Candidosis

- Candida is the most common invasive fungus seen in a patient with hematological disorder, as well as the most common cause of fungemia overall.
- *Candida albicans* is the most important species; though, other species such as *Candida tropicalis, Candida parapsilosis, Candida krusei, Candida glabrata,* and *Candida lusitaniae* are also gaining importance, especially with triazole prophylaxis.

Clinical Features

- Invasive candidiasis can present as oropharyngeal candidiasis, esophageal candidiasis, candidemia, acute disseminated, or chronic disseminated candidiasis (hepatosplenic candidiasis)
- The most common presentation is with fever not responding to broad-spectrum antibacterial drugs.
- Skin lesions mostly involve the trunk and extremities in the form of 5 to 10 mm pink dermal papules; ecthyma gangrenosum-like lesions; or painful folliculitis in hair-bearing areas (in heroin abusers), etc.
- Muscle pain, renal impairment, and endophthalmitis **(Fig. 14)** are other manifestations. Almost any organ can be affected.

Diagnosis

- *Direct microscopy*: It reveals budding yeast and pseudohyphae.
- *Histopathology*: It shows subcorneal pustule, parakeratosis, spongiosis, and invasion of stratum corneum by fungal hyphae and yeasts.
- *Computed tomography (CT) scan*: It may show defects in the liver, spleen, lungs, and other organs.
- *Fungal cultures*: These are often negative.
- *Candida enolase antigenemia (CaEno1)*: It is a useful indicator of invasive candidosis.

Treatment

- Drugs most often used are amphotericin B and fluconazole.
- Fluconazole is useful for mucosal forms in neutropenic patients.
- Echinocandins (anidulafungin, caspofungin, or micafungin) are recommended as initial therapy for invasive candidiasis in neutropenic patients with hematologic malignancies.
- For non-neutropenic stable patients with uncomplicated candidemia, an initial course of echinocandin followed by fluconazole is reasonable if the organism proves to be *C. albicans*.

Mucormycosis

- Mucormycosis, also known as black fungus, is an infection with mucormycetes fungi.
- The fungus is common in natural environments, especially in soil. Although rare, it has been around for decades in patients with comorbidities, or severely

weakened immune systems due to steroid use. It has emerged as the third most common invasive mycosis in immunocompromised patients.
- It is considered an emerging angio-invasive infection caused by the filamentous fungi of Mucorales order of the class zygomycetes. The most common organisms causing human infection are *Mucor*, *Absidia*, *Cunninghamella,* and *Rhizopus*.
- Human infections result from inhalation of fungal sporangiospores or direct inoculation into disrupted skin. More recently, an epidemic-like scenario was seen in patients post coronavirus disease 2019 (COVID-19) disease.

Clinical Features

- *Rhinocerebral mucormycosis* begins as nasal or paranasal sinus infection and spreads as a mass of ischemic necrosis **(Fig. 15)**, through bone to the orbit or the brain. *Symptoms and signs* include painful unilateral facial swelling, proptosis, and ophthalmoplegia, with serosanguineous nasal discharge. *Characteristics* such as black intranasal and palatal eschars are often seen. This was the type most commonly seen as a post-COVID manifestation. In disseminated cases, other visceral organs may be involved.
- *Cutaneous mucormycosis*: It presents as firm thick eschar with surrounding erythema and induration, overlying a deep soft tissue infarction beyond the diameter of the cutaneous lesion. Other manifestations include circinate and targetoid lesions and a cotton-like appearance (resembling bread mold)

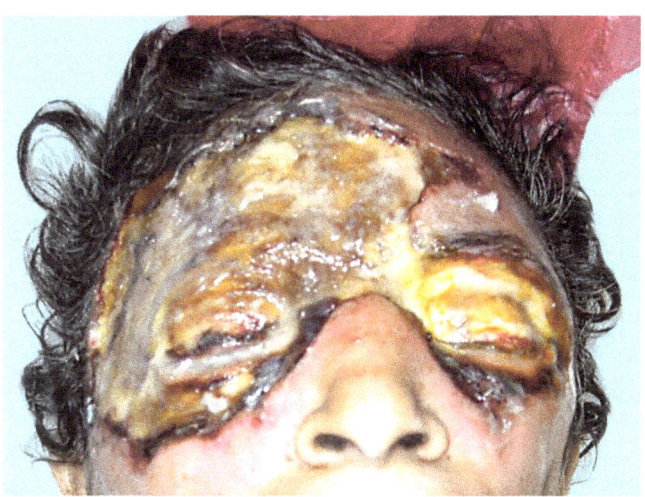

FIG. 15: Mucormycosis involving skin and eyes with cerebral involvement in an uncontrolled diabetic patient that proved fatal despite treatment.

in open wounds. It may also resemble pyoderma gangrenosum and bacterial gangrene.

Diagnosis

Rhinocerebral mucormycosis is a medical emergency confirmed with sinus radiographs, CT scans, and skin smears. Microscopy shows non-septate hyphae with branching at 90° angles.

Treatment

Amphotericin B is the drug of choice followed by triazoles such as posaconazole and echinocandins. Surgical debridement is also necessary.

CHAPTER 6

Herpes Virus Infections

Introduction

Herpesviruses are deoxyribonucleic acid (DNA) viruses, known to cause common cutaneous diseases. They elicit a strong immune response during a primary infection, followed by an evasion of the immune system resulting in latency. Among the herpesviruses, herpes simplex virus type 1 (HSV-1) and herpes simplex virus type 2 (HSV-2), varicella-zoster virus (VZV), *Cytomegalovirus*, human herpesvirus (HHV)-6 and -7 cause clinically overt diseases which are recurrent in nature. Epstein–Barr virus and HHV-8 are oncogenic in nature and result in malignancy. The mainstay of treatment is antivirals; their early initiation and timely duration is essential for a favorable outcome.

Herpes Simplex Virus Infections

The clinical manifestations of herpes infections differ according to the different body areas affected by the virus. Primary HSV infection is defined as an infection occurring in individuals without preexisting antibodies against HSV. HSV-1 infections are acquired through close contact with infected fluids, while type 2 infections mainly occur after puberty and are sexually transmitted.

Clinical Features

Depending on the primary body area affected and the HSV types, there are varying manifestations, as detailed further.

Herpes Gingivostomatitis and Herpes Labialis

- It is a common clinical manifestation of HSV-1 infection, mostly affecting children between the age of 1–5 years and occasionally adults. A primary episode lasts for 2–3 weeks and is characterized by involvement of the buccal and gingival mucosa.
- The affected mucosa appears to be inflamed and erythematous. Superficial vesicles evolving into shallow erosions with yellow pseudomembrane formation, are characteristic. Self-resolution or healing occurs over time **(Figs. 1A and B)**.
- Associated symptoms are common in the primary episode. These include fever, sore throat, malaise, and cervical lymphadenopathy. Following a primary episode, active viral shedding can occur through saliva for a period of 6–12 months.
- Recurrent infection in this site is commonly known as *fever blisters* or *cold sores*. The episode is often heralded by a prodrome of pain, tingling, burning, or itching which lasts for 4–6 hours followed by the appearance of vesicles over the vermilion border of lips that lasts for 48–72 hours **(Figs. 2A and B)**. The lesions evolve into pustules followed by ulceration and crusting within 72–96 hours and completely heal by 8–10 days. However, intraoral lesions are rare in recurrence and occur without a prodrome. These can occur following dental procedures. Recurrences are known to occur in 15–45% seropositive individuals. Rarely, lesions may involve surrounding areas, such as the nose **(Fig. 3)**.

Genital Herpes (Herpes Genitalis)

- Primary genital herpes caused by HSV-2, manifests as macules and papules, followed by vesicles, pustules, and erosions. In women, the lesions tend to be bilateral and symmetrical over the vulva **(Fig. 4)** and cervix. In men, the lesions tend to occur over the glans and penile shaft **(Fig. 5)**.
- Extra genital involvement of areas such as buttocks, perineum skin, and thighs, can occur in both sexes. The primary infection is associated with a prodrome

CHAPTER 6: Herpes Virus Infections

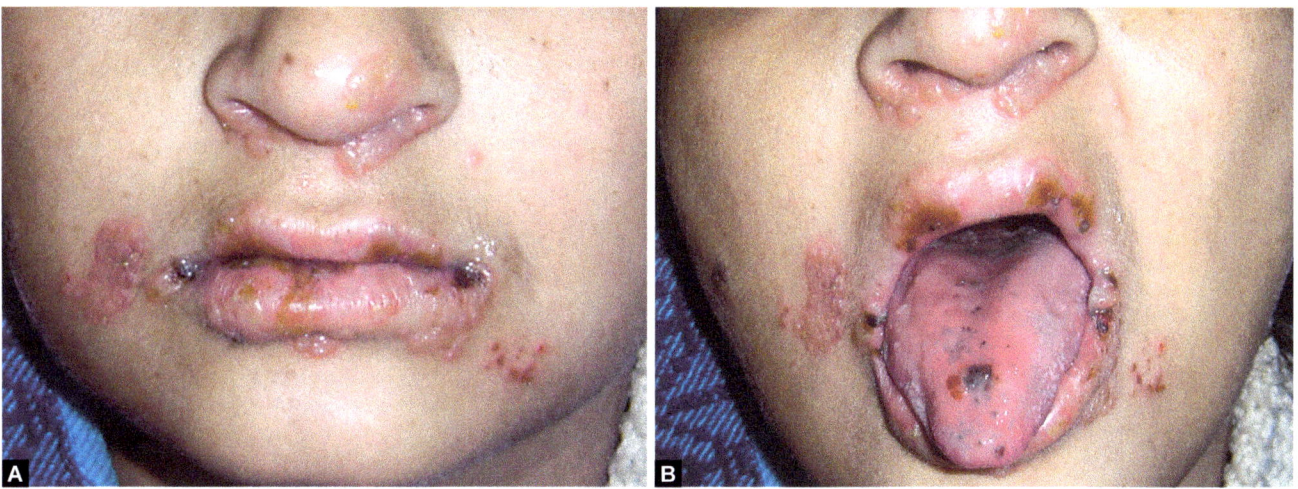

FIGS. 1A AND B: Primary episode of herpes with extensive herpetic cutaneous involvement and gingivostomatitis. Note extensive hemorrhagic blisters on the tongue.

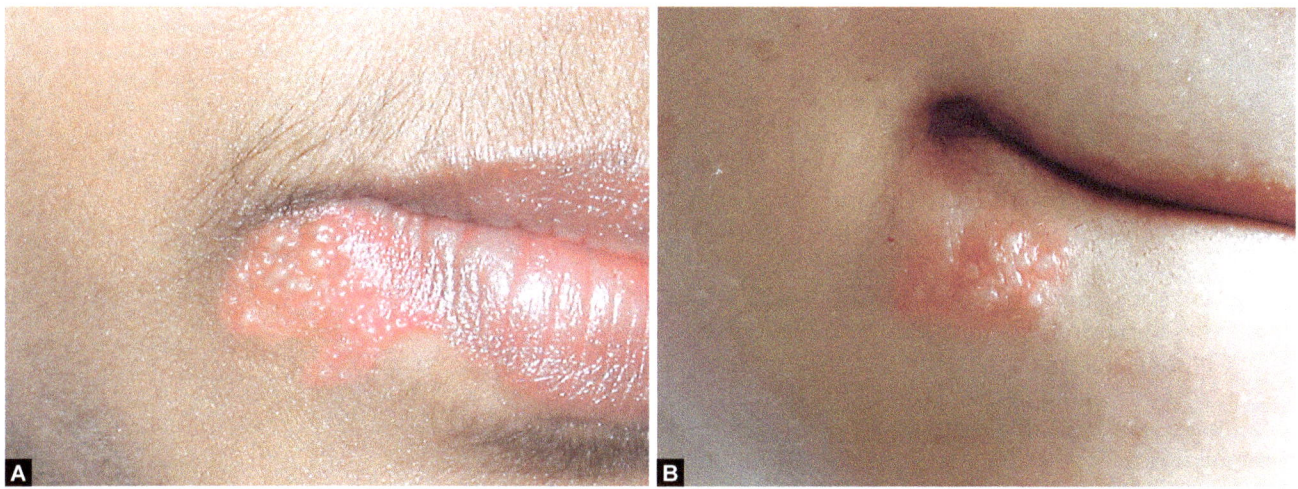

FIGS. 2A AND B: Close-up view of the grouped vesicles seen in herpes labialis.

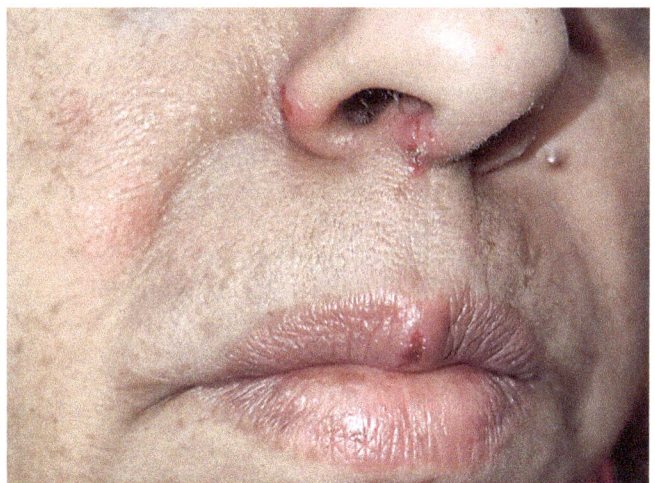

FIG. 3: Recurrent herpes labialis with intranasal involvement.

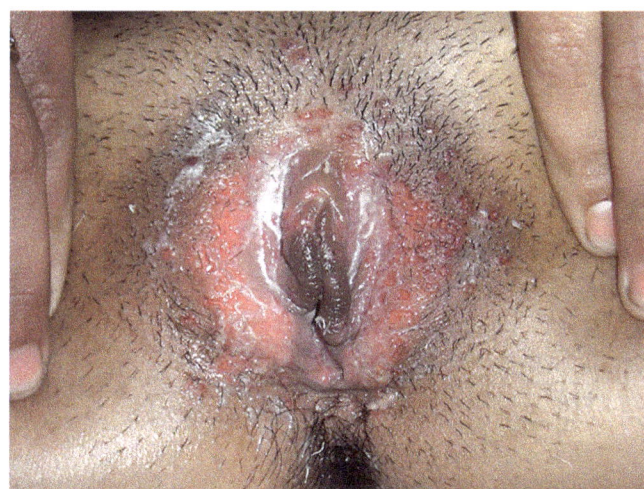

FIG. 4: Herpes genitalis in a female patient. Note the extensive bilateral involvement.

CHAPTER 6: Herpes Virus Infections

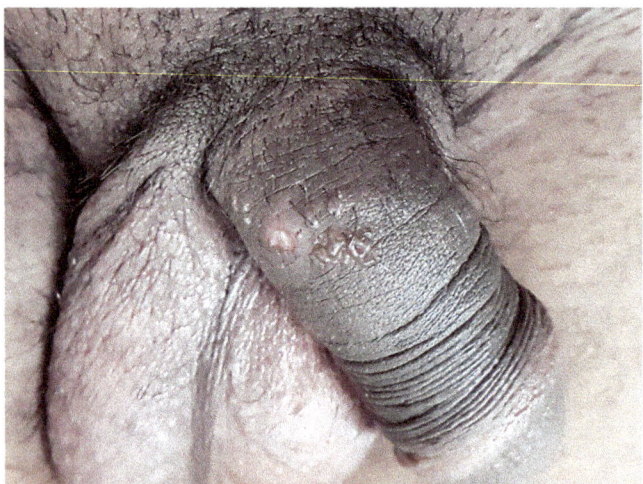

FIG. 5: Herpes genitalis in a male patient.

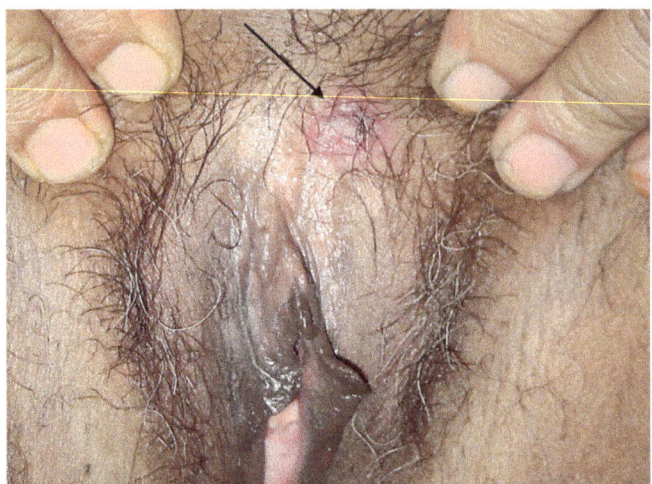

FIG. 6: Recurrent herpes genitalis. Note the limited area of involvement.

of tingling, burning, pain, fever, dysuria, and localized inguinal lymphadenopathy.
- The primary infection is generally more severe and tends to be associated with more complications in women as compared to men. These may include urinary retention syndrome, aseptic meningitis, paresthesia, and dysesthesia over the lower limbs and perineum.
- The lesions generally heal by 3 weeks, while asymptomatic viral shedding may keep on occurring for 6 months to 1 year.
- In recurrent genital herpes **(Fig. 6)**, the lesions are limited to few vesicles over the shaft of the penis. In females, it may be characterized simply by minimal lesions or vulvar irritation, lasting for 8–10 days **(Fig. 7)**.
- During pregnancy, an episode of primary genital herpes, especially if acquired close to term, is associated with a 5–50% risk of subsequent neonatal herpes. This risk is much lower if the primary infection occurs in the first and second trimesters. Elective cesarean delivery is especially indicated if active HSV lesions are present during or within 2 weeks of labor.

Eczema Herpeticum
- It is a secondary viral infection caused by either HSV-1 or HSV-2. It occurs in patients with a pre-existing skin disease, which causes impaired skin barrier function. This could be atopic dermatitis (AD) (commonly), long-term topical or systemic steroid use, or use of calcineurin inhibitors.
- Various other dermatological conditions which can present with eczema herpeticum including contact dermatitis, Darier's disease, pemphigus foliaceus,

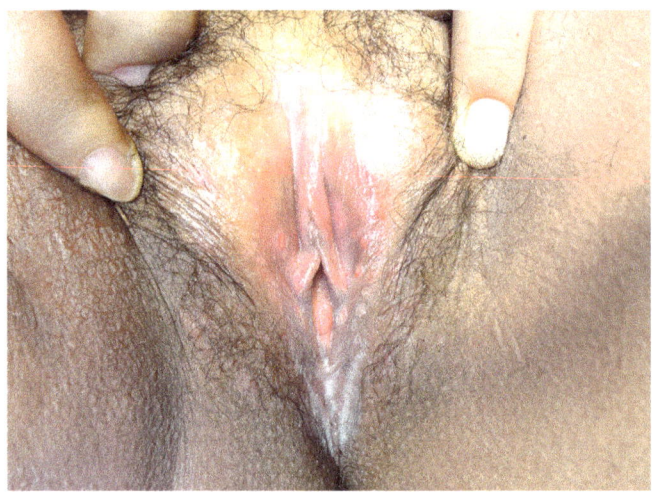

FIG. 7: Recurrent herpes genitalis with vaginal discharge.

Hailey–Hailey disease, ichthyosis vulgaris, psoriasis, or skin postdermabrasion, or laser therapy.
- The affected skin develops multiple, erythematous, small, monomorphic, dome-shaped papulovesicles that rupture to form tiny punched-out ulcers overlying an erythematous base **(Fig. 8)**.
- Such lesions commonly affect the face, neck, and upper trunk **(Fig. 9)**. Constitutional symptoms in the form of fever, malaise, and lymphadenopathy may occur. In most cases, HSV-1 is responsible for this eruption.
- Kaposi's varicelliform eruption is the collective term used for eczema herpeticum (caused by HSV-1), eczema vaccinatum (caused by vaccinia virus), and infections by other viruses like coxsackie A16 in a similar scenario.

CHAPTER 6: Herpes Virus Infections

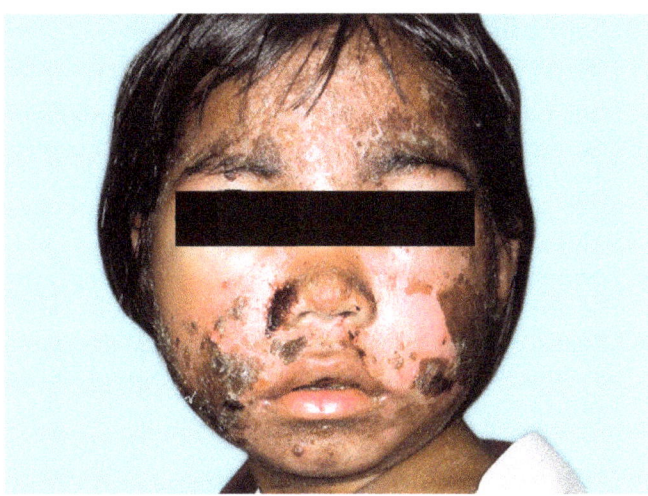

FIG. 8: Eczema herpeticum in an atopic girl child.

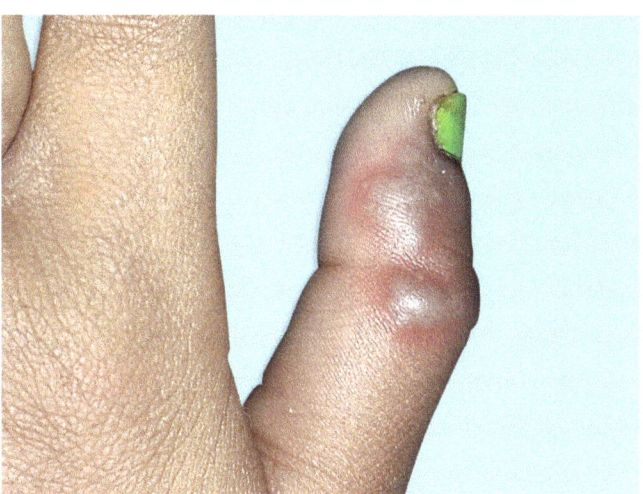

FIG. 10: Severe herpetic whitlow with grouped vesicles, severe pain and digital swelling.

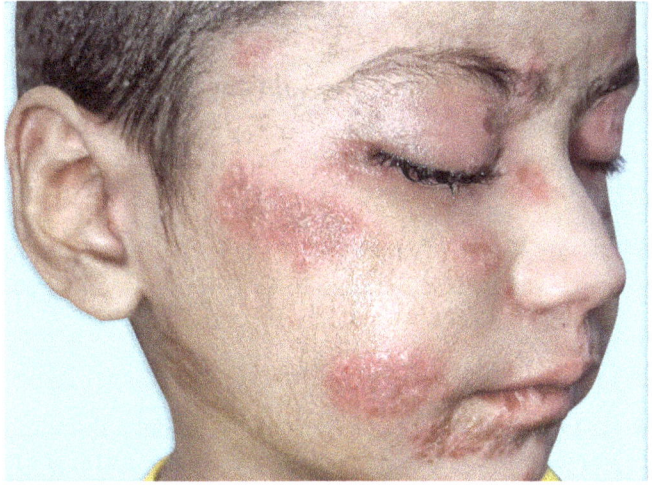

FIG. 9: Eczema herpeticum developing in a child being treated for atopic dermatitis with cyclosporine.

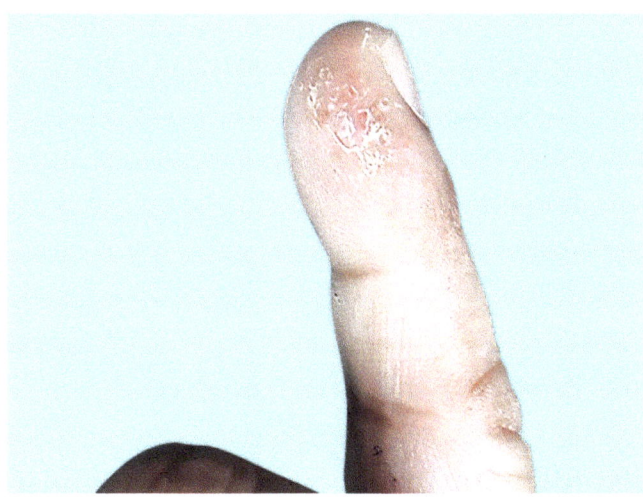

FIG. 11: Herpes whitlow; recurrent lesions.

Herpetic Whitlow
- Herpetic whitlow involves finger pulp, rarely toes.
- It can be caused either by HSV-1/-2 during an episode of primary infection.
- In children, most cases are attributed to autoinoculation of HSV-1 from a focus of herpetic gingivostomatitis; while, autoinoculation of HSV-2 can occur in adolescents and adults including healthcare workers.
- Herpetic whitlow also commonly manifests with a prodrome of burning, pruritus, and/or tingling of the affected finger or the entire limb, followed by erythema, pain, and vesicle formation **(Fig. 10)**.
- Recurrences may be less symptomatic **(Fig. 11)**.

Herpes Gladiatorum
- It is a manifestation, often seen among sport persons involved in contact sports due to close physical contact with an infected person (e.g., wrestlers and rugby players).
- Vesicular eruptions are often seen on the torso but can occur in any location where skin-to-skin contact has occurred **(Fig. 12)**.

Herpetic Keratoconjunctivitis
- It is an HSV infection of the eye presenting with symptoms of eye pain, photophobia, and discharge.
- The pathognomonic finding is dendritic corneal ulcers.
- Failure to recognize early and initiate prompt treatment can result in corneal scarring and loss of vision.

Neonatal Herpes Simplex Virus
- Neonatal HSV infections are uncommon but associated with dreaded complications.

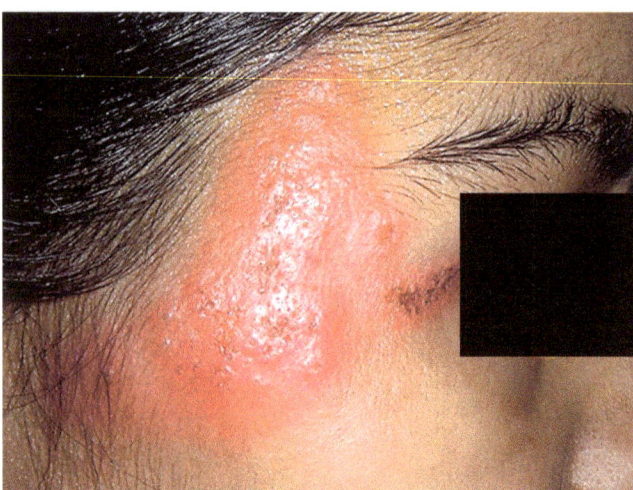

FIG. 12: Herpes gladiatorum.

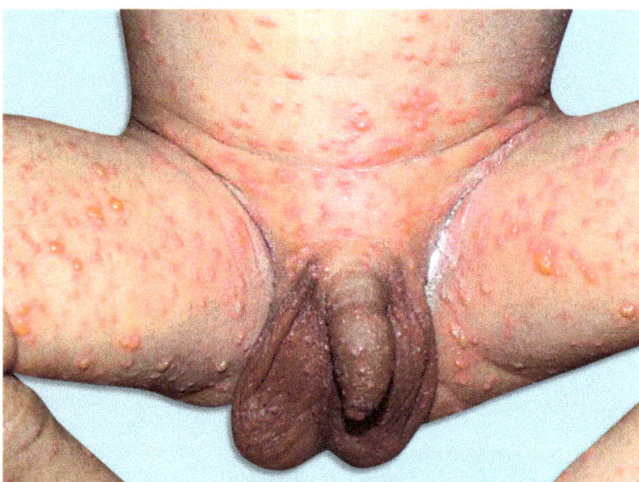

FIG. 13: Neonatal herpes simplex.

- Transmission occurs from the infected mother either during the intrauterine, intrapartum, or postpartum period, especially when the mother suffers from a primary episode of genital herpes close to the time of delivery.
- Recurrent genital herpes carries a lower risk of transmission.
- Neonatal herpes is seen to affect the skin, eyes, neurological system, and multiple internal organs. At or within 10 days of birth, multiple vesicles develop on the skin surface **(Fig. 13)**. Central nervous system involvement usually presents as herpes encephalitis characterized by fever, lethargy, and seizures.
- Disseminated infection usually involves multiple organs, liver, lung, and adrenals causing jaundice, respiratory insufficiency, and disseminated intravascular coagulation.

Complications of Herpes Simplex Virus Infections

- Neurological complications including acute meningitis, autonomic nervous system dysfunction, transverse myelitis, Guillain–Barré syndrome, Bell's palsy, and HSV encephalitis may occur due to latency of the HSV within neurons.
- Lymphedema and leukoderma may develop after recurrent HSV infection.
- Recurrent episodes of urticaria and erythema multiforme have been reported that respond well to antiviral therapy.

Herpes Simplex Infection in Immunocompromised

- Manifestations of HSV in the immunosuppressed patient are usually more severe, extensive, recurrent, and resistant to treatment **(Figs. 14A and B)**. Among patients with human immunodeficiency virus (HIV) infected recurrent and persistent herpetic ulceration is considered an AIDS (acquired immunodeficiency syndrome)-defining illness.
- Anogenital herpes results in persistent shedding of HIV.
- Extensive oropharyngeal **(Fig. 15)** involvement followed by tracheobronchitis, and pneumonitis are known to occur in the immunocompromised.

Diagnosis

- A Tzanck smear, prepared from the vesicular fluid, and stained using Wright–Giemsa stain demonstrates the presence of multinucleate giant cells.
- A skin biopsy reveals ballooning degeneration of cells, intraepidermal bulla formation, and the presence of large multinucleated giant cells with intranuclear inclusions.
- Detection of virus/viral antigen by enzyme-linked immunosorbent assay (ELISA) can be done.
- Viral culture is the "gold standard" for HSV diagnosis. The characteristic viral cytopathic effect appears 2–3 days after inoculation in human diploid fibroblast cultures or green monkey kidney cell cultures. This is generally not used for routine diagnosis.
- HSV-polymerase chain reaction (PCR) has a higher rate of HSV detection and eventually may replace viral culture as the gold standard for the diagnosis of genital herpes.
- Serological tests are useful in diagnosing recurrent lesions, atypical lesions, culture-negative cases, and asymptomatic infections in immunocompromised patients and their sex partners.

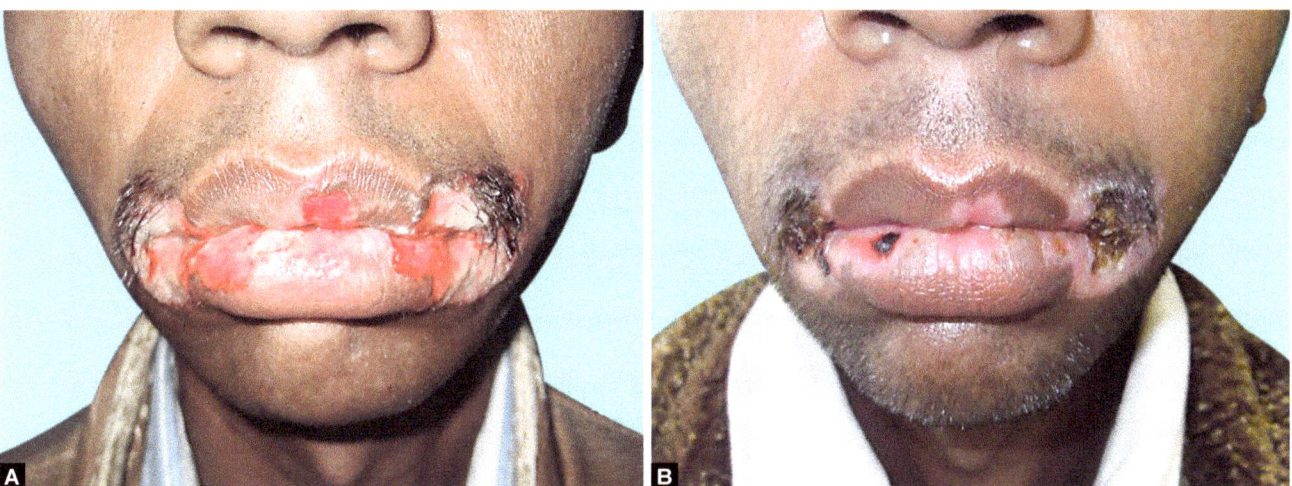

FIGS. 14A AND B: Severe ulcerative herpes labialis in a human immunodeficiency virus (HIV)-positive male. Healing with scarring.

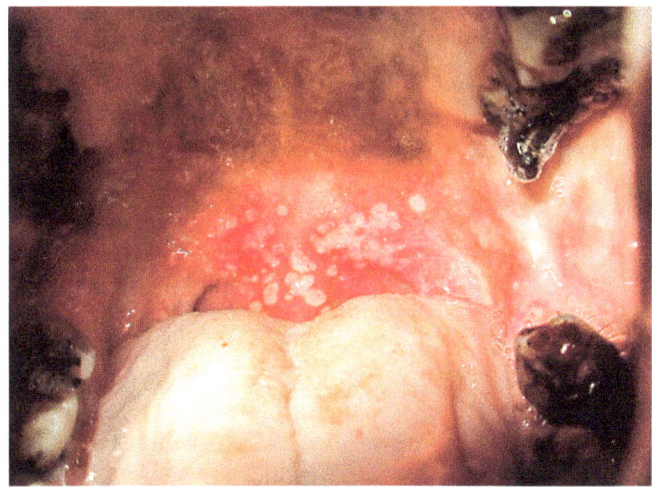

FIG. 15: Oral lesions of herpes simplex involving posterior palate and pharyngeal wall in a human immunodeficiency virus (HIV)-positive female.

Differential Diagnosis

Orolabial Herpes
- Herpangina
- Aphthous stomatitis
- Stevens–Johnson syndrome
- Drug-induced mucositis

Genital Herpes
- Syphilitic chancre
- Chancroid
- Traumatic ulcer
- Lymphogranuloma venereum

Treatment

General Measures

The primary infection is extremely painful and adequate analgesia is required with the use of nonsteroidal anti-inflammatory drugs (NSAIDs). In vesicular lesions, cool compresses with tap water or Burrow's solution are advocated three to four times/day. Cleansing mouthwashes containing anesthetics such as lignocaine and antibacterials soothe the involved mucosa and decrease secondary bacterial superinfections. Genital lesions may be aided by a sitz bath using tepid water.

Specific Measures

- Antiviral therapy is useful when instituted in the first few hours.
- Systemic antivirals are required, especially for primary infection **(Table 1)** and immunosuppressed patients.
- Topical antivirals have a negligible role.
- Systemic antiviral suppressive prophylaxis is considered in cases with frequent recurrences.

Prevention

Due to the chronic and lifelong nature of the infection, it is often said that prevention of transmission is an aspect that needs to be adequately reinforced.

Prevention of Orolabial and Genital Herpes

- Counsel the patient regarding the triggering factors and avoid them.

CHAPTER 6: Herpes Virus Infections

TABLE 1: Systemic antiviral therapy.

Disease	Drug and dosage
• Herpes labialis (first episode) • Herpes genitalis (first episode)	• Acyclovir 200 mg five times/400 mg TDS/day × 7 days • Valacyclovir 1 g BD × 7 days • Famciclovir 250 mg TDS × 7 days
• Herpes labialis (recurrences) • Herpes genitalis (recurrent episode)	• Acyclovir 200 mg five times/400 mg TDS/day × 5 days • Valacyclovir 1 g BD × 5 days • Famciclovir 250 mg TDS × 5 days
Suppressive therapy for recurrent orolabial herpes infection and genital herpes	Acyclovir 400 mg BD × 6–12 months
Neonatal herpes	IV acyclovir 20 mg/kg every 8 hours for 14–21 days
Eczema herpeticum	• Acyclovir 200 mg five times/ 400 mg TDS 14–21 days • Valacyclovir 1 g BD × 14–21 days • IV acyclovir 10–15 mg/kg three times/day—14–21 days

(BD: twice a day, IV: intravenous; TDS: thrice a day)

- Recommend sexual abstinence, use of condoms, or circumcision.
- Sexual partners should be evaluated and treated.

Prevention of Neonatal Herpes

- Serological tests may be considered to identify women at risk of acquiring new infections.
- Recommend abstinence or protective condoms or antiviral prophylaxis in the context of sero-incompatible couples.
- Prophylactic antivirals from the 36th week of gestation in pregnant females at a high risk of HSV outbreaks, may be considered.
- Cesarean delivery is to be considered in women with active lesions at the time of birth.

Varicella Zoster Virus Infections

Varicella-zoster virus causes two clinically distinct forms of disease. The primary infection causes varicella or "chickenpox;" while, herpes zoster (HZ) (shingles) is caused by the reactivation of latent VZV.

Varicella (Chickenpox)

- It is a highly contagious infection, with secondary attack rates of >90% in susceptible individuals. It is a self-limited illness.
- Transmission occurs via aerosolized droplets from nasopharyngeal secretions of an infected individual or by direct skin contact with vesicular fluid.
- The average incubation period is 14–16 days. The period of infectivity lasts from 48 hours before the onset of the rash until all skin lesions have fully crusted.

Clinical Features

- The onset is with a prodrome of fever, malaise, pharyngitis, and loss of appetite.
- A characteristic rash appears in successive crops over several days. The lesions begin as macules and papules, rapidly evolving into vesicles arising from an erythematous base. This is responsible for the classic "dewdrops on rose-petal" appearance **(Fig. 16)**. The lesions have a centripetal distribution with maximum concentration of the lesions over the trunk **(Figs. 17 and 18)**.
- An enanthem involving the oropharyngeal, and conjunctival mucosae may also be seen.
- The lesions dry up to form crusts, which fall off by 1–2 weeks and heal with hypopigmentation.

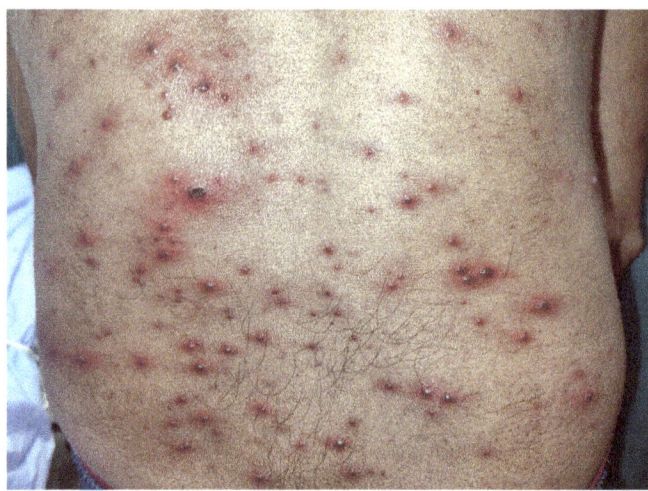

FIG. 16: Varicella in an adult male. The typical vesicles on an erythematous base, showing the "dew drops on a rose petal" appearance can be seen.

- In adults, varicella may be frequently associated with very extensive lesions and the patient is toxic **(Figs. 19A and B)**.
- Mucosal involvement is not common but may occur **(Fig. 20)**.
- Immunocompromised patients may present with multisystem involvement and extensive pustular lesions that take longer to resolve **(Fig. 21)**.
- If the mother contracts the infection close to the time of delivery, the neonate may be born with lesions of varicella or may develop them soon after birth **(Fig. 22)**.

Complications

- The most common systemic complications noted are varicella pneumonitis (in 16–25%) and encephalitis.
- Secondary bacterial infection, usually due to *Staphylococcus aureus,* is the most common complication.

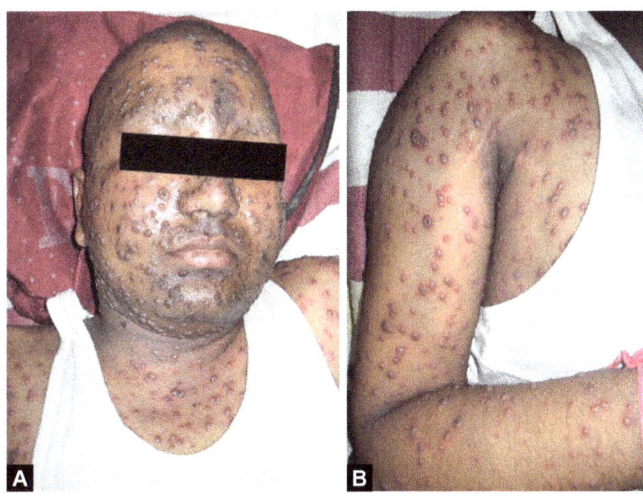

FIGS. 19A AND B: Adult varicella. Note the numerous lesions and a toxic patient.

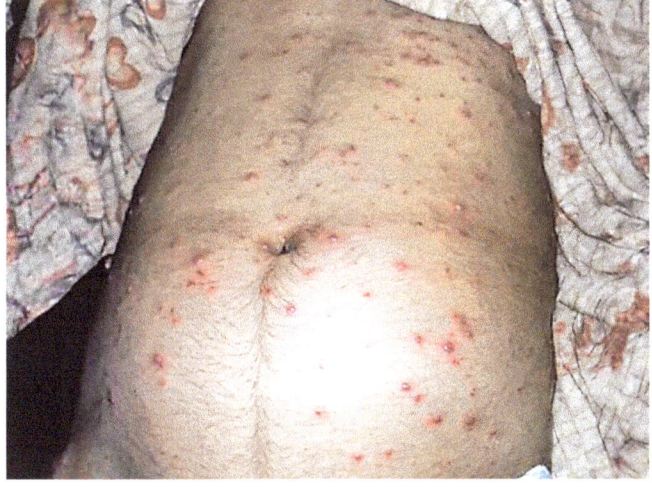

FIG. 17: Vesicles arising from an erythematous base seen in varicella.

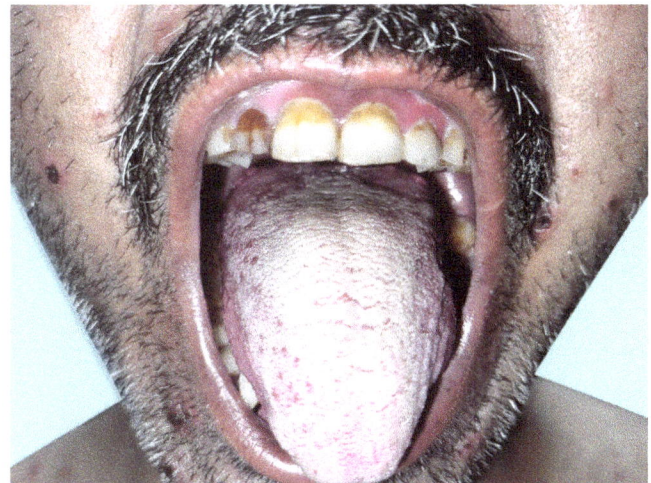

FIG. 20: Mucosal involvement in a patient with severe varicella. Note the extensive gingivitis.

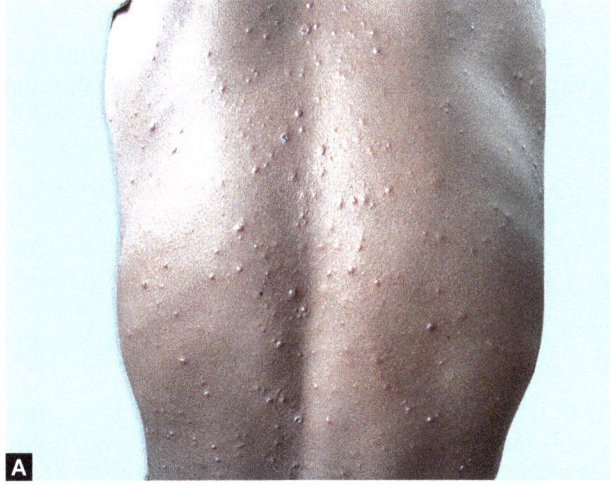

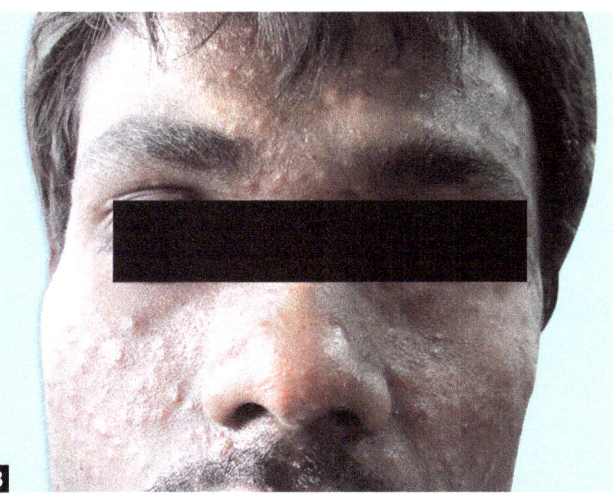

FIGS. 18A AND B: Crops of lesion seen over the head, neck, and trunk in varicella.

CHAPTER 6: Herpes Virus Infections

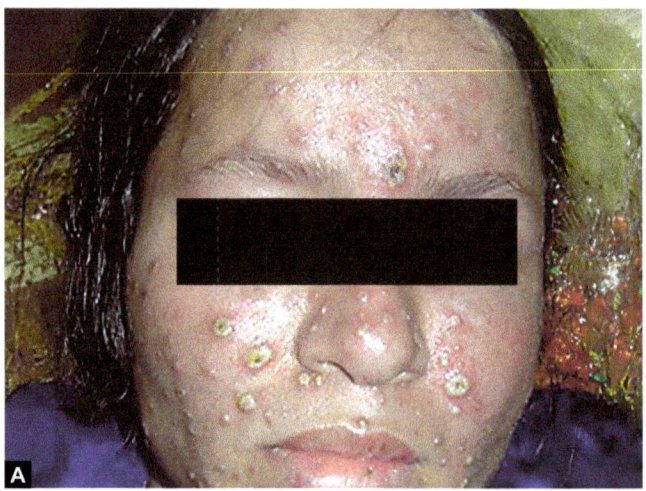 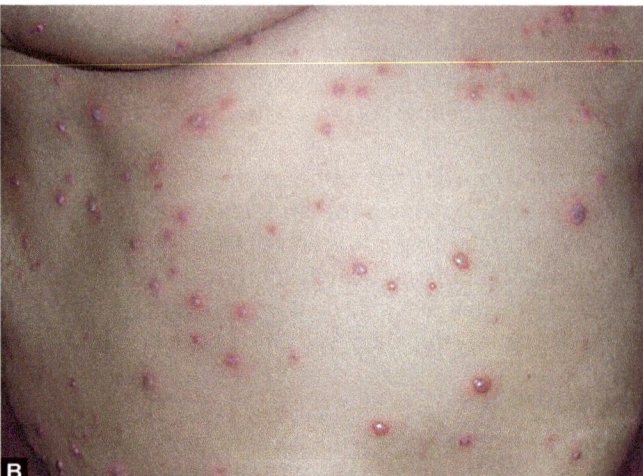

FIGS. 21A AND B: Varicella in immunocompromised patients.

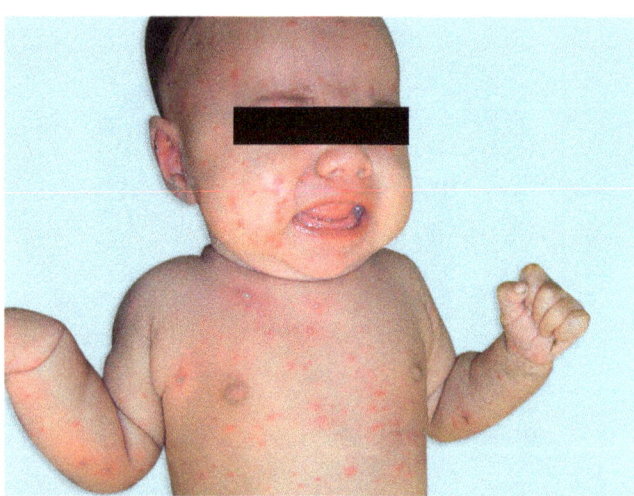

FIG. 22: Neonatal varicella.

- Varicella gangrenosa caused by *Streptococcus pyogenes*, is characterized by rapidly progressive erythema and induration around a single preexisting lesion. Deep ulcerative lesions and regional lymphadenitis may occur.
- Other complications include subclinical hepatitis, thrombocytopenia, acute myocarditis, acute pancreatitis, glomerulonephritis, and disseminated intravascular coagulation.

Differential Diagnosis

- Disseminated herpes simplex infection
- Pityriasis lichenoides et varioliformis acuta
- Insect bite reactions
- Erythema multiforme
- Hand–foot–mouth disease
- Insect bite reaction

Treatment

General Measures

- Isolation is recommended till lesions crust and fall off, to prevent onward transmission to healthy children or adults.
- The patient should be advised to keep nails short.
- Antihistamines should be administered to decrease itching and prevent chances of secondary infection and scarring.
- Antipyretics or acetaminophen may be used to decrease fever.

Antiviral Therapy

- In view of its self-limiting and benign course, antivirals are avoided in healthy children, especially because of their moderate side effects.
- In adults, antivirals are the mainstay of treatment. Antiviral treatment is highly effective if initiated within 24 hours after the onset of the rash.
- Acyclovir is the only United States Food and Drug Administration (US FDA) approved drug; although, famciclovir and valacyclovir are also used frequently. It reduces the number of lesions, and days of fever and accelerates healing.
- Dose (adult with uncomplicated infection):
  - Tablet acyclovir 800 mg (20 mg/kg) five times/day × 7 days
    Or,
  - Tablet valacyclovir 1 g TDS (20 mg/kg TDS) × 7 days
- For immunocompromised adults/children or immunocompetent adults/children with complications: Intravenous acyclovir 10 mg/kg every 8 hours for 7 days.

Vaccination

Varicella is a vaccine-preventable disease.
- US FDA approves the use of live varicella vaccine in individuals 12 months and older. It has 70–90% efficacy in preventing varicella and >95% efficacy in preventing severe varicella.
- The vaccine is administered as 0.5 mL subcutaneous dose in the deltoid region or anterolateral thigh.
- A two-dose regimen is recommended for routine administration. The first dose is given at 12–15 months of age, and the second dose at 4–6 years old.
- In adults, two doses are administered 4–8 weeks apart.
- Vaccine is US FDA-approved for postexposure prophylaxis and outbreak control. It helps prevent or modify disease when given within 3–5 days after exposure.
- Most commonly reported adverse effects include soreness or swelling at the injection site.
- Other rare adverse effects include fever or mild vaccine-associated varicelliform rash.
- After administration of the vaccine, it is recommended to avoid salicylates for 5 weeks due to the risk of Reye's syndrome.
- *Contraindications*: Allergy to constituents including neomycin, immunosuppressed or immunodeficient individuals [severe combined immunodeficiency, lymphoma, leukemia, AIDS, blood dyscrasias, hypogammaglobulinemia, agammaglobulinemia, immunoglobulin A (IgA) deficiency, malignant neoplasms affecting the bone marrow or lymphatic system, patients receiving steroids, chemotherapy, or X-rays as a treatment for cancer], patients with febrile illness, or active, untreated tuberculosis, pregnant or lactating females.
- Women should delay pregnancy for 3 months after vaccination.

Herpes Zoster (Shingles)

Herpes zoster occurs following a reactivation of VZV from the affected sensory ganglion.
- It is often preceded by a prodrome of tingling pain/numbness over the affected dermatome, malaise, fever, and headache.
- A maculopapular erythematous rash in a dermatomal distribution develops within 48–72 hours. It is associated with moderate-to-severe pain and rapidly evolves into vesicular lesions.
- HZ commonly involves the thoracic dermatome between T5 and T10, followed by cranial and lumbosacral dermatomes **(Figs. 23A and B)**.
- Scattered skin lesions (beyond the primary dermatome) are observed occasionally in the healthy host **(Figs. 24A and B)**.
- Disseminated cutaneous zoster is the presence of >20 vesicles outside the primary and adjacent dermatomes. It is seen in 10–40% of immunocompromised hosts and rarely in normal individuals **(Figs. 25A to C)**.
- These vesicles become hemorrhagic, dry to form crusts and fall off in 7–10 days. The affected area heals with pigmentation or scarring depending on the severity of the rash **(Figs. 26A and B)**.

Complications

- Postherpetic neuralgia occurs in 9–19% of patients, especially common in the elderly.
- Neurological complications include encephalitis, cerebral angiitis, peripheral motor neuropathy; Guillain–Barré syndrome, facial palsy **(Fig. 27)**, and hearing defect (Ramsay Hunt syndrome) **(Fig. 28)**.
- Debilitating ocular complications such as dendritic keratitis, iridocyclitis, and panophthalmitis are known

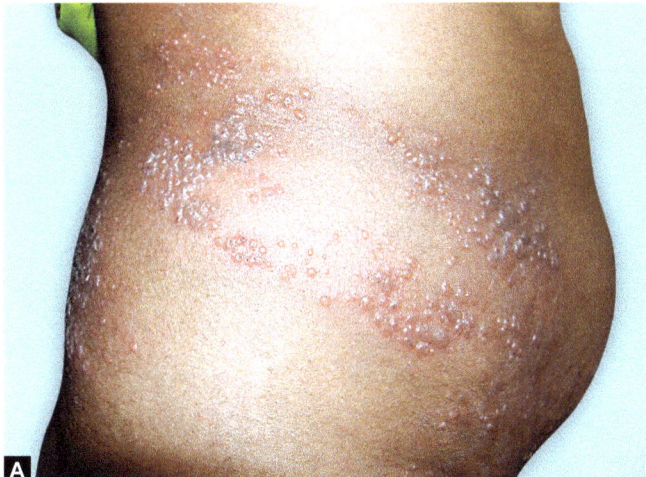
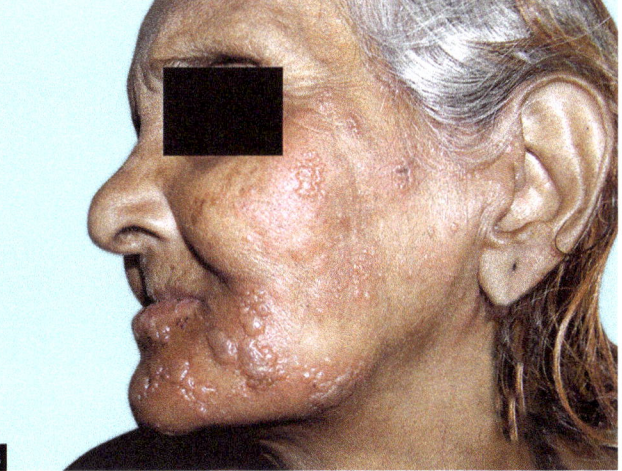

FIGS. 23A AND B: Herpes zoster occurring over thoracic and trigeminal dermatome, respectively.

CHAPTER 6: Herpes Virus Infections

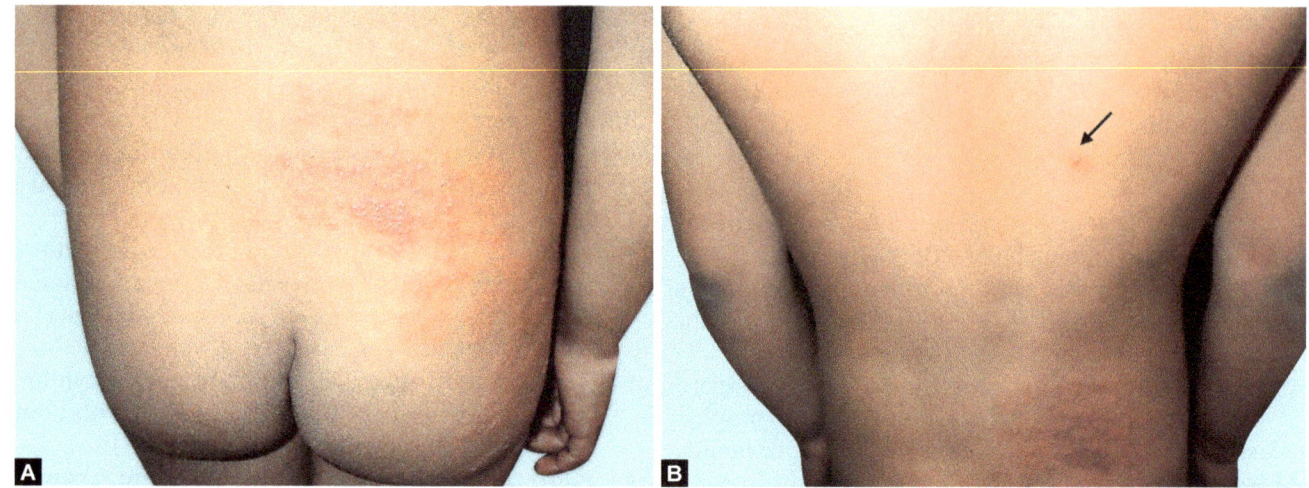

FIGS. 24A AND B: Extradermatomal involvement in herpes zoster.

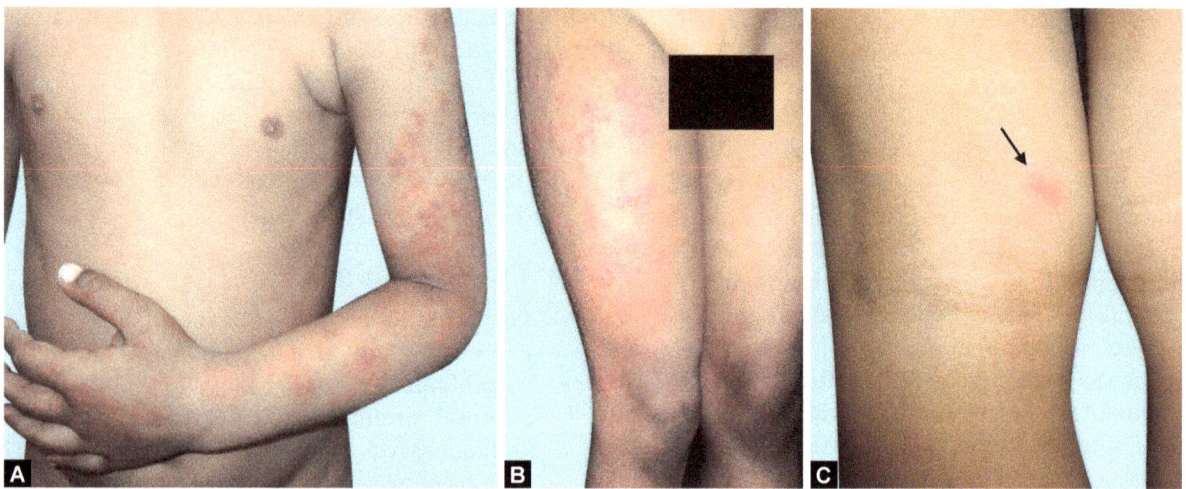

FIGS. 25A TO C: Disseminated herpes zoster.

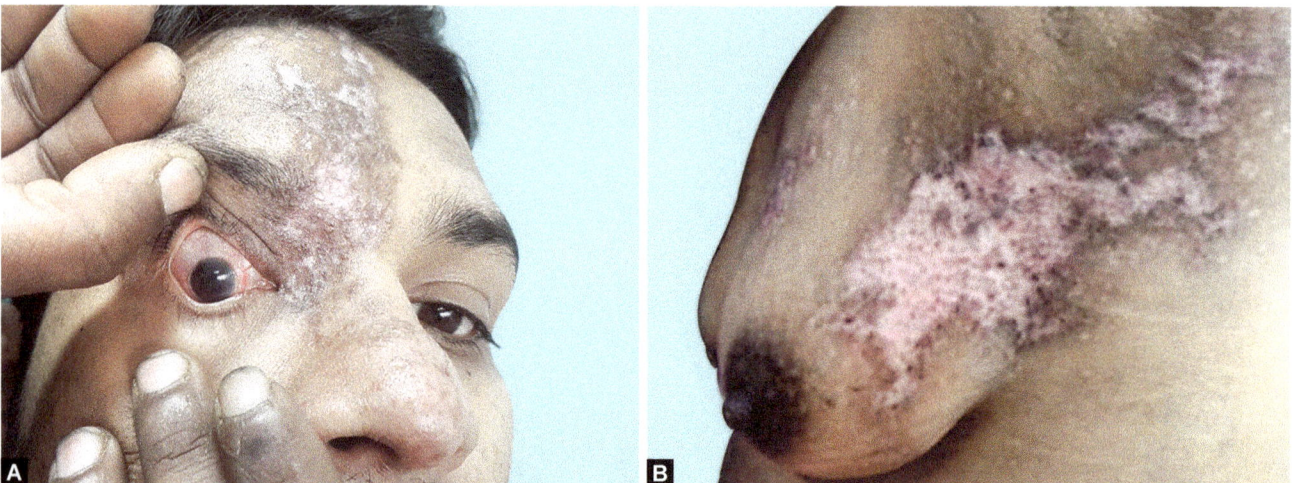

FIGS. 26A AND B: Postzoster depigmentation and atrophy.

CHAPTER 6: Herpes Virus Infections

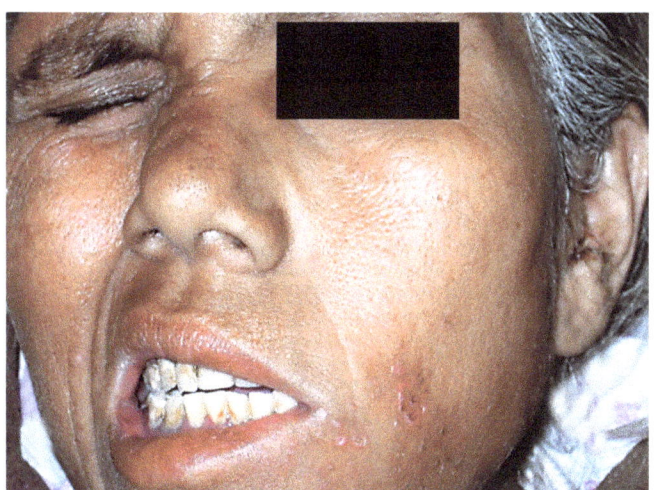

FIG. 27: Facial palsy in a patient with herpes zoster.

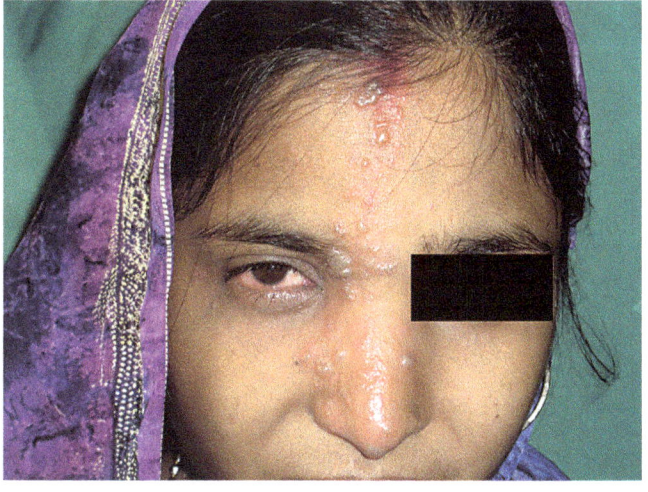

FIG. 29: Herpes zoster ophthalmicus with Hutchinson's sign in the form of involvement of the tip of the nose. This signifies a significant risk of corneal involvement.

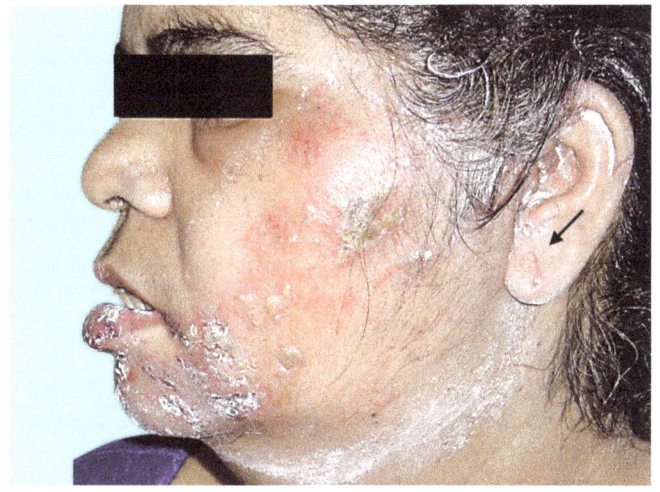

FIG. 28: Ramsay Hunt syndrome; note lesions over left pinna and left facial nerve palsy.

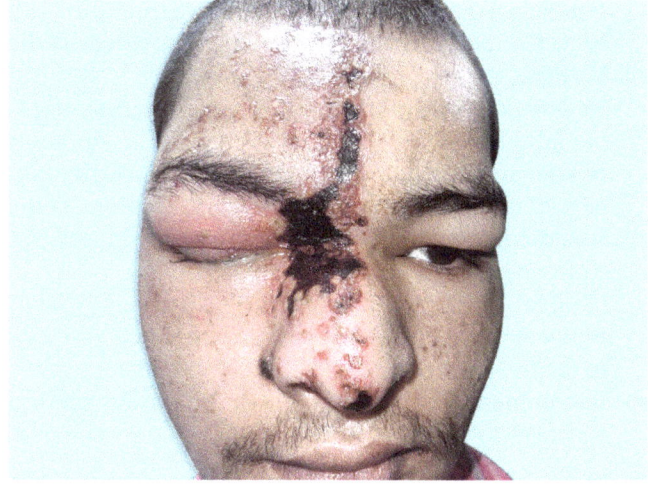

FIG. 30: Necrotic herpes zoster ophthalmicus in an immunosuppressed male.

to occur post-HZ ophthalmicus **(Figs. 29 and 30)**. The involvement of the tip of the nose in HZ ophthalmicus (Hutchinson sign) is considered a harbinger of severe corneal involvement **(Fig. 30)**.
- HIV patients can have recurrent HZ and chronic HZ, and lesions may become hemorrhagic and necrotic **(Figs. 30 and 31)**.

Diagnosis
- A Tzanck smear often reveals the presence of multinucleate giant cells but does not distinguish between HSV and VZV infections.
- Tissue culture and PCR may be performed.

Treatment

General Measures
Patients with localized zosters should avoid contact with susceptible persons at high risk for severe varicella until all the lesions become dry.

Specific Measures
- HZ in otherwise healthy individuals is a self-limiting disease. It may not always require antiviral therapy and can be treated symptomatically. However, in severe acute disease, elderly individuals, or HZ involving cranial nerves, treatment with systemic antivirals is most essential.

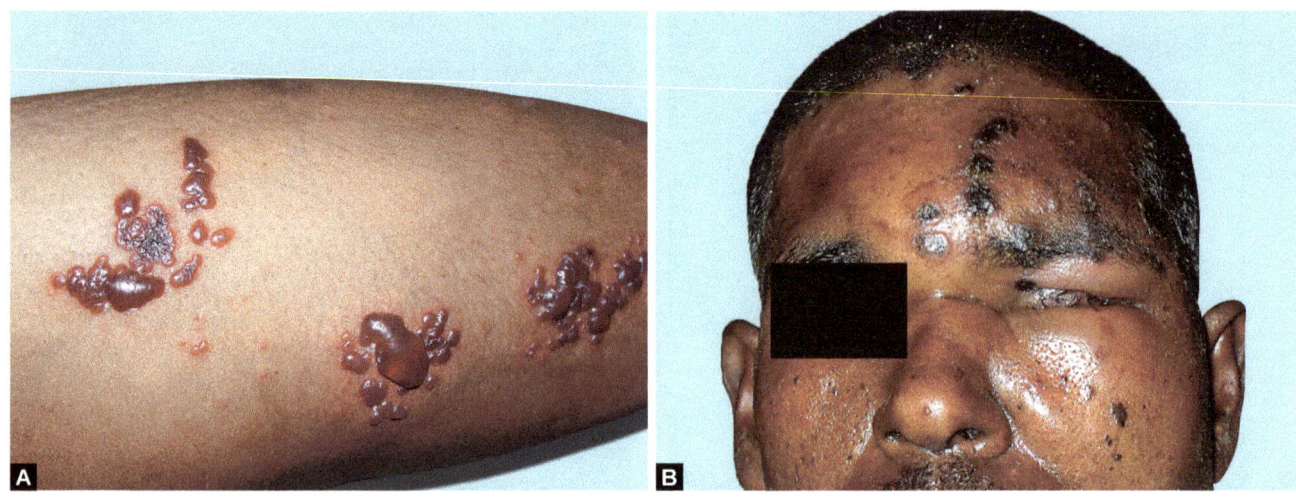

FIGS. 31A AND B: (A) Hemorrhagic blisters in herpes zoster; (B) Necrotic lesions of herpes zoster.

- Systemic antiviral drugs (acyclovir, valacyclovir, and famciclovir) are often used in the treatment of HZ; however, acyclovir is the only drug approved by the US FDA.
- Benefits of antiviral therapy are observed only if it is instituted within 48–72 hours after onset of symptoms or appearance of vesicles. In placebo-controlled trials, acyclovir was observed to shorten the duration of viral shedding, accelerate healing, and reduce the severity of acute pain.
- Clinical studies on famciclovir and valacyclovir indicate equal effectiveness as compared to acyclovir in the treatment of HZ.
- Recommended antiviral regimen in various clinical scenarios is as shown in **Box 1**.

BOX 1	Recommended treatment regimens in herpes zoster.

- Acyclovir 800 mg five times daily for 1 week
- Valacyclovir 1,000 mg three times a day for 1 week
- Famciclovir 500 mg three times a day for 1 week

Vaccination

- Centers for Disease Control and Prevention (CDC) USA, recommends routine vaccination for HZ with recombinant zoster vaccine (RZV, Shingrix) in immunocompetent adults 50 years or older. It is to prevent HZ and related complications.
- Two doses (0.5 mL each) separated by 2–6 months need to be administered, irrespective of prior episode of HZ.
- CDC also recommends two doses of RZV for immunodeficient or immunosuppressed adults ≥19 years of age.
- For patients with a history of HZ, no specific wait time is recommended, though it should not be administered during an acute episode.
- There are currently no recommendations for use in pregnancy and it is preferable to delay vaccination until after pregnancy. No contraindication exists with breastfeeding.
- Vaccine efficacy at preventing HZ is 91–97%; while its efficacy in preventing post-herpetic neuralgia is 88–91%.

Human Papillomavirus

Introduction

Human papillomavirus (HPV) is a small 50–55 nm, double-stranded, non-enveloped deoxyribonucleic acid (DNA) viruses replicating only in fully differentiated keratinocytes. HPV can infect humans and many animal species (cats, rabbits, and nonhuman primates). It produces clinical lesions known as warts, or verrucae, which are benign proliferations of skin and mucosa. HPV virions consist of a protein coat encapsulating a circular DNA molecule of approximately 8,000 base pairs (8 kb) in size. Their viral genome is divided into three domains **(Fig. 1)**.

Papillomaviruses are highly species-specific, exhibiting tropism for epithelial cells causing infections of the skin and mucous membranes. Till date, >150 different HPV types have been recognized. Non-genital warts occur in 7–10% of the general population, with a peak incidence in the 12–16-year age group. Hand is the most common site involved. Anogenital warts affect 1% of the Indian population.

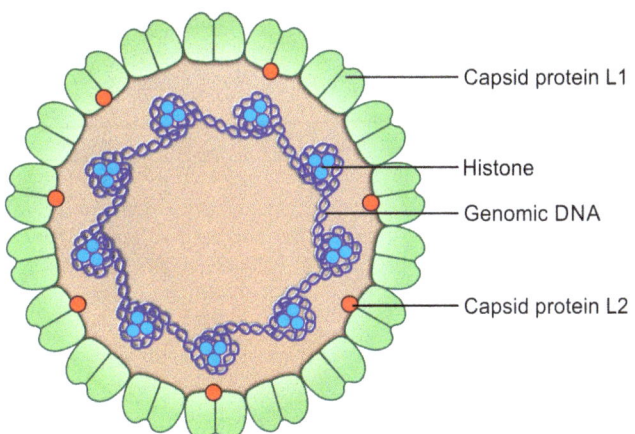

FIG. 1: The structure of HPV.
(DNA: deoxyribonucleic acid; HPV: human papillomavirus)
Source: Adapted from Swiss Institute of Bioinformatics, Viral Zone. *Papillomaviridae*. [Online] Available from http://viralzone.expasy.org/all_by_species/5.html [Last accessed September, 2024].

The source for HPV is the individual with clinical and subclinical infection, or virus present in the environment. Transmission occurs through direct person-to-person contact or indirectly by fomites. Swimming pools and bathrooms are common areas notorious for the spread, especially as skin is macerated and touches rough surfaces. Once HPV has infected the skin, autoinoculation can occur by scratching, shaving, or traumatizing. Occupational handlers of meat, fish, and poultry have a high incidence of hand warts. Anogenital warts are the most common sexually transmitted infection worldwide.

Warts can present with several morphological forms, major determinants being body site, immunological status, and environmental influences. Manifestations can be as benign and pre-malignant or cutaneous and mucosal lesions.

Benign Cutaneous Warts

Verruca Vulgaris

- These present as individualized papules or nodules with a rough surface **(Fig. 2)**. The HPV types most commonly involved are HPV-2, 27, 57, and types 1–4.
- Lesions may be single or multiple **(Fig. 3)**, with varying sizes, and are usually asymptomatic. Confluence can form large masses.
- Warts can occur in any part of the integument but are more common on the back of hands and fingers **(Fig. 4)**.
- The palms and soles are also involved mostly **(Fig. 5)**.
- Isolated warts may remain unaltered for months or years, or a large number of new lesions may develop rapidly in a short period of time. Approximately, 65% of warts disappear spontaneously within 2 years.
- Warts around or beneath the nail (periungual and subungual) are not uncommon and present as therapeutic challenge **(Figs. 6 and 7)**.

CHAPTER 7: Human Papillomavirus

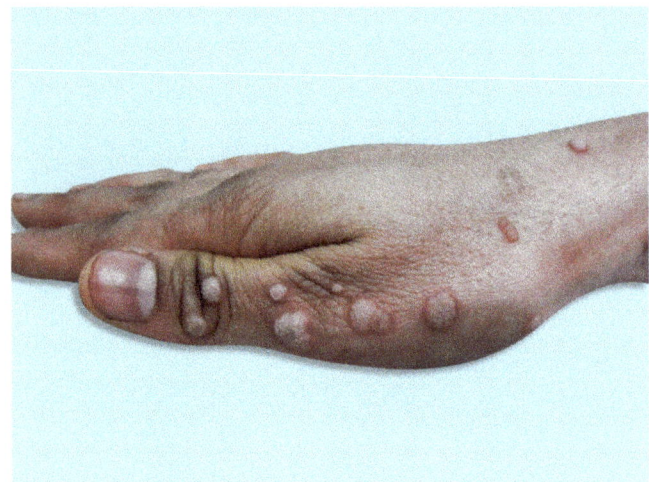

FIG. 2: Verruca vulgaris involving the hand.

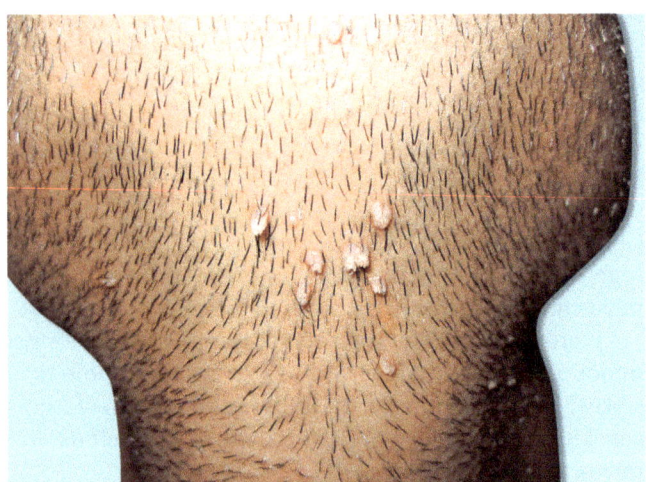

FIG. 3: Multiple verrucae over the neck.

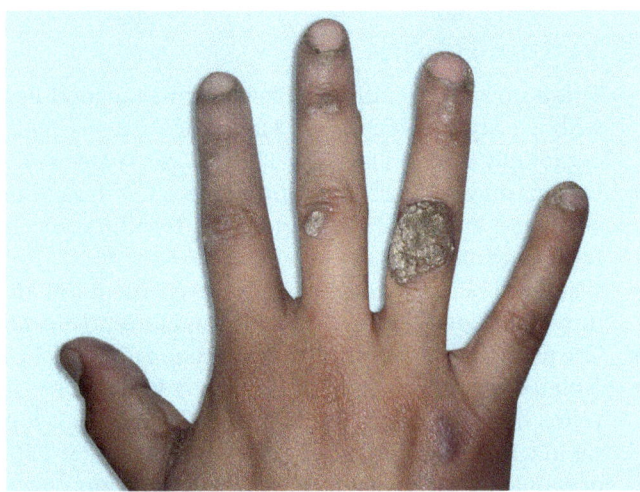

FIG. 4: Multiple warts over the dorsum of the hand, extending to the nail unit.

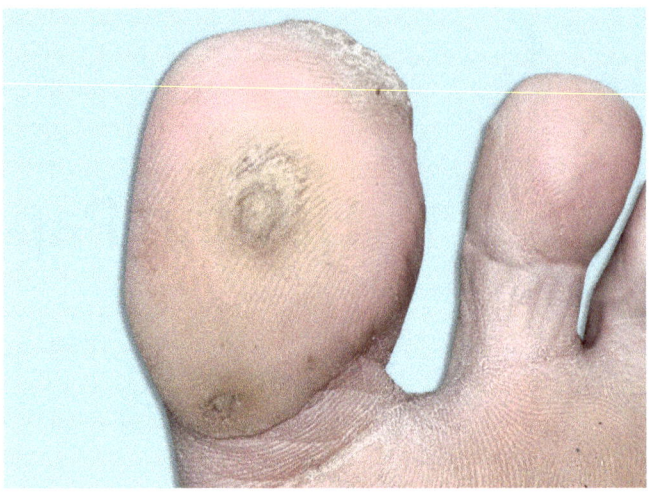

FIG. 5: Multiple warts involving sole.

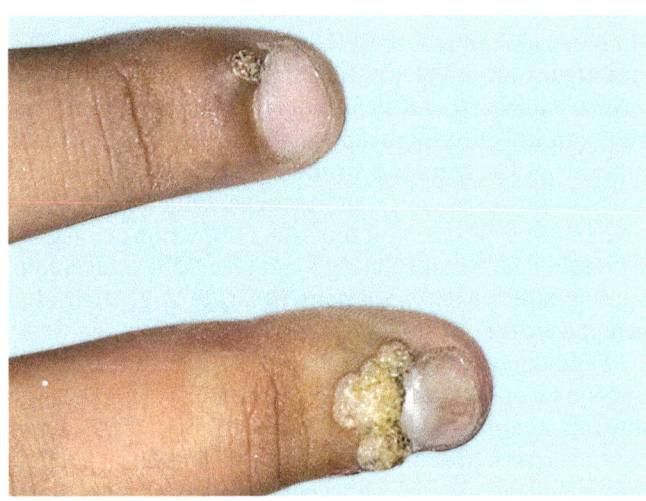

FIG. 6: Periungual warts.

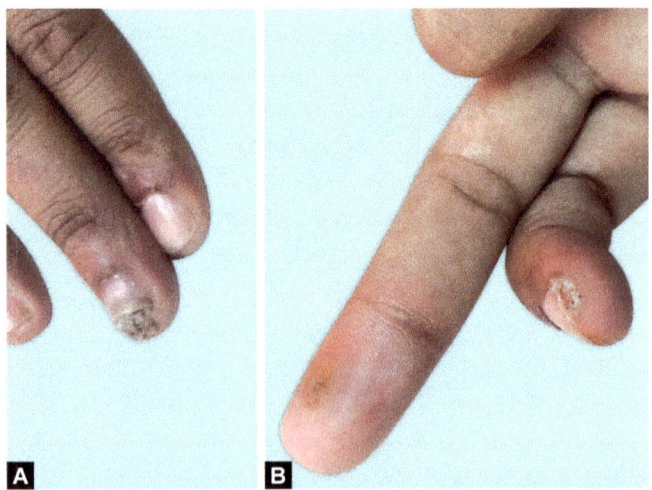

FIGS. 7A AND B: Subungual and palmar warts.

Plantar Warts

- These involve the plantar skin.
- They may lie deep, and this presentation form is known as *Myrmecia*. They are commonly painful and caused by HPV-1 **(Fig. 8)**.
- When developing more superficially, they form hyperkeratotic plaques, called mosaic warts. These are less painful and usually caused by HPV-2 **(Fig. 9)**.
- HPV-4 is also detected in lesions of plantar warts. Most plantar warts occur beneath pressure points.
- Regression of warts is often clinically inflammatory and often culminates in blackening from thrombosed blood before the lesion separates.

Verruca Plana

- Flat warts are slightly raised, skin-colored, or pigmented, with a smooth or slightly rough surface. They are rounded or polygonal, ranging from 1 to 5 mm in diameter or more **(Fig. 10)**.
- Face and back of hands are the most common locations.
- There is often a linear distribution of lesions (pseudo-koebner phenomenon).
- Spontaneous regression is common, usually preceded by inflammation.
- HPV types most frequently detected are HPV-3 and HPV-10, -11, -17.

Filiform Warts

- These are pedunculated, spiculated lesions growing in a perpendicular or oblique fashion with respect to the skin surface **(Fig. 11)**.
- Isolated or multiple lesions affect mainly the face and neck.
- HPV types appear to be the same as for common warts, especially HPV-2.

Pigmented Warts

- These present color variations varying from gray to blackish brown **(Fig. 12)**.
- Histopathologically, they present specific homogeneous cytoplasmic inclusion bodies.
- The HPV types detected in these lesions are HPV-4, -60, and -65.

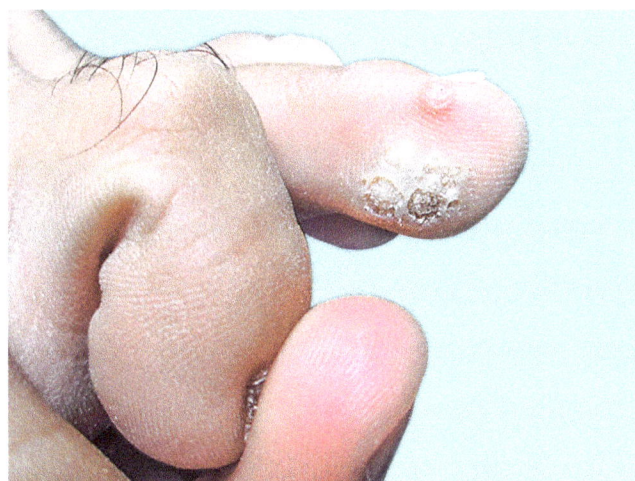

FIG. 8: *Myrmecia* appearance of plantar warts.

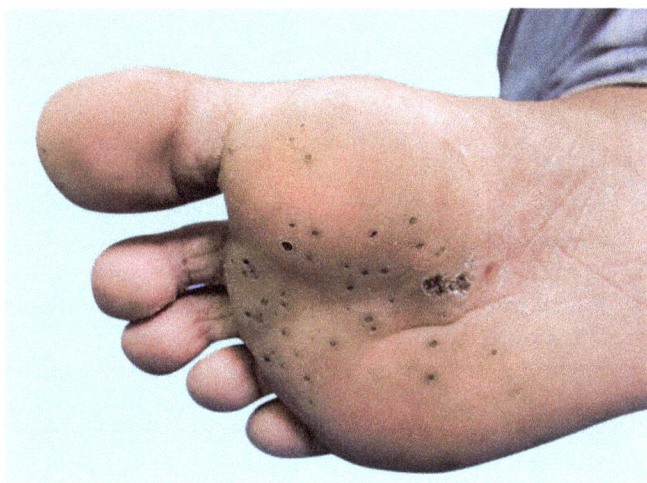

FIG. 9: Plantar mosaic warts.

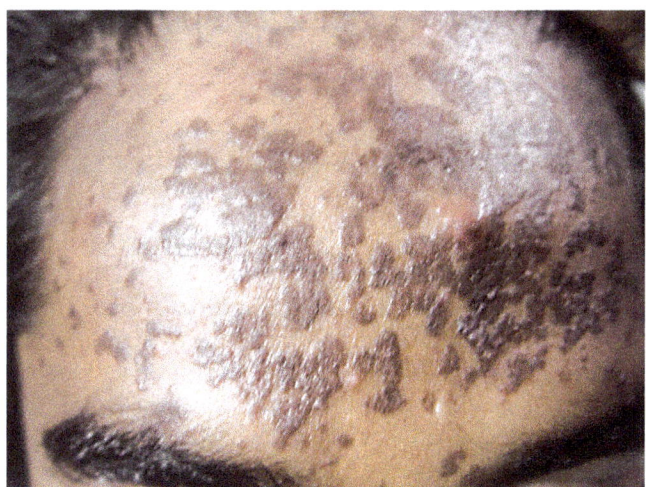

FIG. 10: Verruca plana involving the forehead.

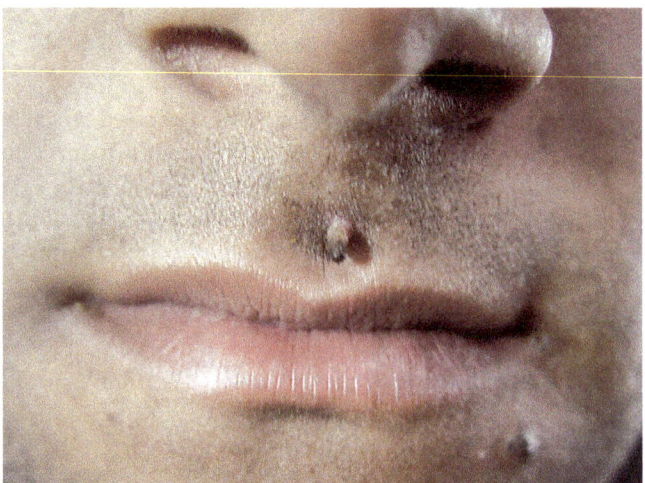

FIG. 11: Filiform wart over the lower face.

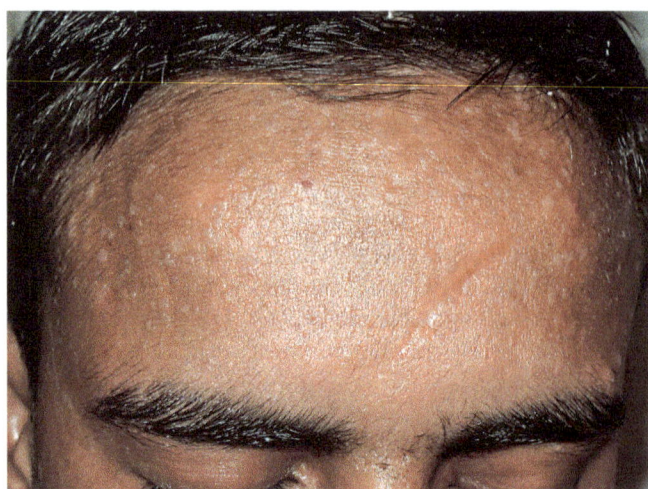

FIG. 13: Verruca plana-like lesions of epidermodysplasia verruciformis (EDV) over the face.

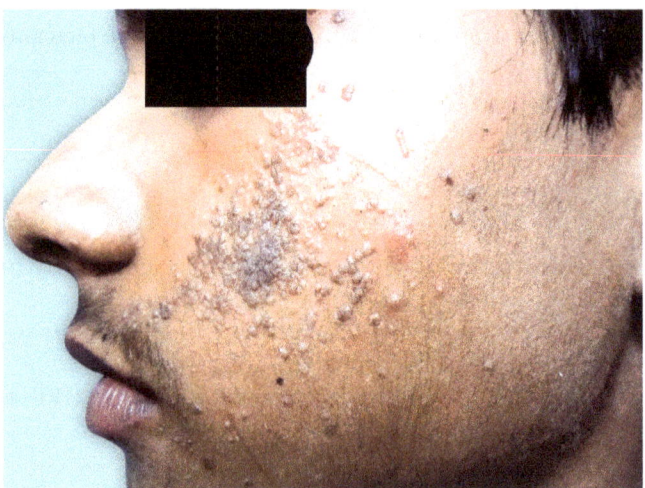

FIG. 12: Pigmented warts involving the face.

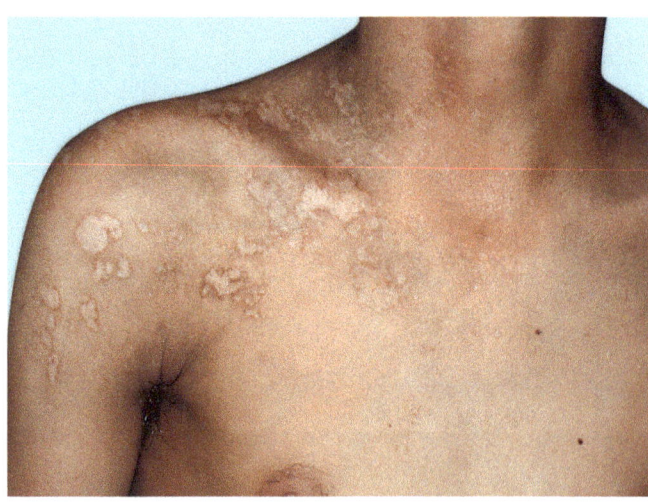

FIG. 14: Pityriasis versicolor-like lesions of epidermodysplasia verruciformis (EDV) on the trunk.

Epidermodysplasia Verruciformis

- It is a rare, usually autosomal recessive, genetic disorder due to a defect in cellular immunity and high susceptibility to skin cancer induced by HPV.
- Patients with epidermodysplasia verruciformis (EDV) are highly predisposed to infection by specific HPV types and are at a high risk of developing cutaneous malignancy due to the oncogenic effects of the viruses.
- Skin lesions appear early in childhood and are polymorphic, practically indistinguishable from flat warts **(Fig. 13)**.
- Scaly hypo or hyperpigmented erythematous macules, similar to pityriasis versicolor, may occur. These are especially present on the trunk and limbs **(Fig. 14)**.
- Thicker, pink, or violet plaques, similar to seborrheic keratosis, are also found.
- Malignant transformation generally begins in the fourth and fifth decade of life and predominates in sun-exposed areas.
- Premalignant lesions, e.g., actinic keratoses, and malignant lesions, e.g., Bowen's disease or squamous cell carcinoma (SCC) are observed.
- The HPV types (HPV-EDV) most commonly found are types 5, 8, 9, 12, 14, 15, 17, 19–25, 28, 29, 36–38, 47, 49, and 50.

Benign Mucosal Lesions

Condylomata Acuminata

- Anogenital warts, or condylomata acuminata are the most common manifestations of HPV in the genital area **(Figs. 15A and B)**.
- They present as papules, nodules or soft, filiform, pinkish, sessile, or pedunculated growths.
- These are asymptomatic, exophytic growths similar to a cauliflower **(Fig. 16)**.
- Occasional bleeding or crusting may be seen **(Fig. 17)**.
- The low-risk HPVs, HPV-6 and HPV-11, are the most detected ones.

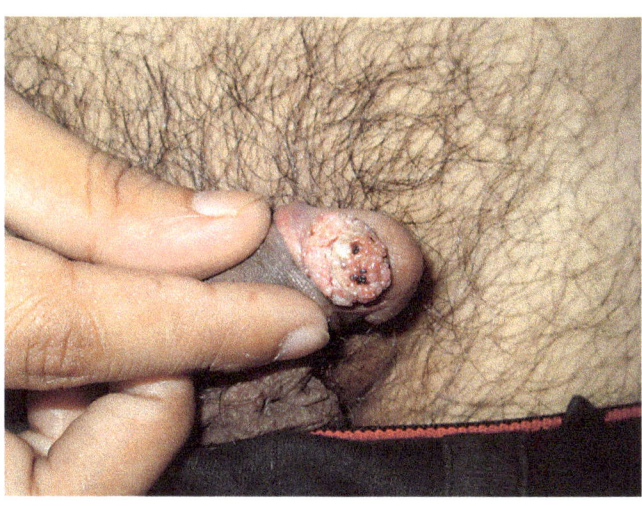

FIG. 17: Penile warts showing superficial hemorrhagic crusting.

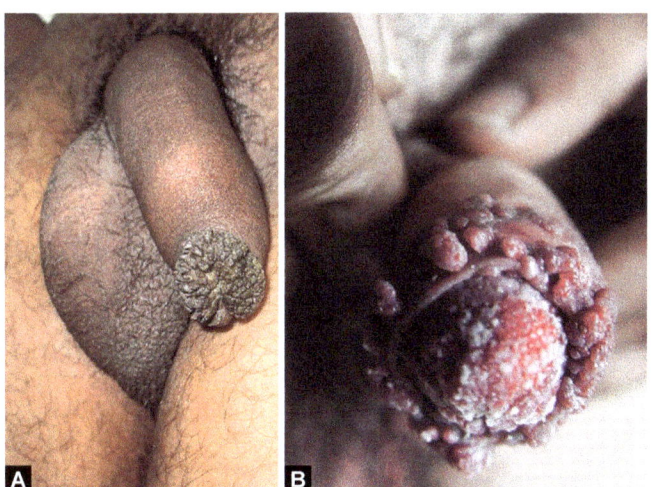

FIGS. 15A AND B: Condylomata acuminata lesions in men.

Buschke–Löwenstein Tumor

- It is also known as giant condyloma acuminatum or verrucous carcinoma of the anogenital region **(Fig. 18)**.
- It is a clinically aggressive tumor, with ulcerated cauliflower-like lesions.
- It is often associated with fistulas and abscesses or surrounding maceration and inflammation **(Fig. 19)**.
- It can present as exophytic or endophytic growth, with local invasion and high recurrence rates, though metastases are very rare.
- This lesion is associated with HPV-6 and -11.

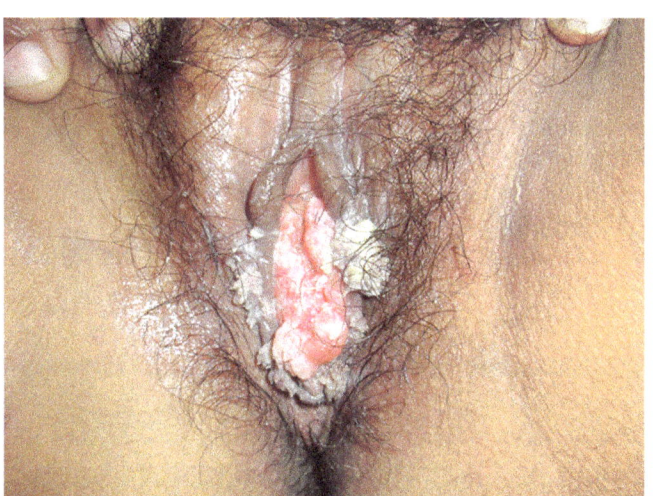

FIG. 16: Exuberant genital warts covering the whole vaginal os in a human immunodeficiency virus (HIV)-positive female.

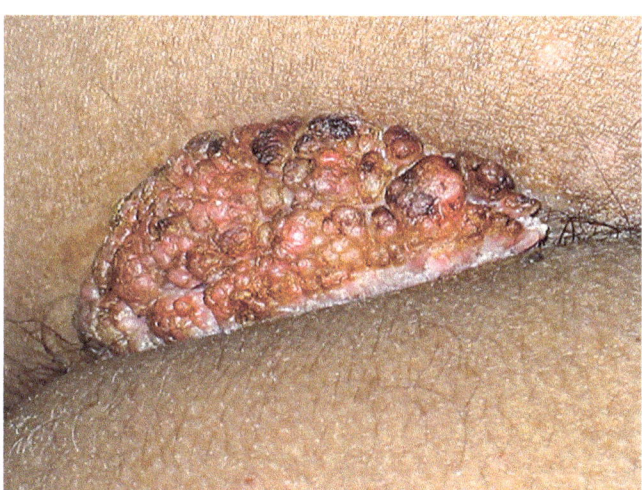

FIG. 18: Giant condyloma acuminate of Buschke–Löwenstein.

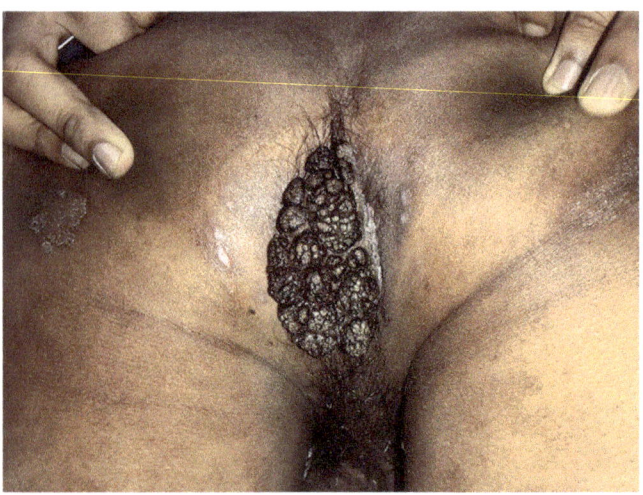

FIG. 19: Pigmented Buschke–Löwenstein tumor in the perianal location with maceration and surrounding inflammation.

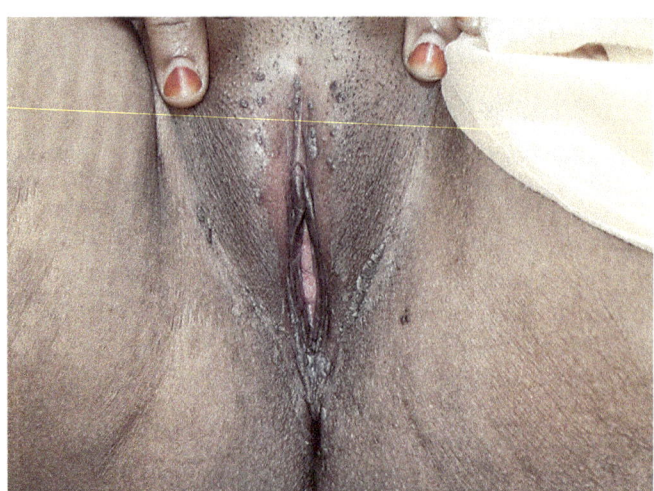

FIG. 21: Bowenoid papulosis simulating common warts.

Bowenoid Papulosis

- It presents as multifocal papular lesions on the genitalia with histological features similar to SCC in-situ **(Fig. 20)**.
- It is characterized by multiple brownish or erythematous papules located in the anogenital region, affecting mostly young adults with an active sex life.
- Clinically, it must be differentiated from seborrheic keratosis, melanocytic nevus, and common warts **(Fig. 21)**.
- Bowenoid papulosis is strongly associated with HPV type 16.

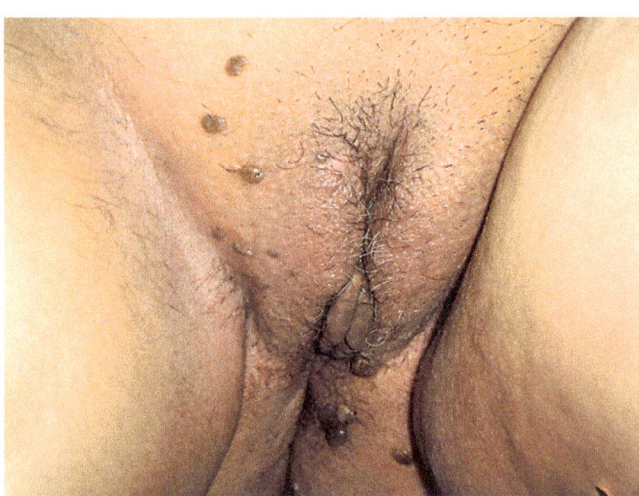

FIG. 20: Pigmented lesions of bowenoid papulosis.

Malignant Cutaneous Lesions

Bowen's Disease of Genitalia

- Carcinoma-in-situ or Bowen's disease of genitalia is associated with high-risk HPVs, especially type 16.
- Clinically, it presents as a plaque, usually single, without a tendency for regression **(Fig. 22)**.
- It has the potential to progress to invasive SCC in 10% of cases.

Extragenital Bowen's Disease

- HPVs, particularly the high-risk mucosal types, are frequently found in lesions of extragenital Bowen's disease.
- The lesions occur especially in the periungual region, on hands, and more rarely on feet **(Fig. 23)**, probably due to autoinoculation from genital lesions
- Similar lesions can be present in the perigenital area as well **(Fig. 24)**.
- The lesions are generally well-defined, crusted plaques **(Fig. 25)**.
- The role of HPV is not fully clarified in extragenital forms.

Basal Cell Carcinoma and Squamous Cell Carcinoma

- HPV has an important potential to induce skin carcinogenesis, both in immunocompetent and immunocompromised patients **(Fig. 26)**.

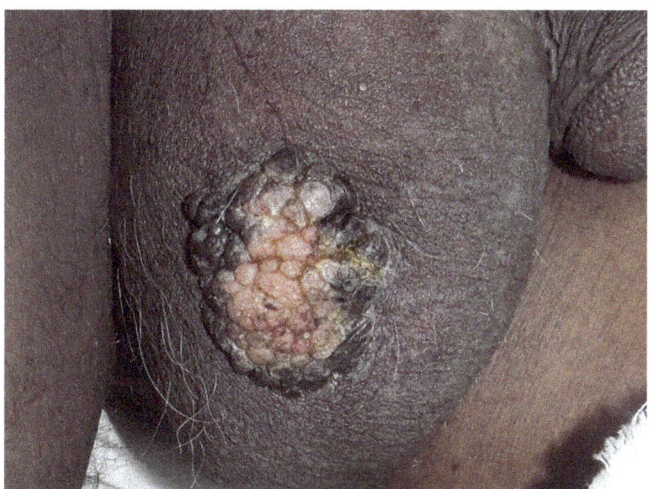

FIG. 22: Bowen's disease involving the scrotum.

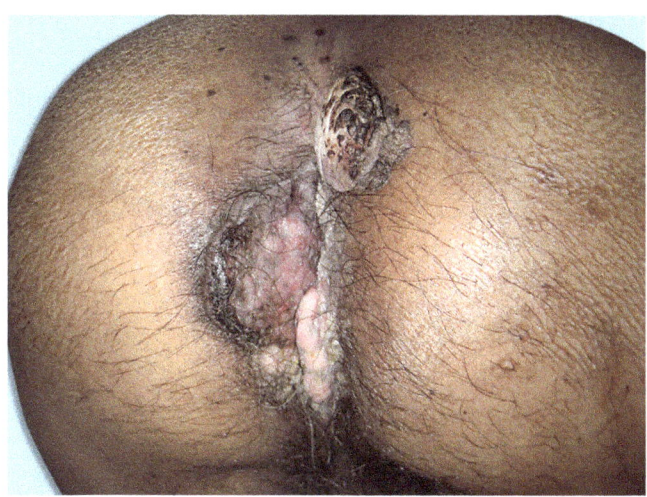

FIG. 25: Bowen's disease in a male.

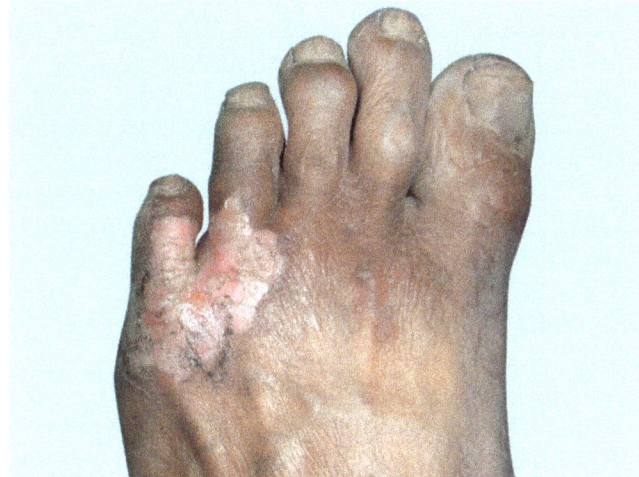

FIG. 23: Bowen's disease involving the dorsum of the foot.

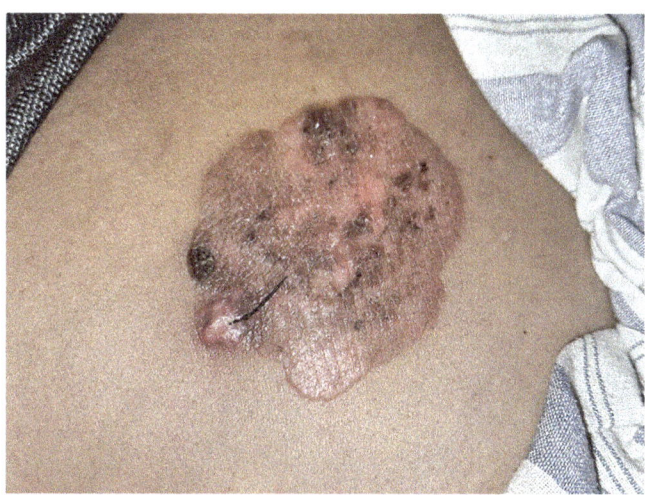

FIG. 26: Squamous cell carcinoma (SCC) in a male with a long-standing Buschke–Löwenstein tumor in the perianal location.

- The exact role of HPV in the development of nonmelanoma skin cancer (NMSC), especially SCC and basal cell carcinoma (BCC), is not yet fully defined.

Penile Cancer

- Clinically, the lesions are hardened, nodular, ulcerated, or erosive and may present with a verrucous surface **(Figs. 27 and 28)**.
- HPV is detected in 40–70% lesions of penile cancer. It is the most frequent HPV type 16.

Cervical Cancer

- Lesions of the cervix associated with HPV may range from incipient cytological abnormalities, and dysplasia of varying degrees, to frank cervical cancer **(Figs. 29 and 30)**.

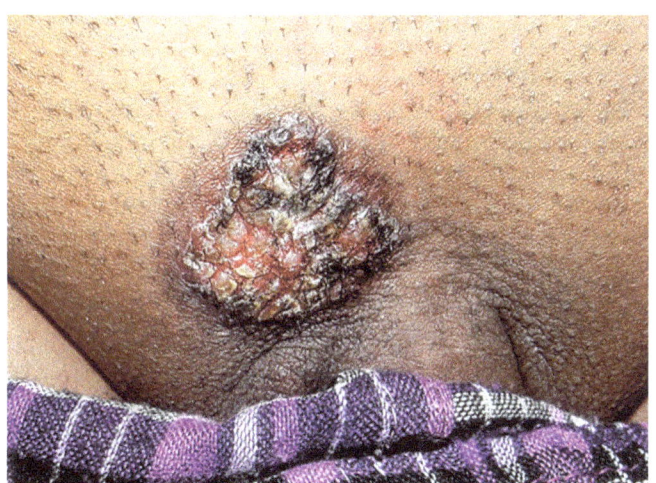

FIG. 24: Extragenital Bowen's disease at the base of the penis.

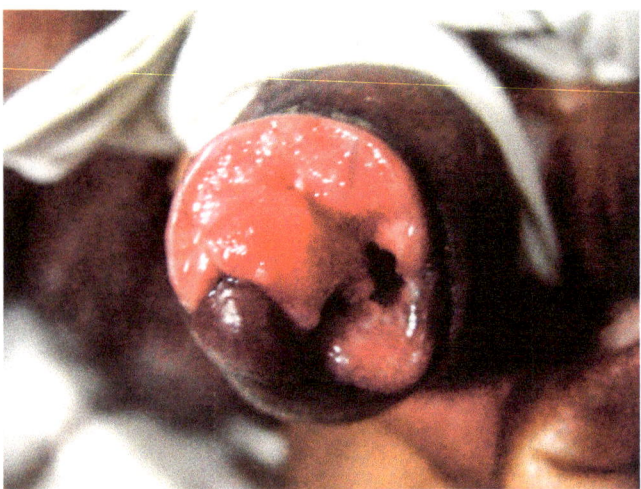

FIG. 27: Ulcerative lesion of penile squamous cell carcinoma (SCC).

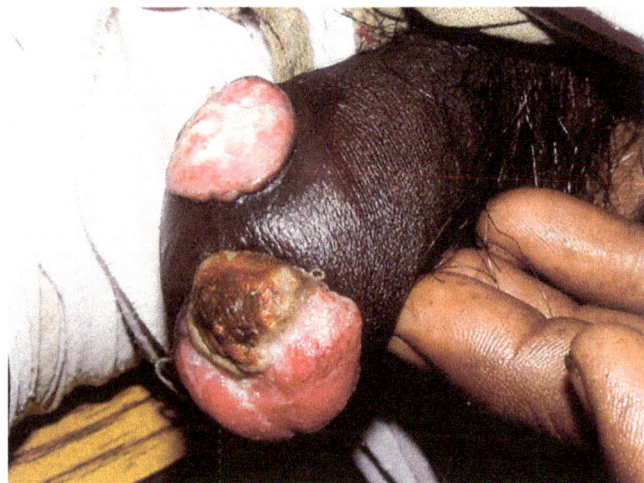

FIG. 28: Indurated ulcerative lesion of penile squamous cell carcinoma (SCC).

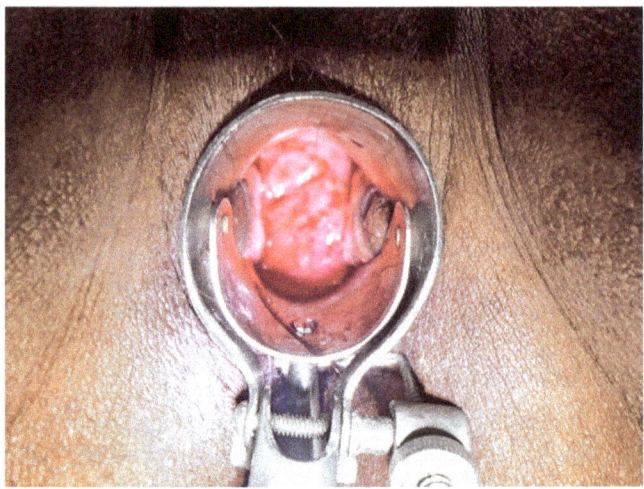

FIG. 29: Ulcerated cervix with intense acetowhitening suggestive of carcinoma cervix.

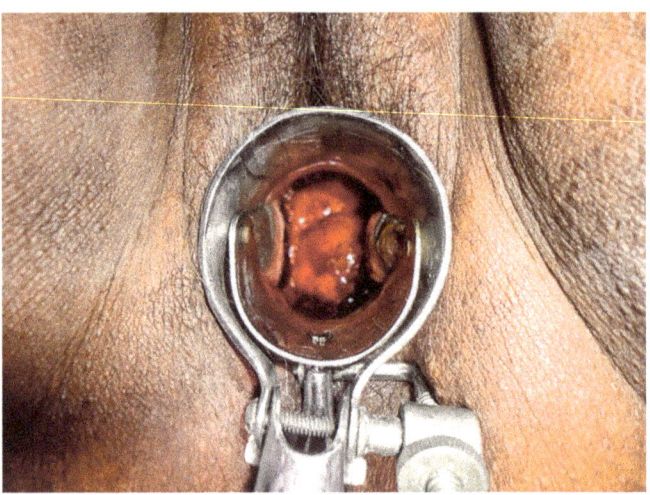

FIG. 30: Iodine nonuptake in anterior and posterior lips of the cervix: Suspect invasive cancer.

- A causal relationship between HPV and cervical cancer has been observed in 90–100% of cases.
- Cervical infection caused by some HPV types is a precursor for the genesis of cervical cancer, though other cofactors do contribute.
- HPV types 16 and 18 are the two most important carcinogenic types. Others include HPVs 31, 33, 35, 39, 45, 51, 52, and 58.

Diagnosis

- Diagnosis of warts is usually clinical. Rarely, one may require a biopsy for confirmation.
- Other techniques include polymerase chain reaction (PCR), in situ hybridization, Southern blot analysis, blot hybridization, or hybrid capture assays.
- Biopsy and histopathology are indicated for long-standing or poorly responsive lesions, especially to rule out malignancy.

Management

Managing warts is a challenge and no single therapy is proven effective in achieving a complete remission. As a result, many different medical and surgical approaches exist. Treatment decisions should be made on a case-to-case basis. Factors determining the treatment choice include the physician's experience, the patient's preference, and the application of evidence-based medicine. Depending on the patient-specific factors, treatment options may need to be individualized **(Table 1)**.

Almost half of cutaneous warts resolve spontaneously within 1 year, and about two-thirds within 2 years. However, treatment may be requested because of social stigma or discomfort. Indications for the treatment of warts are summarized in **Box 1**.

CHAPTER 7: Human Papillomavirus

TABLE 1: Special considerations.

	Pregnancy	Small children	Immunosuppressed
Small asymptomatic lesions	No treatment required	• Keratolytics • Cryotherapy • Chemical cauterization • Immunotherapy	• Topical immunotherapy • Imiquimod • Topical chemotherapy
Large and multiple lesions	• Keratolytics • Cryotherapy • TCA • Surgical excision after the first trimester	Immunotherapy	Oral retinoids
Contraindication	• Interferon, podophyllin, and 5-FU • Imiquimod should not be used in pregnancy	Painful destructive therapies should be avoided	Painful destructive therapies that are difficult to heal should be avoided

(5-FU: 5-fluorouracil; TCA: trichloroacetic acid)

BOX 1 Indications for the treatment of warts.
- Patient's desire for therapy
- Symptoms of pain, bleeding, itching or burning
- Disabling or disfiguring lesions
- Large number or large size of lesions
- Patient's desire to prevent the spread of warts to unblemished skin of self or others
- Immunocompromised condition

Treatments commonly employed can be grouped as discussed further.

Destructive Modalities

- *Salicylic acid (SA)*: It is a keratolytic agent causing mild irritation, thus generating an immune response. Over-the-counter preparations are available as flexible collodion base (17% SA with lactic acid) or plaster patch (40% SA). The affected warts should be soaked in warm water for 5 minutes, surface abraded and then SA paint should be applied every day. SA is used for palmar and plantar warts, but never for facial warts, due to the risk of severe irritation, and the potential for scarring. It is reasonably effective, cheap, and causes minimum pain. Disadvantages are slow response and occasional contact dermatitis due to colophony in the collodion base.
- *Cantharidin*: It is derived from the blister beetle, *Cantharis vesicatoria*. It causes epidermal cell death, and blister formation which heals in 1–2 weeks. This process is repeated at 1–3 week intervals.
- *Caustics*: Monochloroacetic acid, trichloroacetic acid, silver nitrate, and phenol can be used with effect, but they may cause painful reactions. These are physician-applied therapies *only*.
- *Formic acid*: It is a chemical irritant found in the stings and bites of bees and ants. Topical 85% formic acid/needle puncture technique results in high clearance.
- *Cryotherapy*: It is one of the most commonly used modalities that causes necrotic destruction of HPV-infected keratinocytes, inducing local inflammation, and triggering an effective cell-mediated response. The most commonly used cryogen is liquid nitrogen (–196°C) applied using a cryogun or swab stick, until a 2 mm white halo forms around the wart. Adverse effects include hyper- or hypopigmentation, blistering, and damage to underlying tissue.
- *Radiofrequency ablation*: Both localized heating with radiofrequency heat generators as well as surgical excision with radiofrequency electrosurgical knives have been found useful in warts.
- *Laser ablation*: Various lasers can be used for the treatment of water. Carbon dioxide laser (CO_2 laser) causes non-selective thermal tissue destruction and is useful for periungual and subungual warts. Erbium-doped yttrium aluminum garnet (Er:YAG) laser emits a shorter wavelength (2,940 nm) causing a smaller zone of thermal damage allowing more precise thermal ablation. Pulsed dye laser acts through yellow light absorption (585 nm) by oxyhemoglobin, causing selective microvascular destruction of dilated capillaries in warts. It is particularly used for facial warts and perianal warts in children.
- *Surgical measures*: Excision is usually avoided because of the risk of scarring and recurrence. It may be used for extremely large lesions though. Curettage and cautery/electrocoagulation, usually in combination, may be used for filiform and resistant warts.

Antimitotic Therapy

- *Podophyllin*: Podophyllin resin causes blockage of cell division by binding to the mitotic spindle. It is used extensively in the treatment of anogenital warts, but it is less effective in cutaneous warts. It is available as a 10–25% solution in compound tincture of benzoin. Podophyllin should be applied accurately

and carefully to the affected area by the clinician and then allowed to be dried for a few minutes. The resin should be washed thoroughly with water after 4 hours. Applications are repeated weekly. It is teratogenic and contraindicated in pregnancy. Common adverse effects include local irritation and a burning sensation. It should not be used over extensive areas.
- *Podophyllotoxin*: It is available as 0.5% solution or cream to be applied at home twice daily for three consecutive days each week for 4 weeks.
- *Bleomycin*: It is derived from *Streptomyces verticillus* and stimulates immune response by causing acute tissue necrosis. It is reserved for the treatment of recalcitrant warts failing other therapies. It is especially useful for periungual, subungual, and palmoplantar warts. Being an antimitotic agent, it should not be used in pregnant women, children, immunosuppressed patients, or patients with vascular disease.
- *5-fluorouracil (5-FU)*: It is used topically as an ointment. Intralesional injection of 40 mg/mL 5-FU weekly for up to 4 weeks has also produced clearance.

Immunotherapy

It works by manipulating the immune system to achieve an HPV-targeted immune reaction, leading to a delayed-type hypersensitivity response to wart tissue. Various agents used are as follows:
- *Imiquimod*: It is a 5% cream that stimulates various cytokines, including tumor necrosis factor-alfa, Interferon-alpha (IFN-α), interleukin-1 (IL-1), interleukin-6 (IL-6), granulocyte-macrophage colony-stimulating factor (GM-CSF), and granulocyte colony-stimulating factor (G-CSF). It is licensed for use in anogenital warts by the United States Food and Drug Administration (US FDA), but cutaneous wart may also respond.
- *Interferon-alpha*: It is used for recurrent or recalcitrant genital warts. It is injected intralesionally twice weekly for up to 8 weeks.
- *Contact sensitizers*: Dinitrochlorobenzene (DNCB) is no longer used now because of mutagenicity. Diphencyprone (DCP) is nonmutagenic agent with good efficacy. Squaric acid dibutyl ester (SADBE) is used in the treatment of recalcitrant warts but it is more expensive and less stable than DCP.
- *Intralesional immunotherapy*: Various antigens either singly or in combination have been tried with variable success in the management of recalcitrant warts. These include mumps, *Candida*, Bacillus Calmette-Guérin (BCG) vaccine, MMR (measles, mumps, and rubella) vaccine, and *Mycobacterium w*. Intralesional injections of these antigens induce a localized, cell-mediated, and HPV-specific response affecting the target, as well as distant warts. These are administered as 0.1–0.3 mL injection into the largest wart and repeated every 3–4 weeks up to three treatments.
- *Autoimplantation therapy*: It involves harvesting donor tissue by paring a verrucous lesion and then, autografting on the non-dominant flexural forearm or the upper anteromedial thigh by giving a subcutaneous deep stab incision of about 3–5 mm. Margins of the wound are approximated by pressure and a micropore plaster is applied.
- *Oral immunomodulators*: These include retinoids, oral levamisole, oral zinc, cimetidine, etc.
- *Photodynamic therapy*: Systemic or topical aminolevulinic acid is metabolized to protoporphyrin which is then photoactivated to produce a damaging effect on viral infected cells.

Virucidal Therapy

- Virucidal properties of glutaraldehyde and formaldehyde can be used in wart treatment.
- Cidofovir can be used systemically by infusion (5 mg/kg once weekly) or locally as 1% gel/cream or by intralesional injection (2.5 mg/mL). It is quite effective in various types of warts, even in immunodeficiency.

Alternative Modalities

- These include local heat therapy, occlusive duct tape, garlic extract, green tea extract, homeopathy, etc.
- There are sporadic reports of clearance of warts after hypnosis or autosuggestive therapy.

Human Papillomavirus Vaccines

These are an important approach in cancer control strategies aimed at reducing the global incidence of cervical cancer. Vaccination is recommended at 11–12 years of age, though can be given as early as 9 years of age. These are recommended even in teens and young adults (<26 years age) who have already not received them.

As per Centers for Disease Control and Prevention (CDC) recommendations, 11–12-year-olds should receive two doses of HPV vaccine 6–12 months apart. Only two doses are needed if the first dose is given before 15 years of age. For those older than that, three doses of HPV vaccine will be needed. Vaccination is not recommended for everyone older than age 26 years. However, unvaccinated adults aged 27–45 years may be given depending on their risk for new HPV infections and the possible benefits of vaccination. Vaccination is less beneficial in this age group as most have already been exposed to HPV. The vaccine is contraindicated in those with a life-threatening allergic reaction to any ingredient, allergy to yeast (Gardasil and Gardasil 9), or those pregnant. People with a moderate or severe illness should wait until they are better.

Three HPV vaccines are licensed by the US FDA. All three HPV vaccines protect against HPV types 16 and 18 which cause most HPV cancers:

1. *9-valent HPV vaccine (Gardasil 9, 9vHPV)*: It is protective against nine HPV types (6, 11, 16, 18, 31, 33, 45, 52, and 58).
2. *Quadrivalent HPV vaccine (Gardasil, 4vHPV)*: It is composed of four HPV type-specific virus-like particles (VLPs) from the capsid protein of HPV-6, 11, 16, and 18 combined with an aluminum adjuvant. It is recommended for females 9–26 years, administered intramuscularly according to a three-dose schedule at 0, 2, and 6 months.
3. *Bivalent HPV vaccine (Cervarix, 2vHPV)*: It is composed of two VLPs of HPV-16 and 18 and is recommended for females 10–25 years through intramuscular injection according to a 3-dose schedule at 0, 1, and 6 months.

Human papillomavirus vaccination works extremely well and has the potential to prevent >90% of HPV-attributable cancers. Since the start of its usage in 2006, infections with HPV types that cause most HPV cancers and genital warts have dropped 88% among teen girls and 81% among young adult women. It has also reduced the number of cases of precancers of the cervix in young women. The protection provided by HPV vaccines lasts a long time.

CHAPTER 8

Pox, Rubella, Coxsackie, and Other Viral Cutaneous Disorders

Introduction

With the advent of the human immunodeficiency virus (HIV) pandemic, ease of global travel, and mass migrations, dermatologists need to be aware regarding the various cutaneous presentations of both deoxyribonucleic acid (DNA) and ribonucleic acid (RNA) viruses. With recent reports of outbreaks of various earlier known zoonotic infections crossing over into humans, such as monkeypox (Mpox) and *buffalopox*, the need to mass educate healthcare providers becomes paramount to identify, manage and control such infections at the earliest. This chapter covers viral cutaneous disorders caused by miscellaneous viruses including pox, rubella, and coxsackie viruses.

Poxviruses

- Poxviruses are brick-shaped (240 × 300 nm) viruses, which are relatively larger.
- They have a complex internal structure including a double-stranded DNA genome (130–260 kb) and associated enzymes.

Smallpox

Smallpox has been eradicated since 1976, following worldwide vaccinations. However, remnants of the disease on the skin can still be seen in patients who suffered before that **(Fig. 1)**. Smallpox is caused by the *Variola virus*; a double-stranded deoxyribonucleic acid (dsDNA) linear enveloped virus that has been divided into two major groups:
1. *Variola major*: The severe and most common form of smallpox, which caused an extensive rash and high fever.
2. *Variola minor*

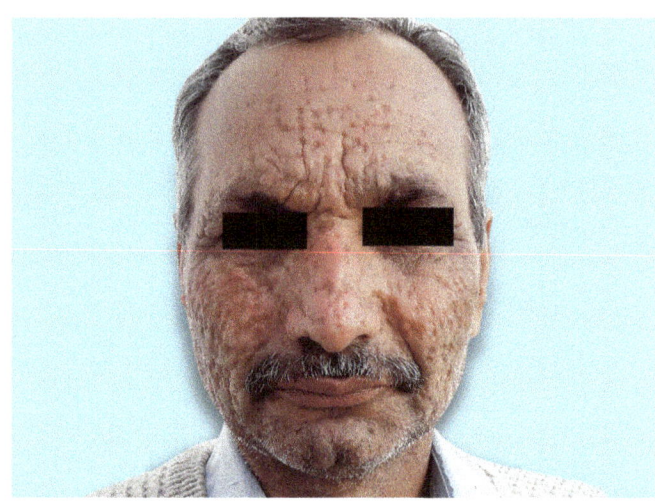

FIG. 1: Disfiguring well-defined hyperpigmented pitted scars (pockmarks) on the face of a patient post-smallpox. On the face due to larger and numerous sebaceous glands, scarring is the most prominent.

The disease transmission used to occur via respiratory droplets from an infected individual. It was seen more in winter and early spring (low humidity and temperature). Very young, elderly, and pregnant women used to develop severe infections.

Clinical Features

- High fever, myalgia, and severe headache develop within an average of 7–17 days of exposure.
- A rash (enanthem) emerged first as small red spots on the tongue, mouth, and oropharynx and broke open to discharge large amounts of the virus into the mouth and throat. At this time, the person was most contagious.
- Then rash (exanthem) appeared on the skin, starting on the face and spreading to the arms and legs and then to the hands and feet (centrifugal distribution),

CHAPTER 8: Pox, Rubella, Coxsackie, and Other Viral Cutaneous Disorders

within 24 hours. As the rash appeared, the fever usually resolved.
- By the third day of disease, the rash transformed into papular lesions that subsequently became varioliform. The palms and soles were frequently affected.
- By the end of 1 week, the scabs formed and were shed off leaving behind pockmarks as a disfiguring sequel of the infection **(Fig. 1)**.

Differential Diagnosis
- Varicella
- Disseminated herpes zoster
- Impetigo
- Erythema multiforme
- Secondary syphilis
- Molluscum contagiosum

Diagnosis
Characteristic intracytoplasmic Guarnieri bodies may be seen apart from ballooning degeneration of the epidermis. Papillary dermal edema and perivascular lymphohistiocytic infiltrate may be seen in histopathology. Electron microscopy and polymerase chain reaction (PCR) also can be done.

Treatment
Treatment is mainly supportive. Maintenance of general hygiene, management of fever, body ache, calamine/bland emollient application over lesions, and oral antihistamines.

Mpox (Monkeypox)

The Monkeypox virus is a zoonotic orthopoxvirus, incidentally causing disease in humans, which is similar to but much milder than smallpox. The first confirmed human case was in 1970 from a child in the Democratic Republic of Congo. The virus was endemic to western and central Africa, with outbreaks in Europe related to exotic pet trade and international travel. However, recent outbreaks have been reported with sexual transmission, more commonly in men having sex with men (MSM) population. Earlier coincidental immunity to the Mpox virus achieved with vaccinia vaccination has been ebbing with its discontinuation after the eradication of smallpox, making Mpox clinically relevant.

Transmission
- Mpox is a zoonosis, spreading from animals to humans. Animal reservoirs include squirrels, rats, monkeys, primates, prairie dogs, hedgehogs, pigs, and mice.
- Ongoing epidemic (since 2022) is driven by human-to-human transmission through respiratory droplets, fomites, and direct contact with lesions.
- Sexual transmission is a major route, with a presentation involving predominantly genital lesions. The ongoing outbreak may have a newly emerging clade.

Clinical Features
- Initial symptoms include fever, headache, myalgia, or fatigue.
- Lymphadenopathy is present, which helps differentiate it from smallpox.
- Mucosal lesions develop after 1–2 days **(Fig. 2)**.
- These are followed by cutaneous lesions involving the face **(Fig. 3)**, neck and extremities **(Fig. 4)**, palms, and

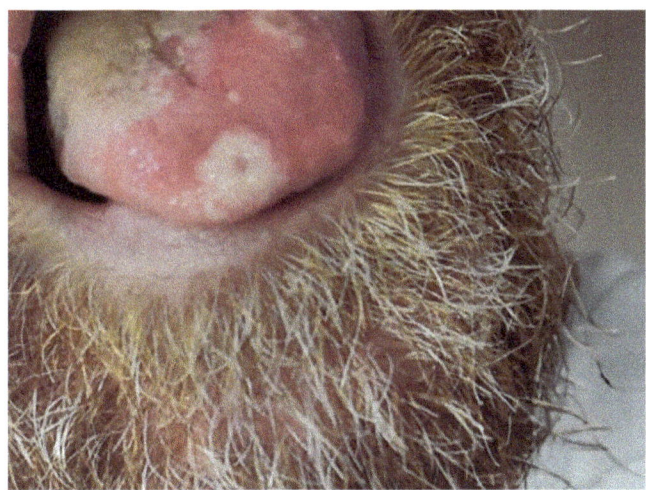

FIG. 2: Oral mucosal lesions in a patient with Mpox.
Courtesy: Dr Rajasekhar Reddy Rangareddy MD (DVL), Specialist Dermatologist, Lifecare Hospital, Abu Dhabi, UAE.

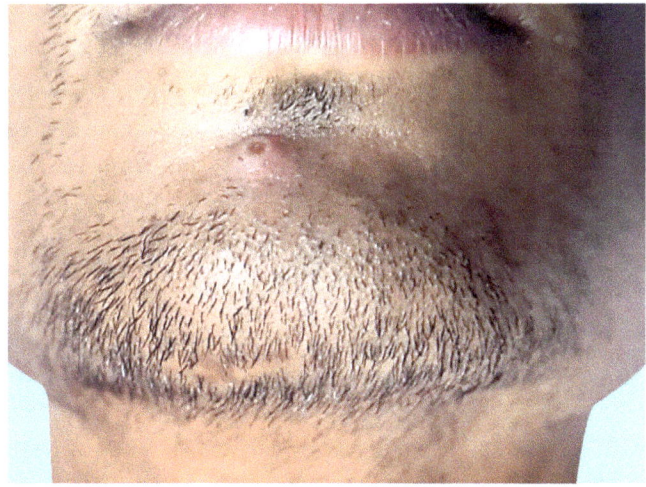

FIG. 3: Facial lesions in a patient.
Courtesy: Dr Rajasekhar Reddy Rangareddy MD (DVL), Specialist Dermatologist, Lifecare Hospital, Abu Dhabi, UAE.

soles **(Fig. 5)**, and are centrifugal in distribution. They may or may not spread.
- The number of lesions is also highly variable **(Fig. 6)**, and they keep evolving over 2-4 weeks in 1-2-day increments.
- Initial macular lesions evolve through papular, vesicular, and pustular phases, synchronously **(Fig. 7)**.
- They tend to be firm, deep-seated, and 2-10 mm in size.
- The pustular phase lasts for 5-7 days before crusting and desquamation over 7-14 days, rendering the patient non-infectious over 3-4 weeks **(Fig. 7)**.
- Umbilicated and pseudopustular lesions are classical **(Fig. 8)**.
- Genital **(Figs. 9 and 10)** and perianal area **(Fig. 11)** are commonly involved with lesion clustering and lymphadenopathy. The current epidemic is especially presenting with lesions in the genital area, especially in MSM.

Differential Diagnosis

- Smallpox and generalized vaccinia
- Disseminated zoster and chickenpox
- Eczema herpeticum and disseminated herpes simplex
- Syphilis and yaws
- Scabies
- Rickettsialpox

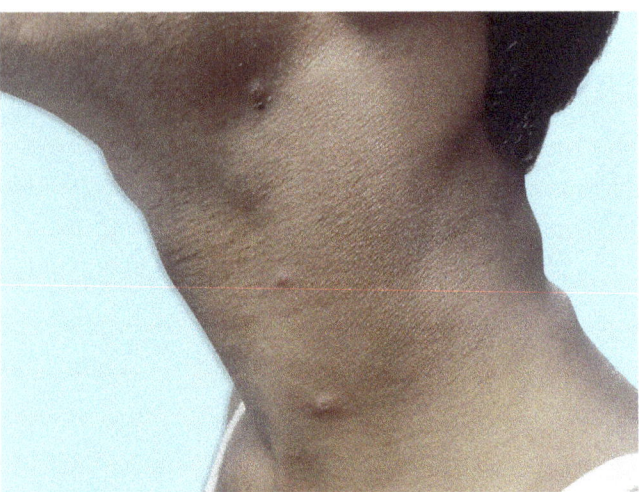

FIG. 4: Neck lesions, scarcely distributed.
Courtesy: Dr Rajasekhar Reddy Rangareddy MD (DVL), Specialist Dermatologist, Lifecare Hospital, Abu Dhabi, UAE.

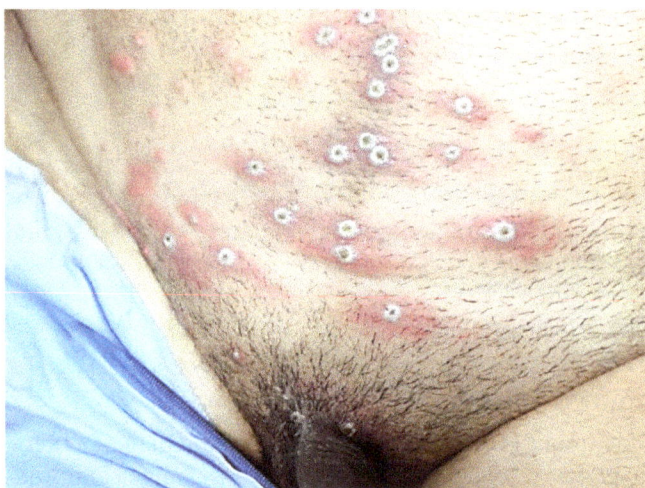

FIG. 6: A large number of lesions in an immunosuppressed patient with Mpox.
Courtesy: Dr Rajasekhar Reddy Rangareddy MD (DVL), Specialist Dermatologist, Lifecare Hospital, Abu Dhabi, UAE.

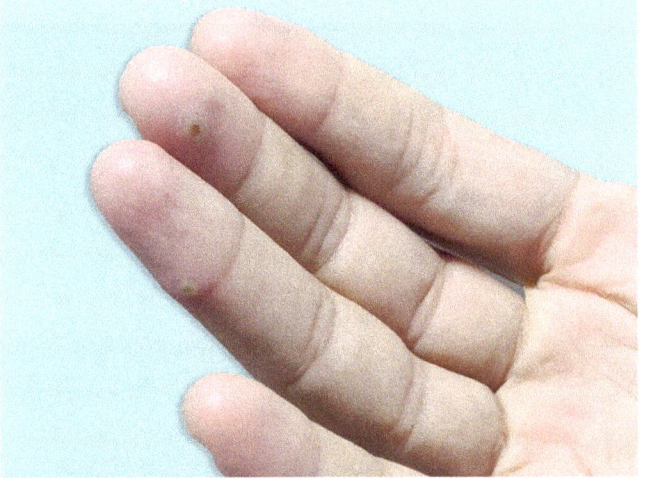

FIG. 5: Palmar lesions in a patient with Mpox.
Courtesy: Dr Rajasekhar Reddy Rangareddy MD (DVL), Specialist Dermatologist, Lifecare Hospital, Abu Dhabi, UAE.

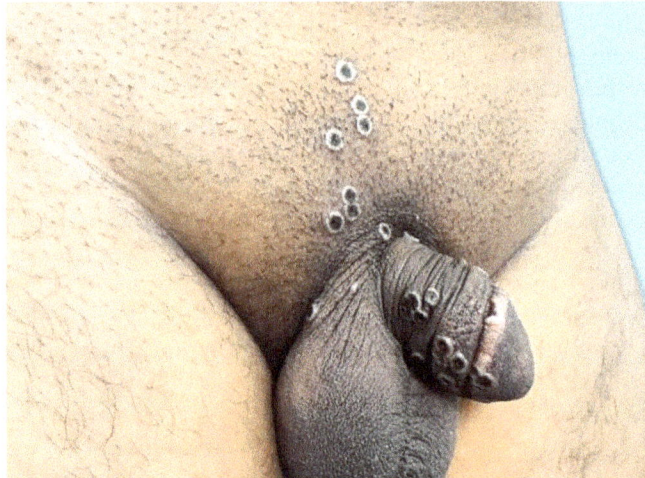

FIG. 7: Typical umbilicated and pseudopustular lesions progressing to crusting and desquamation.
Courtesy: Dr Rajasekhar Reddy Rangareddy MD (DVL), Specialist Dermatologist, Lifecare Hospital, Abu Dhabi, UAE.

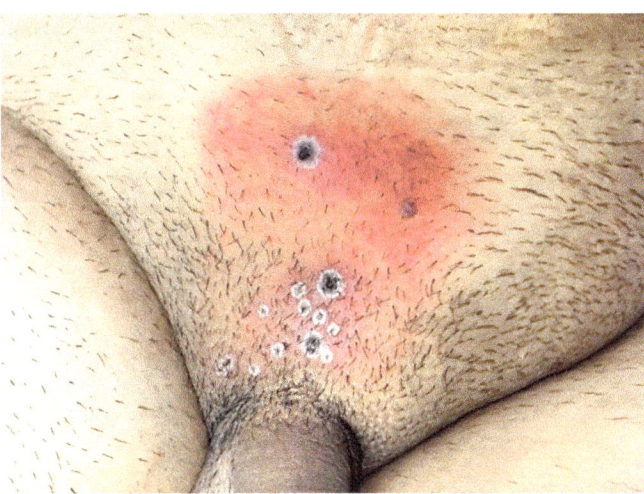

FIG. 8: Umbilicated lesions with peripheral erythema and significant inflammation, involving the genital area.
Courtesy: Dr Rajasekhar Reddy Rangareddy MD (DVL), Specialist Dermatologist, Lifecare Hospital, Abu Dhabi, UAE.

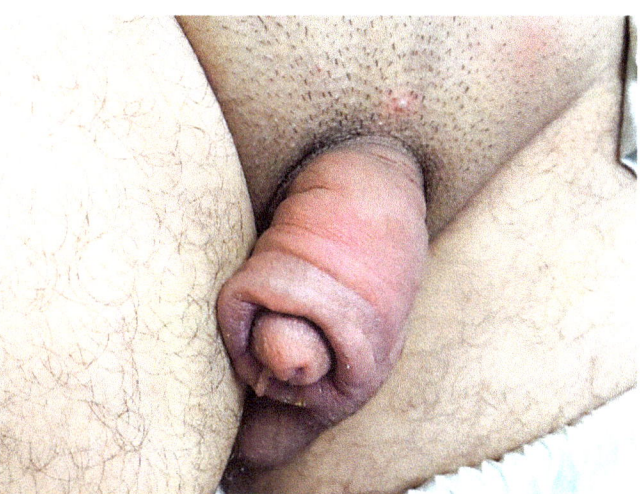

FIG. 10: Reactive edema due to multiple lesions in the same patient.
Courtesy: Dr Rajasekhar Reddy Rangareddy MD (DVL), Specialist Dermatologist, Lifecare Hospital, Abu Dhabi, UAE)

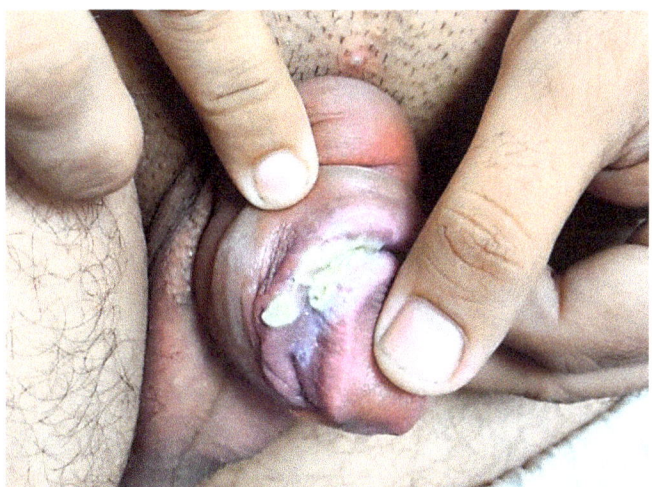

FIG. 9: Mpox lesions involving the coronal sulcus.
Courtesy: Dr Rajasekhar Reddy Rangareddy MD (DVL), Specialist Dermatologist, Lifecare Hospital, Abu Dhabi, UAE.

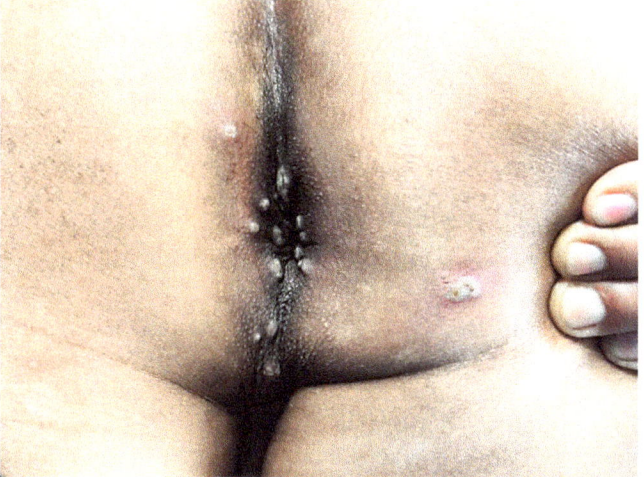

FIG. 11: Perianal lesions in a patient with Mpox.
Courtesy: Dr Rajasekhar Reddy Rangareddy MD (DVL), Specialist Dermatologist, Lifecare Hospital, Abu Dhabi, UAE.

- Measles
- Bacterial skin infections
- Drug rash

Diagnosis

The "Acute, Generalized Vesicular or Pustular Rash Illness Protocol" by the Centers for Disease Control and Prevention (CDC) is followed. Lymphadenopathy is a required primary criterion to determine the need for testing.

- Testing for the presence of *Orthopoxvirus* by electron microscopy, immunohistochemical staining for orthopoxvirus antigens, or serology for anti-orthopoxvirus antibodies can be sufficiently diagnostic if the clinical setting suggests so.
- Confirmation is based on isolation in viral culture or by PCR for Mpox virus DNA.

Complications

These include bacterial superinfection of lesions, scarring, loss of vision (corneal scarring), pneumonia, dehydration (poor oral intake or fluid loss due to lesions), sepsis, encephalitis, and death.

Management

- Treatment is largely supportive
- No specific antivirals exist. In severe cases, investigational use of drugs with benefits against

orthopoxviruses in animal studies or severe vaccinia vaccine complications, can be considered. These include
- *Brincidofovir*: Oral DNA polymerase inhibitor. It is approved for the treatment of smallpox. Normal saline and probenecid should be given concurrently.
- *Tecovirimat*: Oral intracellular viral release inhibitor. It inhibits viral envelope protein VP37, thus blocking viral maturation and release from infected cells.
- *Intravenous vaccinia immunoglobulin (VIG)*: It is licensed by the Food and Drug Administration (FDA) to treat complications of vaccinia vaccination.

Prevention and Postexposure Prophylaxis

- Infected individuals should remain in isolation, wear a surgical mask, and keep lesions covered till crusts fall off and epithelialization occurs.
- For individuals exposed to the virus, temperature and symptoms should be monitored twice daily for 21 days (upper limit of Mpox incubation period). Isolation is not needed as infectiousness starts with symptom onset.
- *Ankara vaccine*: It is replication-defective modified vaccinia (two shots, 4 weeks apart) and has a superior safety profile compared to first and second-generation smallpox vaccines. It does not create a skin lesion or pose a risk of spread. Postexposure vaccination is recommended, especially for high-risk exposure, defined as contact with broken skin or mucous membranes, infected patient's body fluids, respiratory droplets, or scabs. Vaccination within 4 days of exposure may prevent disease onset, and within 14 days may reduce disease severity.

Camelpox

Camelpox is an infectious and economically important contagious skin disease of camelids (members of the biological family Camelidae) caused by the *Camelpox virus* (CMLV). CMLV outbreaks have been reported from India, Pakistan, Middle East countries, Afghanistan, and North-East Africa **(Fig. 12)**. The incubation period of CMLV varies from 3 to 15 days.

Clinical Features

- In humans, lesions are mainly noticed on the hands.
- Initial signs include fever, itching with slight pain, and erythema at the affected site.

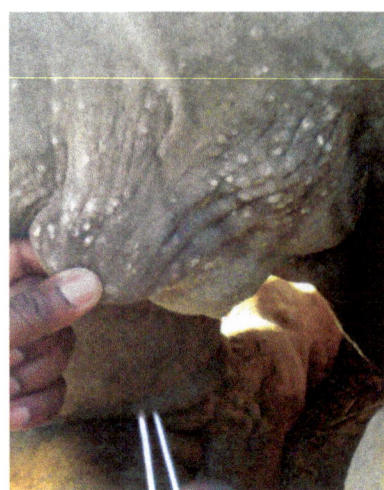

FIG. 12: Lesions of camelpox on a camel, multiple ulcerated papulovesicular lesions on hindquarters of a camel.

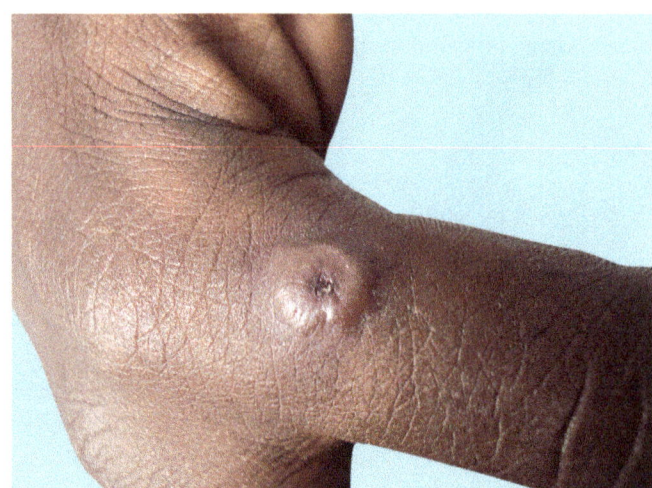

FIG. 13: A papulovesicular lesion on the finger showing central crusting, peripheral edema, and erythema.

- Local edema and vesicle may appear 4–7 days after infection **(Fig. 13)**.
- About 7–10 days later, these vesicles may rupture leaving a deep ulcerated wound surrounded by a red zone of inflammation.
- Subsequently, 2 weeks after the infection, lesions gradually heal by the development of crusts which later slough leaving a central residual scar.

Buffalopox

It was first described in 1934 in India. The causative agent *Buffalopox virus* (BPXV) was first isolated in 1967. BPXV is associated with sporadic outbreaks in Asian buffalos and cows in India, Pakistan, Bangladesh, Russia,

CHAPTER 8: Pox, Rubella, Coxsackie, and Other Viral Cutaneous Disorders

Indonesia, and Egypt. The incubation time in animals is about 2–4 days and in humans, it is 3–19 days. Humans can become infected by contact with diseased animals and infections are mainly noticed in animal attendees, milkers, and veterinarians.

Clinical Features

The symptoms are comparable to those of infections with cowpox virus (CPXV).
- In humans, the lesions are mostly confined to the hand, wrist, finger, face, forehead, buttock, and legs.
- Constitutional symptoms such as fever, axillary lymphadenopathy, general malaise, and an erythematous rash over the chest and abdomen may also be noted.
- Lesions are characterized by progressive stages of macules, papules, vesicles, and pustules **(Figs. 14 and 15)**. Lesions may even involve eyes **(Fig. 16)**. The disease is self-limiting, and lesions may heal within 3–6 weeks leaving a black eschar at the site of lesion.

Diagnosis

- It is mostly based on characteristic clinical features in appropriate settings.
- Swab and serum samples from cattle and humans can be subjected to viral isolation, cell culture, and plaque reduction neutralization test
- PCR may be undertaken.
- *Histopathology*: From the maculopapular stage, stratum malpighii shows multilocular vesicles due to cell vacuolization. Cytoplasmic eosinophilic inclusion bodies are seen. Reticulated vesicles and dilated capillaries, along with necrosis and dense inflammatory infiltrate are also seen **(Figs. 17 and 18)**.

Treatment

- No definite treatment is available.
- Washing the infected lesions with 1% potassium permanganate followed by topical broad-spectrum antibiotics is advisable.
- If symptoms are severe, oral antibiotics and paracetamol are advisable.

Prevention

Isolation of affected animals and wearing of gloves by animal handlers during washing or caring for infected animals is recommended.

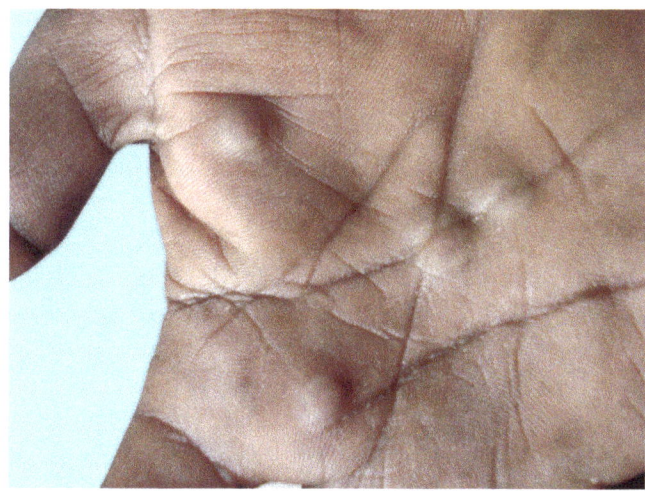

FIG. 15: Lesions on palms of the same patient, a relatively unusual site without a history of prior trauma.

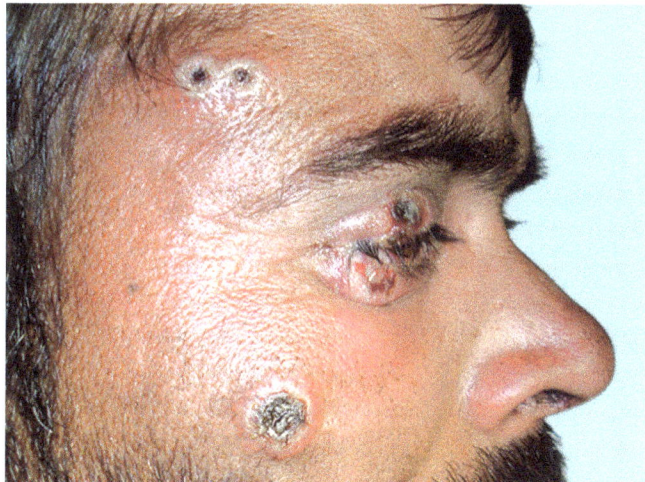

FIG. 14: Multiple well-defined centrally crusted papulovesicular lesions of buffalopox on the face of an infected individual with peripheral edema. Note the lesions on the lid margins.

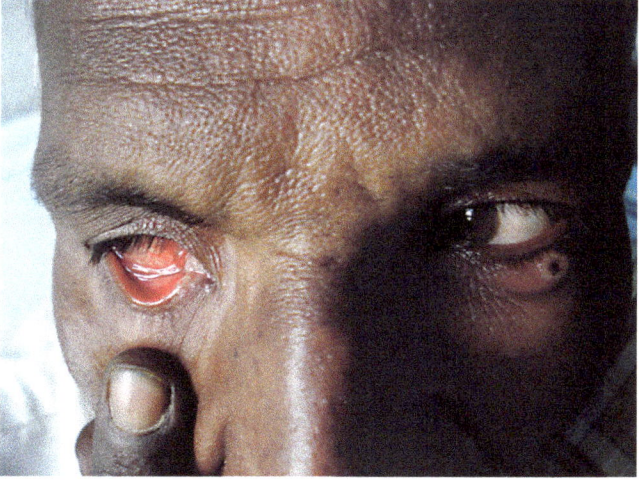

FIG. 16: Conjunctival involvement of the right eye with a lesion on the lower lid margin of the left eye.

CHAPTER 8: Pox, Rubella, Coxsackie, and Other Viral Cutaneous Disorders

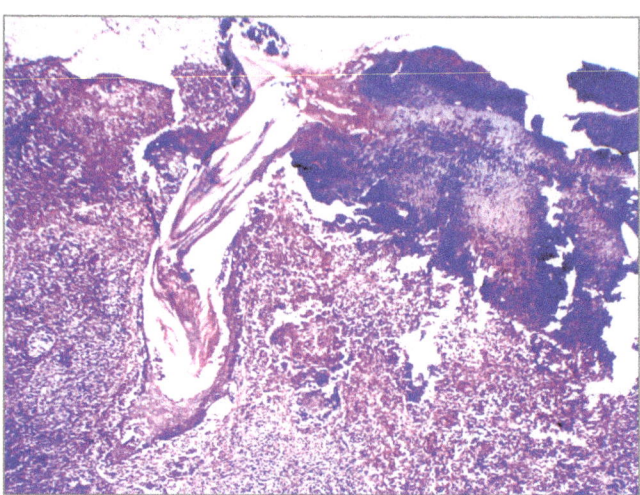

FIG. 17: Hematoxylin and eosin (H&E) (4 × 4) histopathological image of target stage section showing crusting, central hemorrhage, tissue necrosis, and edema. Inflammatory infiltrate in epidermis and dermis.

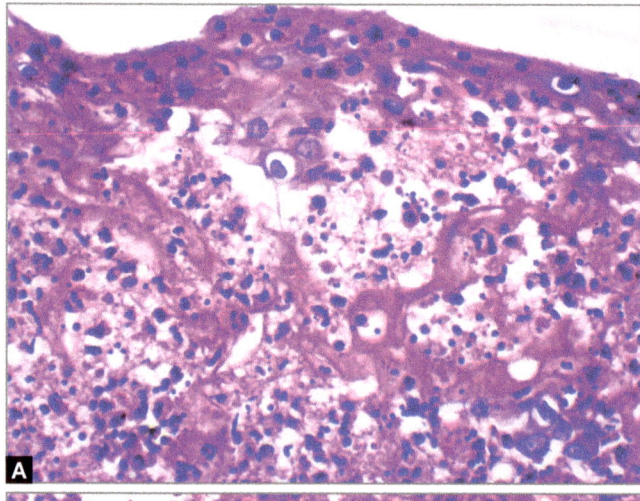

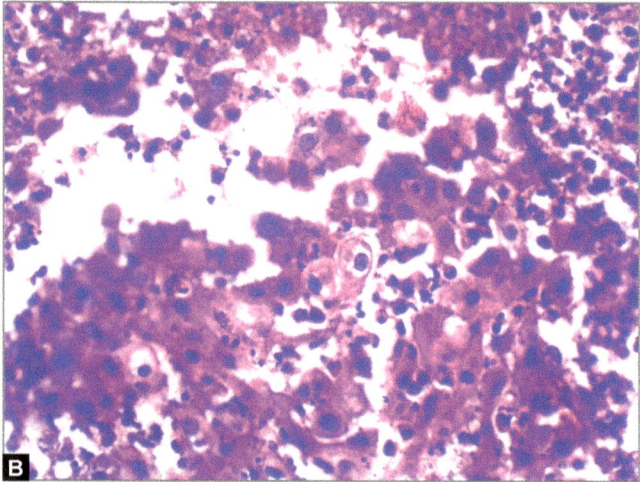

FIGS. 18A AND B: Hematoxylin and eosin (H&E) (4 × 10) magnification view showing Reticulated vesicles (a characteristic feature of viral infection of the epidermis), mixed infiltrate, and eosinophilic inclusion bodies in the cytoplasm of vacuolated epidermal cells.

Orf

It is caused by the dsDNA virus. It is also known as *contagious* ecthyma, sore mouth, or scabby mouth in sheep and goats. It has been reported from most sheep- or goat-raising areas including those in Europe, the Middle East, USA, Africa, Asia, Alaska, South America, Canada, New Zealand, and Australia.

Infection in humans occurs by direct contact or through fomites during contact with infected animals. It is more frequent among milkers, veterinarians, butchers, and people who come in contact with infected animals.

Clinical Features

- At 3–7 days, solitary papules are formed, usually on the hands.
- These are followed by vesicles, and finally wart-like nodules, which subside after 4–6 weeks with little or no scarring.
- The vesicular stage has a characteristic "target" appearance with a red center, white ring, and red halo which progresses to a weeping nodule **(Fig. 19)**.
- The nodule eventually dries creating small black dots on the surface and as it heals, papillomas may develop over the lesion surface.
- Symptoms such as pain, fever, lymphangitis, and erythema have been observed.
- Generalized disease and large progressive lesions ("giant" orf) have been reported in immunocompromised individuals.

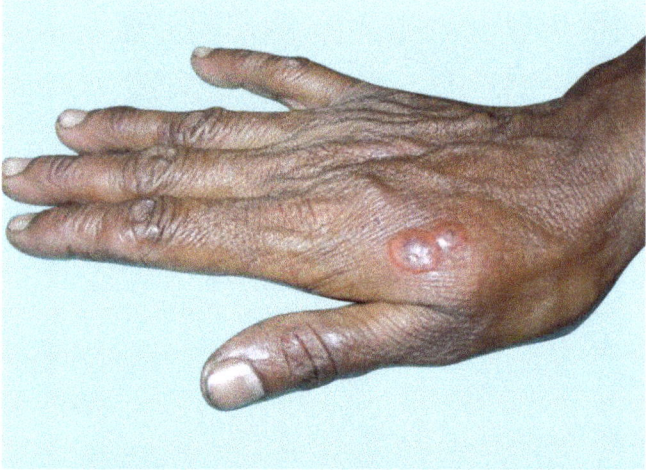

FIG. 19: Lesions of orf on the dorsum of right hand showing well-circumscribed nodular lesions with central dusky center and peripheral erythema and edema.

Diagnosis

The clinical signs are often typical. Laboratory diagnosis by electron microscopy, histology, and PCR offers the most accurate approach.

Treatment

- Moist dressings, local antiseptics, and finger immobilization are done for the lesions.
- Antibiotics, both topical and systemic to prevent bacterial superinfection.
- Topical imiquimod and cidofovir cream have also been used, successfully.

Prevention

The best preventive measure for animals is orf vaccination in every 6–8 months.

Milker's Nodule/Pseudocowpox/Paravaccinia

Milker's nodule is caused by the *paravaccinia* virus. It is a localized benign cutaneous eruption known to occur in milkers, farm workers, butchers, and veterinary students, particularly new to their occupation with no previous immunity. It is prevalent worldwide, including in India. Transmission of disease within the cattle herds occurs by direct and indirect contact including calf suckling of multiple cows, flies, and milking equipment. The incubation period varies between 5 and 15 days.

Clinical Features

- A well-characterized clinical course progresses through the stages of macules, papules, vesicles, pustules, and scabs, lasting approximately 10–15 days.
- Skin lesions become opaque and grayish with small crusts and central depression.
- Some patients may develop lymphangitis or erythema multiforme secondary to the infection.
- Clinical signs spontaneously resolve in 6–8 weeks, leaving no scars.

Differential Diagnosis

- CPXV
- Herpes virus infection
- *Mycobacterium marinum* infection
- Orf
- Pyogenic granuloma
- Occasionally, syphilis and sporotrichosis

Diagnosis

In addition to typical clinical settings, viral culture, DNA hybridization, and PCR can be done for confirmation of diagnosis. The "pan-pox" assay (PCR assay) can be used for screening and diagnosis of human and animal poxvirus infections.

Treatment

Antiviral medications are not effective, only symptomatic treatment is given.

Prevention

Isolation of infected animals and wearing protective gear by their caretakers.

Molluscum Contagiosum

Molluscum contagiosum (MC) is caused by the dsDNA virus; *Molluscipoxvirus* (MCV). MCV commonly infects keratinized skin and infundibular portion of the hair follicle and mucosae, generating the characteristic Henderson–Patterson (HP) cytoplasmic inclusion bodies. The virus entry is facilitated by mechanical trauma to the skin and the incubation period is 2–7 weeks.

Clinical Features

The MCV affects three distinct populations: children, sexually active adults, and immunocompromised individuals.

- In children, the characteristic skin lesions are single or, more often, multiple, rounded, dome-shaped, pink, waxy papules that are 2–5 mm in diameter. The papules are umbilicated and contain a caseous plug **(Fig. 20)**. The common sites involved are the face, extremities, trunk, and chest.
- In immunocompetent adults, molluscum contagiosum most commonly is a sexually transmitted disease. Healthy adults tend to have few typical lesions, limited to the perineum, genitalia, lower abdomen, or buttocks **(Fig. 21)**.
- MC lesions in HIV-positive individuals, or immunosuppressed patients, are numerous, more widespread, larger (giant > 10 mm in diameter), and resistant to conventional therapy. The lesions most often involve the face, neck, and trunk. Disease states associated with widespread MC lesions include sarcoidosis, use of immunosuppressants, topical steroids, and also topical calcineurin inhibitors, suggesting a role of cell-mediated immunity.

CHAPTER 8: Pox, Rubella, Coxsackie, and Other Viral Cutaneous Disorders

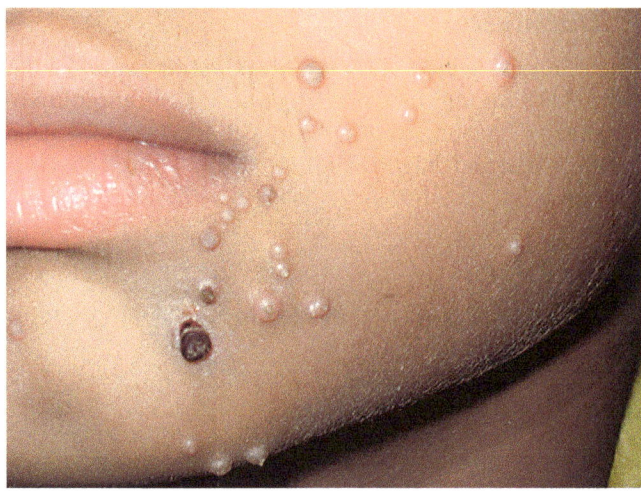

FIG. 20: Pearly white and umbilicated papular lesions of molluscum contagiosum on the face and back of a child.

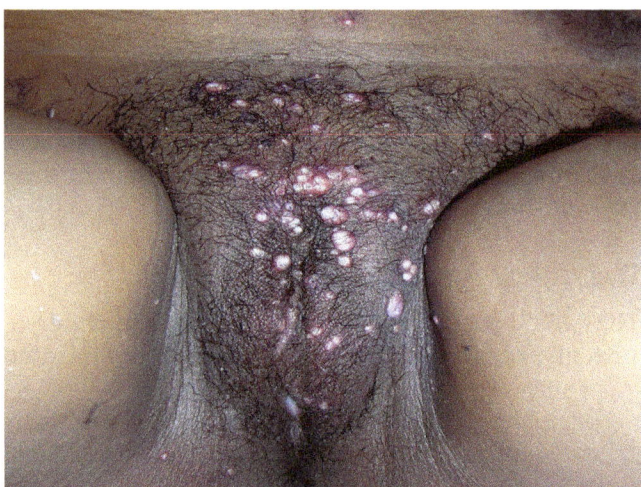

FIG. 21: Numerous papulonodular lesions of molluscum contagiosum (MC) on the vulva showing characteristic central umbilication and inflammation at places.

- Molluscum dermatitis refers to the erythema and eczematous changes occurring around the molluscum lesions. It is often seen in children with atopy.

Differential Diagnosis

- Cryptococcosis
- Histoplasmosis
- Coccidioidomycosis
- *Penicillium marneffei* infection
- Epitheliomas
- Basal cell carcinoma
- Sebaceous hyperplasia

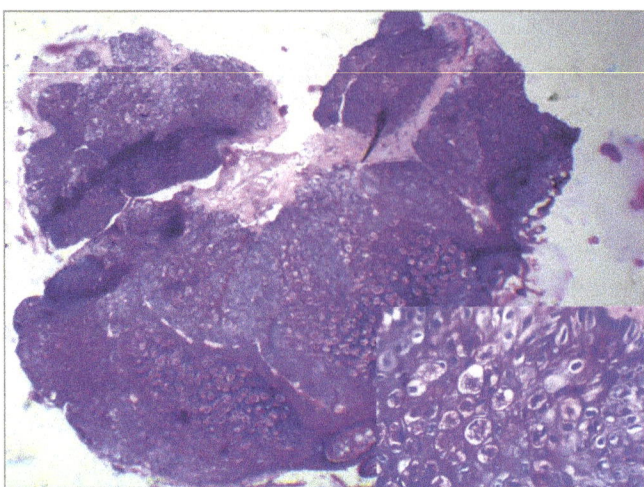

FIG. 22: Histopathological examination showing acanthosis, down the growth of infected epidermal cells having large eosinophilic intracytoplasmic inclusion bodies [Henderson–Paterson (HP) bodies] (H&E 40×). Inset: Close up higher magnification view of the HP bodies (H&E 100×).
(H&E: Hematoxylin and eosin)

Diagnosis

- Diagnosis of MC is mainly clinical.
- However, in atypical cases, squash preparation can be made. It involves a microscopic examination of cellular exudates prepared by manually extracting the cellular material from the lesion, crushing it between two glass slides, and staining with Giemsa.
- *Histopathology* reveals epidermal acanthosis with shells containing intracytoplasmic inclusion bodies (molluscum bodies) **(Fig. 22)**.
- Molecular diagnostics by in situ hybridization and PCR and MCV enzyme-linked immunosorbent assay (ELISA) are additional tools used for unclear cases.

Treatment

Molluscum contagiosum can be treated with various modalities that are discussed in **Table 1**.

Measles

Measles is caused by the single-stranded ribonucleic acid (ssRNA) virus of the genus *Morbillivirus* and family Paramyxoviridae. It is a common disease, for which the first live attenuated vaccine was licensed in the United States in 1963. In India, the measles, mumps, and rubella (MMR) vaccine (a live attenuated strain of Edmonston–Zagreb measles virus propagated on human diploid cell culture) is a part of the universal immunization program. The average incubation period is 10 days.

CHAPTER 8: Pox, Rubella, Coxsackie, and Other Viral Cutaneous Disorders

TABLE 1: Therapeutic modalities for molluscum contagiosum.	
Destructive therapy	Curettage, trichloroacetic acid, 10% KOH application, cryotherapy, and CO_2 laser
Cytotoxic agents	Podophyllotoxin and 5-fluorouracil
Antiviral agents	Topical and systemic cidofovir and intralesional interferon-α
Immunomodulator	Topical imiquimod
Others	Photodynamic therapy, electron beam therapy, introduction of HAART can normally elicit resolution in HIV/AIDS patient

(AIDS: acquired immunodeficiency syndrome; HAART: highly active antiretroviral therapy; HIV: human immunodeficiency virus; KOH: potassium hydroxide)

Clinical Features

- There is a prodrome of high fever (often > 104°F), conjunctival congestion, and Koplik's spots, which appear as bluish-gray specks or "grains of sand" on a red base, on the buccal mucosa opposite the second molars.
- Fever typically lasts 4–7 days followed by a classic triad of conjunctivitis, cough, and coryza (the "3 Cs").
- This is followed by the appearance of a maculopapular rash that lasts 3–5 days. It is generalized, maculopapular, erythematous, and starts on the back of the ears. After a few hours, it spreads to the head and neck region and then covers the entire body, often associated with itching **(Figs. 23 and 24)**.
- Immunocompromised patients may not develop a rash.
- The entire course of uncomplicated measles lasts for 7–10 days. Natural immunity is then known to last as long as 65 years.

Complications

These include diarrhea, pneumonia, acute measles panencephalitis, subacute measles encephalitis, subacute sclerosing panencephalitis, and corneal ulceration. Case fatality rates are higher in malnourished individuals, vitamin A deficiency, pregnancy, and immunocompromised states.

Diagnosis

Clinical diagnosis may be aided by:
- *Microscopy of nasopharyngeal secretions*: It may reveal multinucleate giant cells with inclusion bodies, pathognomonic for measles.
- *Immunofluorescence*: Direct immunofluorescence (DIF) and indirect immunofluorescence (IIF).
- *Virus isolation*: It can be done from the throat or conjunctival washings, sputum, urinary sediment cells, and lymphocytes.
- *Serology*: A fourfold rise between the acute and the convalescent phase, in the measles-specific

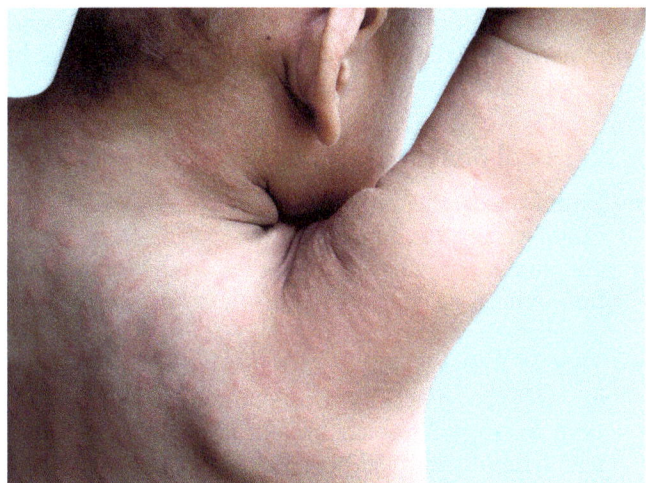

FIG. 23: A typical rash of measles in a child. The rash is typical maculopapular erythematous (morbilliform) in nature.

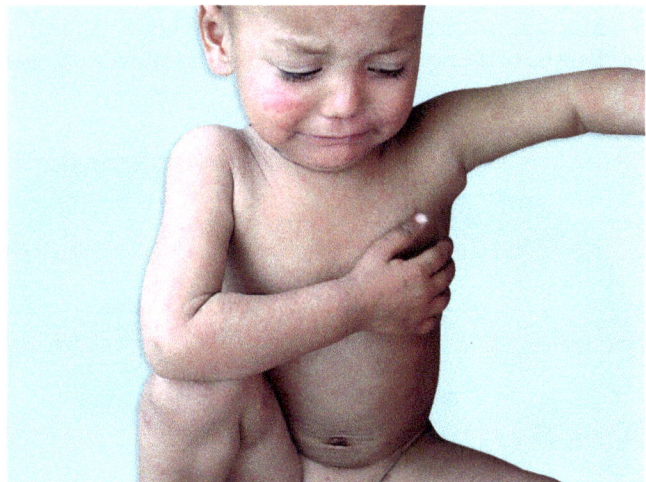

FIG. 24: The same patient with a generalized rash.

immunoglobulin M (IgM) antibodies, is diagnostic and is a commonly performed test.

Treatment

Most of the patients with uncomplicated measles will recover with rest and supportive treatment.

Prevention

The best way to avoid contracting measles is to have the MMR vaccine. A patient hospitalized with measles should be isolated.

Hand, Foot, and Mouth Disease

It is a viral infection occurring as outbreaks mostly in spring and summer. In India, disease activity has been reported from different parts since 2004. It is a distinctive eruption of children caused by *Coxsackievirus* A16 and *Enterovirus* 71. It is highly contagious, and the route of spread is feco-oral, oral, and contact with skin lesions.

Clinical Features

- Initial prodrome consists of sore throat, dysphagia, mild fever, and abdominal pain.
- The enanthem consists of papules on the tongue and buccal mucosa which break down to form ulcers with an erythematous base.
- This is followed by exanthema with the sudden appearance of erythematous papulovesicular eruptions in crops. These are initially filled with clear fluid which rapidly turns turbid.
- The lesions are 2–10 mm in size with characteristic perilesional erythema appearing on the face, sides and dorsal surfaces of hands and feet, and perineum **(Figs. 25 and 26)**.
- Mucosal involvement is also known **(Figs. 27A to C)**.
- Palms, soles, proximal extremities, and trunk may also be involved.

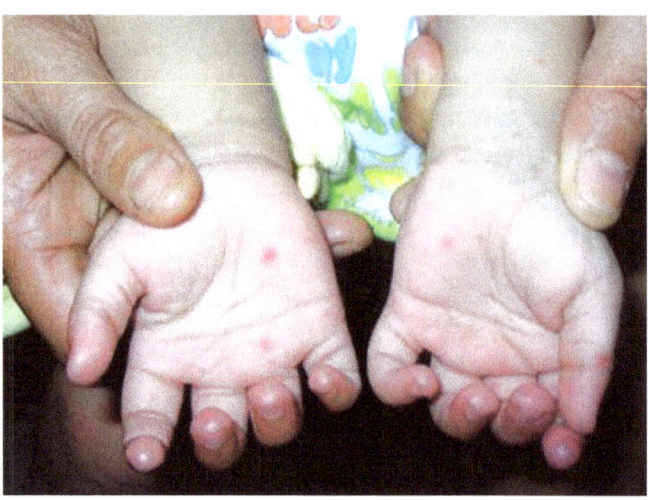

FIG. 26: Lesions on palms and soles of the child with hand, foot and mouth disease (HFMD).

- Lesions heal within 7–10 days without any major complications.
- Rare but fatal complications include cardiac and neurological complications, such as encephalitis, aseptic meningitis, and acute flaccid paralysis.
- Orange-yellow nail discoloration, Beau's lines, and onychomadesis may be seen in one-third to one-fourth of children 3–6 weeks after the lesions have subsided **(Fig. 28)**.

Differential Diagnosis

- Herpangina (lesions being more on the soft palate and tonsils here)
- Varicella
- Herpes stomatitis
- Drug eruptions
- Erythema multiforme
- Aphthous ulcers

Diagnosis

Mainly clinical but PCR is currently the diagnostic method of choice.

Treatment

There is neither an effective antiviral therapy nor a vaccine against HFMD. Good hygiene with proper cleaning of hands, safe drinking water, and avoiding direct contact with patients is of paramount importance.

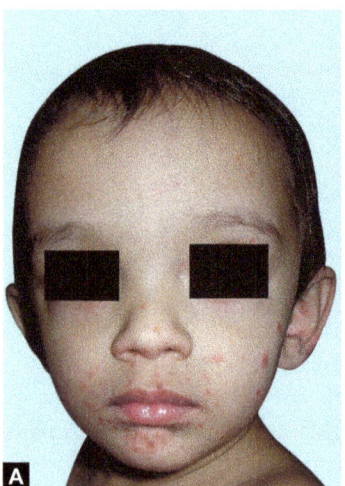 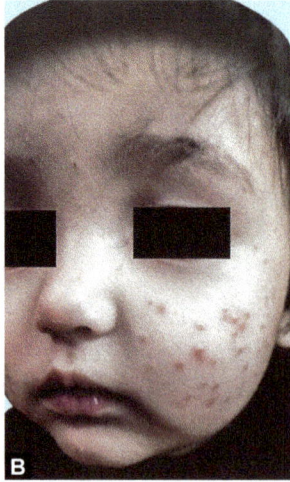

FIGS. 25A AND B: Lesions of hand, foot and mouth disease (HFMD) on the face of children.

CHAPTER 8: Pox, Rubella, Coxsackie, and Other Viral Cutaneous Disorders

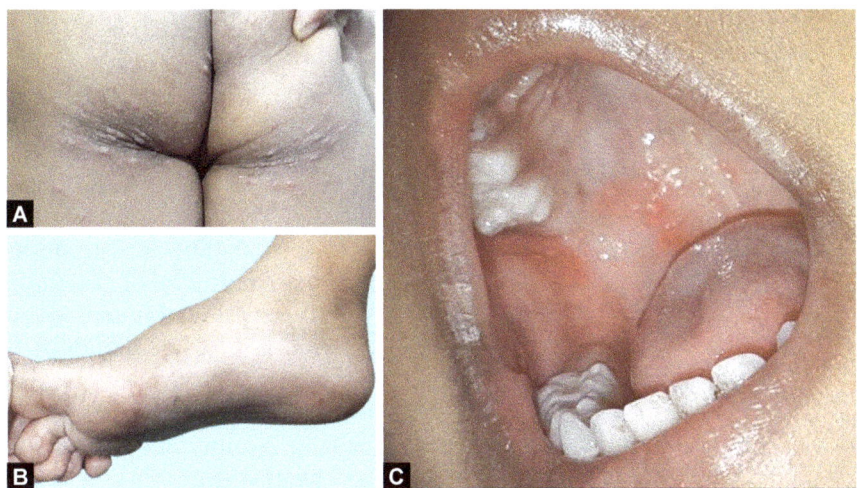

FIGS. 27A TO C: Lesions on the buttocks, sole, and hard palate in a child with hand, foot and mouth disease (HFMD).

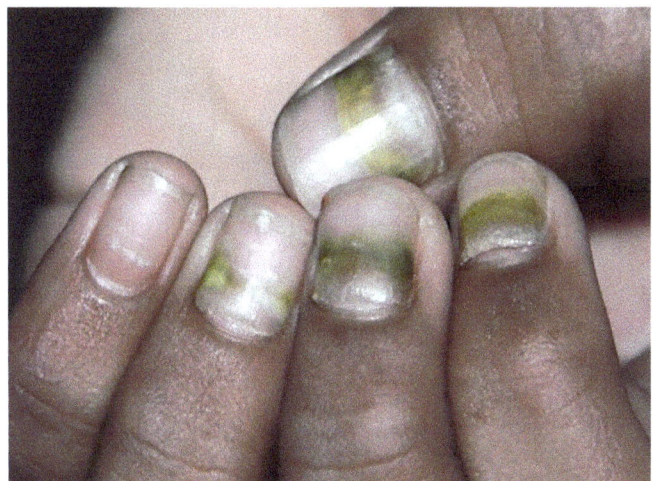

FIG 28: Orange to greenish discoloration of the nail plate, onychomadesis, and Beau's lines post hand, foot and mouth disease (HFMD).

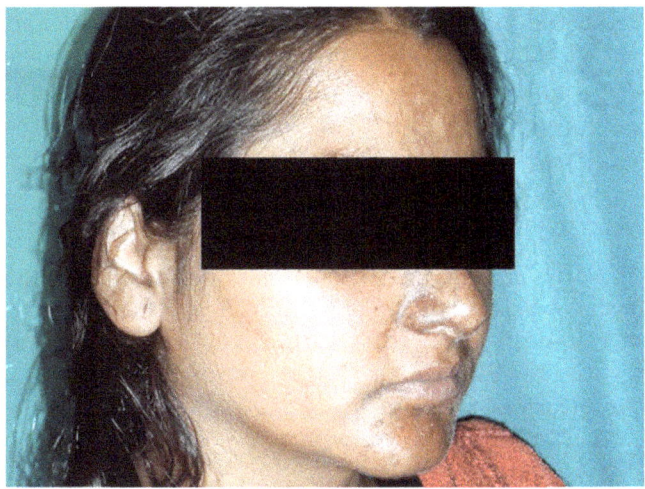

FIG. 29: Melasma-like pigmentation in a patient of chikungunya.

Chikungunya Virus

It was first isolated in India from Kolkata in 1963, followed by an outbreak in 1971 which disappeared in a few years. Recently, there has been a resurgence of this virus. The vector involved in the transmission of this virus is *Aedes aegypti*. Currently, it is an endemic disease in India, Africa, and South-East Asia. The incubation period is 2–12 days.

Clinical Features

- Acute phase manifests as high-grade fever with chills which lasts for 2–3 days. The fever remits for 1–2 days and then reappears.
- Severe polyarticular, migratory arthritis may occur predominantly affecting the small joints of the hand, wrist, ankle, and feet.
- Associated systemic features include nausea/vomiting, fatigue, headache, photophobia, or retro-orbital pain.
- Maculopapular skin rash affecting trunk and limbs manifests in over 50% of the cases. Pruritus occurs in 20–85% of cases. Palmoplantar peeling may occur in a few cases. Oral mucosa may be involved in the form of aphthous ulcers and gingivitis.
- Facial pigmentation may occur in various patterns, including malar, midfacial, and flagellate in up to 30% of cases with characteristic involvement of the nose (Chik sign) **(Figs. 29 and 30)**.
- Various unusual features include urticarial and purpuric rash, photosensitivity, edema of feet and legs, scrotal dermatitis, erythema multiforme-like lesions, diffuse pigmentation, etc.

CHAPTER 8: Pox, Rubella, Coxsackie, and Other Viral Cutaneous Disorders

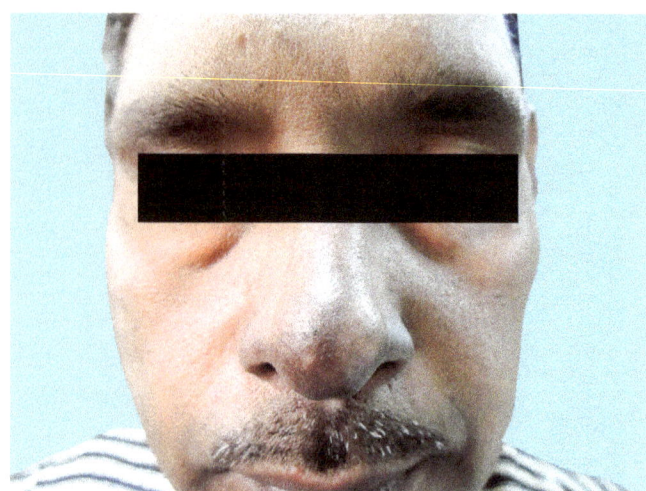

FIG. 30: Residual pigmentation of the nose in a patient of chikungunya (Chik sign).

Differential Diagnosis
- Dengue and dengue hemorrhagic fever
- Rubella
- Parvovirus

Diagnosis
Viremia is present in most patients during the first 48 hours of the disease. The antibodies appear with the cessation of viremia. Virus-specific IgM antibodies are detected by captured ELISA in patients recovering from infection. Virus isolation may also be done.

Treatment
The management is mainly symptomatic and supportive. Aspirin must be avoided in the acute phase.

Dengue

Dengue is perhaps the most important mosquito-borne viral disease in humans, affecting 50–100 million people annually worldwide. The principal vector is *Aedes aegypti*. Humans and mosquitoes both act as reservoirs of the virus. A temperature of >20°C and stagnant water, especially in artificial containers favor epidemic transmission. The incubation period ranges from 3 to 10 days.

Clinical Features

Dengue Fever
The patient presents with high-grade fever and chills, intense headache, and characteristic severe muscle and joint pains (bone-breaking fever). Fever remits for a few hours to 2 days to appear again (biphasic curve) and lasts for 5–7 days.
- A transient, generalized, blanchable macular rash may be seen during the first 24–48 hours of fever.
- A second skin eruption appears during the second febrile phase (in 80%) and lasts for 2 hours to several days.
- The lesions are maculopapular/morbilliform in approximately 50% of cases which appear confluent with the sparing of islands of normal skin sometimes referred to as "white islands in a sea of red."
- It may start on the legs and spread caudally or on the chest and trunk and spread to limbs. The rash is usually asymptomatic or mildly itchy. Facial flushing and hemorrhagic crusting of the lips may be seen in a few cases.
- Unusual clinical features include exfoliative dermatitis (palmoplantar), lymphadenopathy, jaundice, and encephalitis.

Dengue Shock Syndrome and Hemorrhagic Fever
Mucocutaneous features are present in approximately one-third of patients.
- Ecchymosis and petechiae are present in 30% and 13% of patients, respectively **(Fig. 31)**.
- Circumoral cyanosis is another characteristic feature.
- Conjunctival injection and hemorrhagic crusting of lips may be present.
- Hemorrhagic manifestations generally appear 4–5 days after onset of fever and include bleeding phenomenon (epistaxis, petechiae, and gingival bleeding) and rarely menorrhagia and gastrointestinal bleeding.

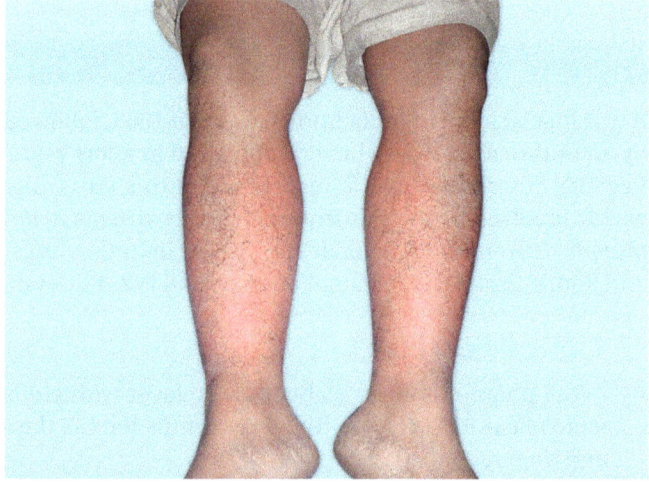

FIG. 31: Petechiae involving bilateral legs in a patient with dengue hemorrhagic fever.

CHAPTER 8: Pox, Rubella, Coxsackie, and Other Viral Cutaneous Disorders

Differential Diagnosis
- Chikungunya fever
- Measles
- Rubella
- Erythema infectiosum
- Exanthem subitum

Diagnosis
It is based on IgM antibody detection, which appears within 2–5 days of onset of illness and persists for 1–3 months. Nonstructural protein-1 (NS-1) antigen detection method is also available.

Treatment
Treatment is mainly symptomatic. Avoidance of aspirin is important. Dengue hemorrhagic fever and dengue shock syndrome are managed with appropriate intravenous fluids and oxygen along with close monitoring of vitals and laboratory parameters.

Chapter 9: Leprosy

Introduction

Leprosy (Hansen's disease) is a chronic infection of low transmissibility caused by acid-fast *Mycobacterium leprae* that has not yet been cultured in vitro. India contributes approximately 65% to the total global leprosy cases. The disease primarily affects skin and nerves. Early diagnosis and treatment of leprosy is important to prevent unsightly deformities.

Transmission usually occurs from infected person to others through nasal droplet infection. Another possible route is through prolonged skin-to-skin contact. Incubation period is long, generally 2–5 years though it ranges from few weeks to as long as 20 years.

Classification

Leprosy presents as a spectrum of clinical manifestation depending upon the host immunity. On one pole are patients with good immunity presenting as paucibacillary (PB) tuberculoid leprosy (TT), borderline tuberculoid (BT), and on the other pole are patients with poor immunity presenting as multibacillary (MB) lepromatous leprosy (LL) **(Flowchart 1)**, depending upon whether the slit skin smears demonstrate any bacilli or not.

Pure neuritic leprosy and indeterminate leprosy are included in the Indian classification.

In 1998, the World Health Organization (WHO) proposed a simpler clinical classification depending on the number of leprosy lesions in the patient:
- PB: Up to five lesions (including maximum 1 nerve).
- MB: More than five lesions (skin lesions and nerve) qualify as MB leprosy.

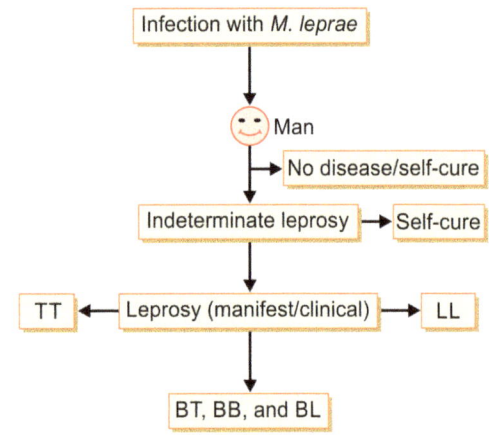

FLOWCHART 1: Spectrum of leprosy.
(BB: mid borderline; BL: borderline lepromatous; BT: borderline tuberculoid; TT: tuberculoid leprosy; LL: lepromatous leprosy; *M. leprae*: *Mycobacterium leprae*)

Clinical Features

Indeterminate Leprosy

It is an early and transitory stage of leprosy, usually seen in children in whom immunological status has not yet been determined. One or few vague hypopigmented or faintly erythematous, slightly dry macules with impaired sensations are present on face, limb, or buttocks **(Fig. 1)**. Hair growth and nerve functions are usually not affected. The diagnosis is confirmed on biopsy that shows the presence of typical perineural infiltration; Acid fast bacilli (AFB) are not demonstrable both on biopsy as well as on slit skin smear examination. Perhaps three out of four indeterminate lesions undergo self-healing and the rest become determinate.

Differential Diagnosis
- Pityriasis alba, pityriasis versicolor, polymorphic light eruption (PMLE), vitiligo (incipient lesion)
- Nevus anemicus/achromicus, postinflammatory hypomelanosis (psoriasis, eczema, etc.).

Tuberculoid Leprosy

This type of leprosy is seen in individuals with good cell-mediated immunity (CMI). 1–3 lesions with well-defined and raised margins, variable sized (<10 cm), very dry surface, anesthesia, and loss of surface hair **(Figs. 2 and 3)** are present. A nerve is usually thickened in the vicinity of the skin lesion. On slit skin smear examination, often no AFBs are found.

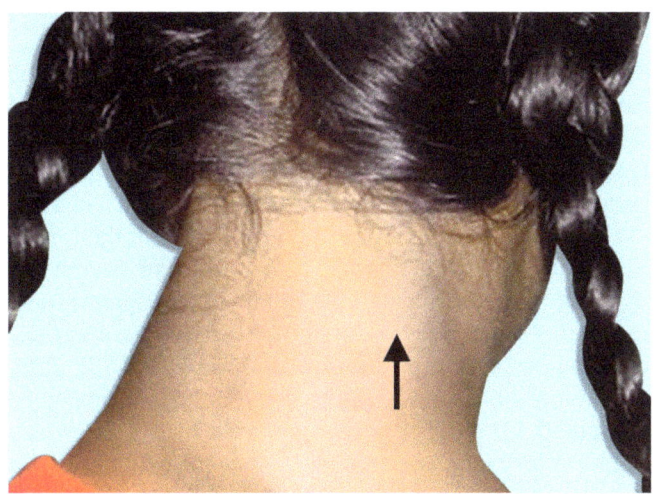

FIG. 1: Vague hypopigmented macule over nape of neck.

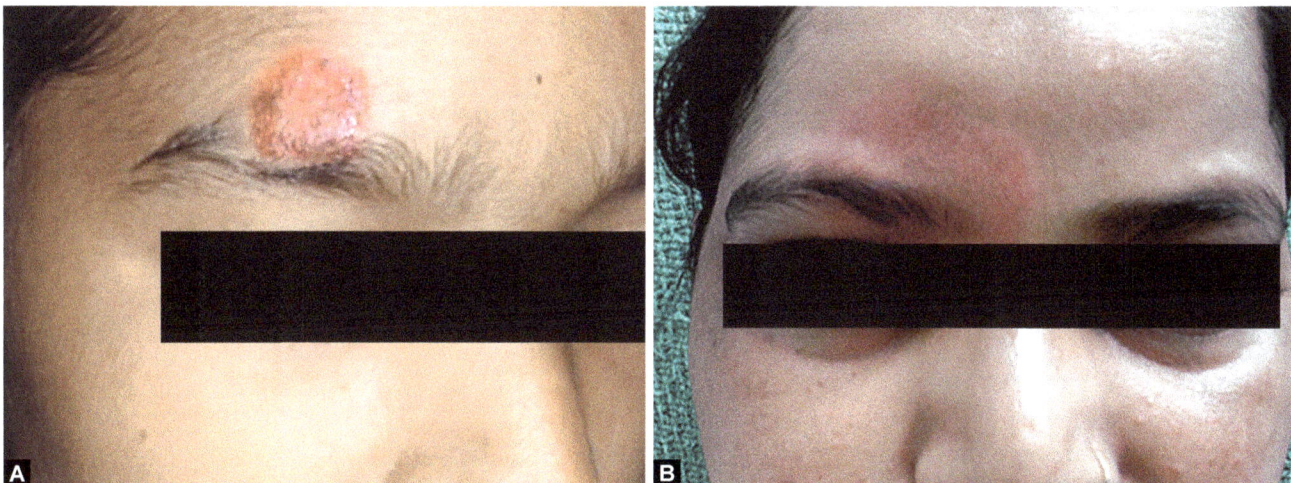

FIGS. 2A AND B: (A) Well-defined plaque of tuberculoid leprosy Hansen; (B) A plaque of tuberculoid leprosy subpolar Hansen around right eye.

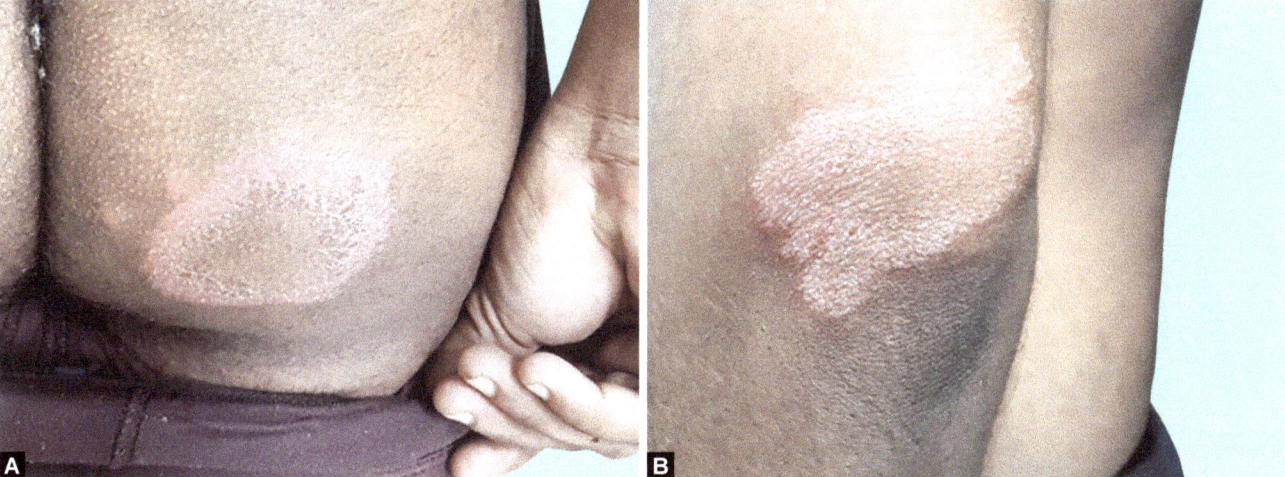

FIGS. 3A AND B: Well-defined dry plaque of borderline tuberculoid (BT) Hansen with satellite lesions: (A) Over right buttock in a child; and (B) BT lesion on left elbow in an adult male.

Differential Diagnosis

- Lupus vulgaris
- Sarcoidosis
- Cutaneous leishmaniasis
- Granuloma annulare (localized variant)
- Discoid lupus erythematosus

Borderline Leprosy

In subjects with borderline leprosy, immunity lies between tuberculoid and lepromatous pole and is unstable with many cases showing upgrading and downgrading (shifting up or down in the spectrum). So, one often finds features suggestive of two forms of leprosy. BT patients have a higher degree of immunity compared to borderline lepromatous (BL) patients. Mid borderline (BB) lies in between the two and shares features of both. The lesions increase in number and they gradually lose their definition (well-defined to ill-defined) as one moves from BT to BL. BT lesions are drier and hypoesthetic as compared to smooth shiny BL lesions with hypoesthesia or may be normoesthesia in BL. The plaques may look annular, punched out, or bizarre looking **(Figs. 4A and B)**. Nerve thickening is asymmetrical and occurs early in the disease.

Differential Diagnosis

- Cutaneous sarcoidosis
- Leishmaniasis
- Lupus vulgaris
- Tinea corporis
- Erythema annulare centrifugum
- Necrobiosis lipoidica

Lepromatous Leprosy

Majority of LL patients (>75%) are slowly downgraded from borderline leprosy (referred as subpolar LL) when they remain untreated for a long time. Patients showing features of LL at the onset are called as polar LL. LL patients have significantly deficient leprosy specific CMI. In early phase, the patient develops diffuse mild-to-marked shiny brownish infiltration, or small ill-defined erythematous to hypopigmented innumerable bilateral and symmetrical macules and nodules with intact sensations, over the ear lobules, face, and extensor aspects of the body (arm, elbow, lower back, lower limbs, etc.) **(Fig. 5)**. An advanced untreated LL patient is recognizable by his face with thick ear lobes, collapsed nose, lost eyebrows, and upper

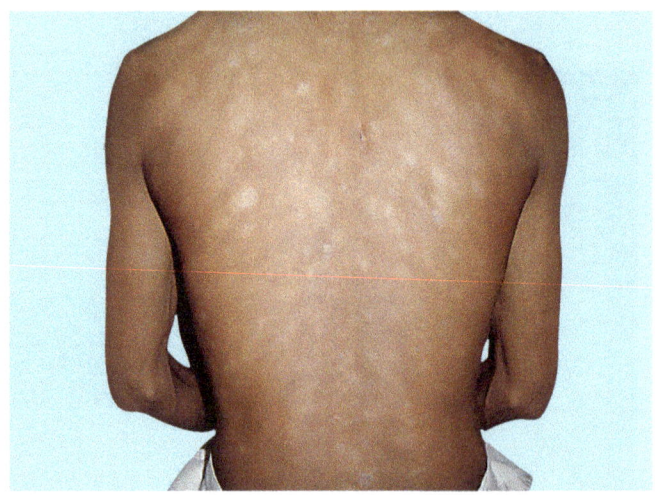

FIG. 5: Bilateral symmetrical hypopigmented macules of lepromatous leprosy.

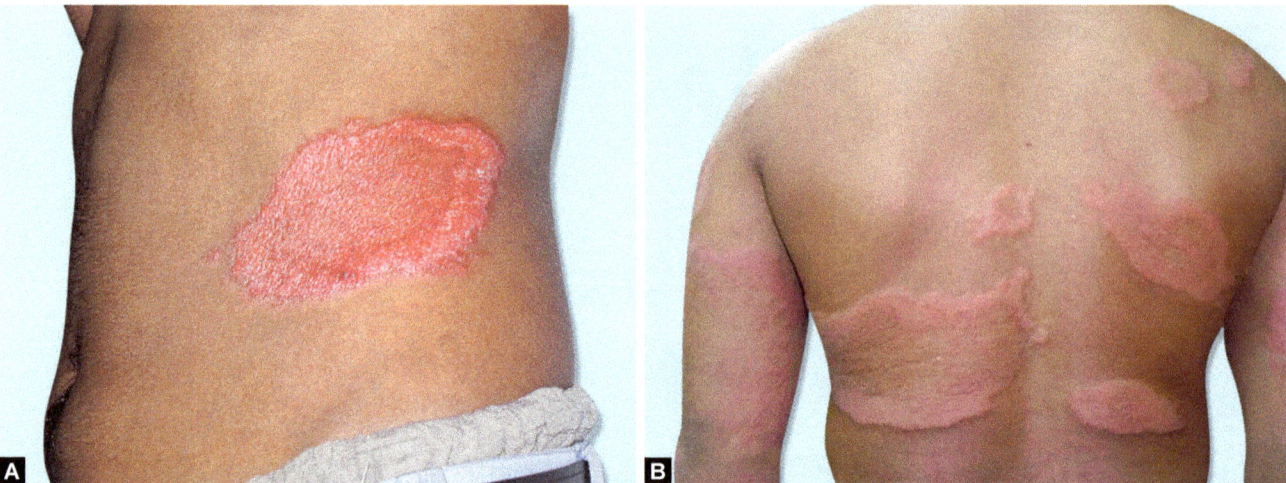

FIGS. 4A AND B: (A) A large dry erythematous annular plaque of borderline tuberculoid Hansen. Note the central clearing; (B) Multiple annular and punched out lesions of mid borderline.

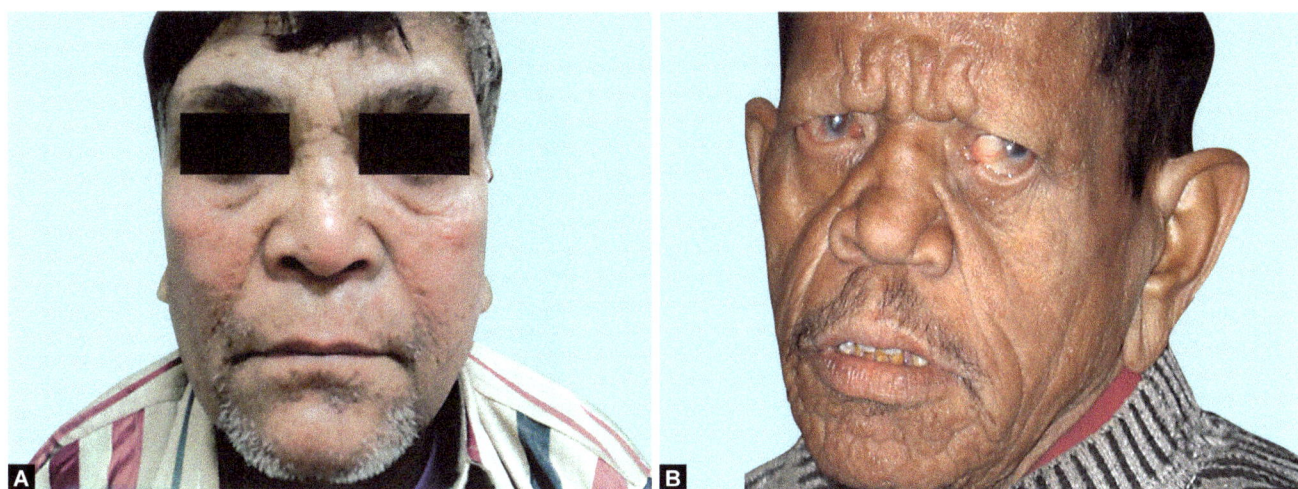

FIGS. 6A AND B: Leonine facies of lepromatous leprosy. Note the depressed nasal bridge.

incisor teeth, thickened skin of forehead (due to leprous infiltration) causing leonine facies **(Figs. 6A and B)**. Multiple peripheral symmetric nerves thickening occurs. Glove and stocking anesthesia is seen late in the disease. These patients may have ichthyosis like skin specially over lower limbs.

Differential Diagnosis

- *Madarosis*: Hypothyroidism, follicular mucinosis, alopecia areata
- *Skin lesions*: Disseminated cutaneous leishmaniasis, reticulohistiocytosis, lichen myxedematosus, cutaneous T-cell lymphoma, post kala-azar dermal leishmaniasis (PKDL)
- *Neuropathy*: Nutritional deficiencies, alcoholism, diabetes, heavy metal effects, and primary amyloidosis of peripheral nerves.

Pure Neuritic Leprosy

In this form of leprosy, one or a few enlarged peripheral nerves **(Fig. 7)** with features of nerve damage are seen but without any skin lesions. This form is seen most frequently but not exclusively in India and Nepal, where it accounts for 5–10% of all patients with leprosy. Histology of affected nerve reveals an infiltrate, characteristic of leprosy.

Differential Diagnosis

- Diabetes mellitus
- Neurofibromatosis
- Amyloidosis
- Hereditary sensory neuropathy
- Autosomal dominant hypertrophic neuropathy

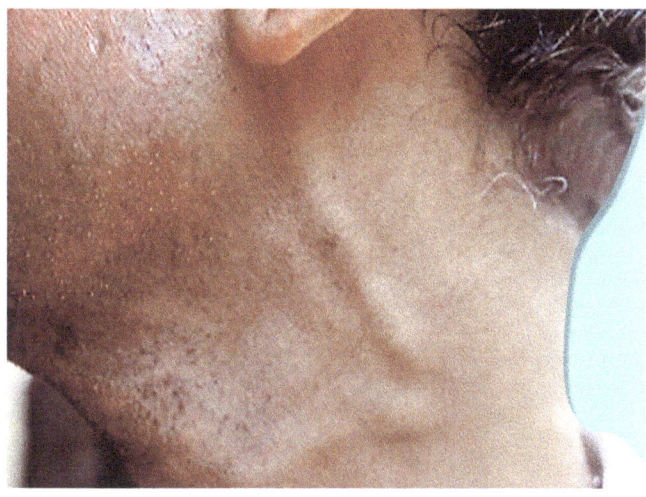

FIG. 7: Enlarged greater auricular nerve in a man with no skin lesions.

Uncommon Variants

Histoid Leprosy

Histoid leprosy is an expression of MB leprosy, characterized by typical well-demarcated cutaneous and/or subcutaneous nodules **(Fig. 8A)** and plaques present over an apparently normal skin with unique histopathology and bacterial morphology. Typical young lesions are firm, reddish or skin colored, succulent, and dome-shaped papules/nodules with shiny and stretched overlying skin **(Fig. 8B)**. It was thought to be due to the development of drug resistance to dapsone, however, de novo cases are known to occur.

A prominent histological feature is the circumscribed nature of the lesion, predominance of spindle shaped

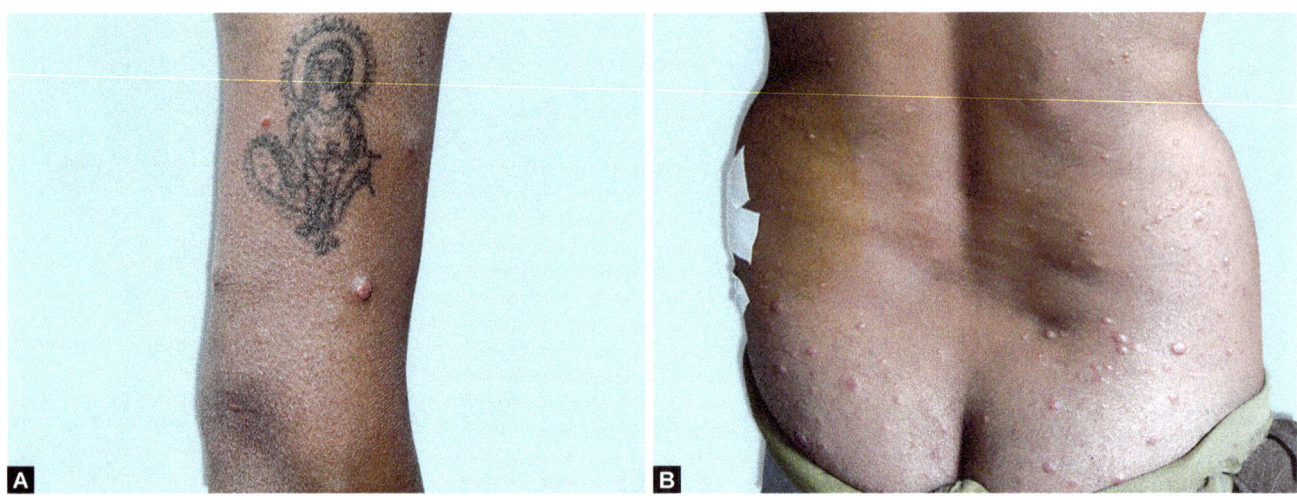

FIGS. 8A AND B: (A) Well-defined succulent cutaneous nodule of histoid Hansen; (B) Multiple dome-shaped shiny lesions of histoid Hansen.

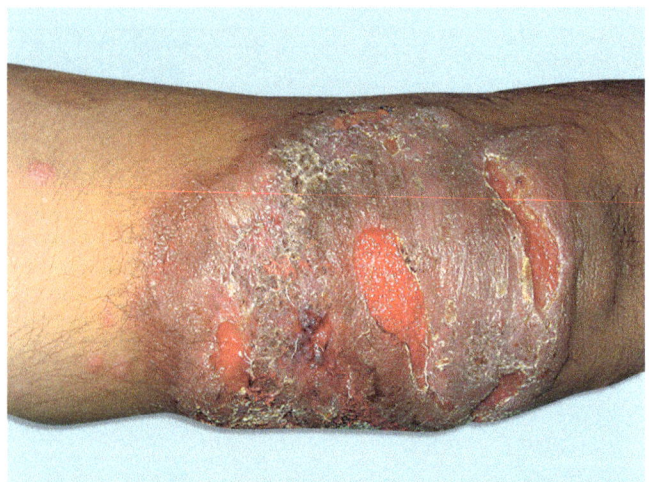

FIG. 9: Ulcerated lesion of borderline tuberculoid (BT) lazarine leprosy.

histiocytes forming interlacing bands, whorls, and unusually large number of AFBs that are uniformly stained long rods with tapering ends, longer than the ordinary lepra bacilli.

Differential Diagnosis

- Lepromatous leprosy
- Sarcoidosis
- PKDL
- Neurofibromatosis type I
- Dermatofibroma

Lazarine Leprosy

An unusual expression of BT leprosy is spontaneous ulceration of skin lesions **(Fig. 9)** resulting presumably from the exaggerated hypersensitivity in type 1 reactions (T1Rs). Rarely, it occurs in the absence of preexisting skin lesions or coexistent nerve pathology. Histopathology shows necrosis due to extreme cellular hypersensitivity. Systemic corticosteroids are necessary for the treatment in addition to antileprosy treatment (ALT). If the disease remains untreated, patient subsequently manifest typical skin lesions and nerve involvement.

Systemic Manifestations in Leprosy

Systemic manifestations are mainly seen in MB patients.

Eye

Madarosis, i.e., loss of eyebrows, drooping (upper eyelid) or ectropion (lower eyelid) may occur due to heavy infiltration of the eyelids. Corneal reflex is impaired and there is conjunctival/corneal anesthesia or hypoesthesia if the trigeminal nerve is involved. Involvement of zygomatic branch of facial nerve produces lagophthalmos **(Figs. 10A and B)** resulting in exposure keratitis due to inability to approximate both eyelids. Anterior structures of eye may be involved leading to superficial punctuate keratitis. Acute iridocyclitis (during reaction) is a dreaded complication. With slit-lamp examination the lepromata are seen as iris "pearls" in iridocyclitis. Ocular defects are seen mostly in smear positive individuals with long-standing disease which is often associated with other deformities.

Upper Respiratory Tract

The nose is the portal of entry for *M. leprae* and is the earliest site of involvement in LL. It becomes heavily bacillated. Edema and mucosal thickening, hemorrhagic crusting, and epistaxis are frequent complaints. Perforation of nasal septum and nasal collapse may occur.

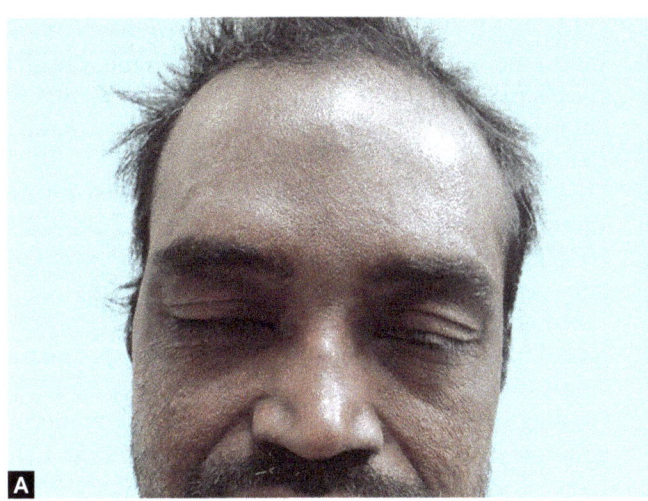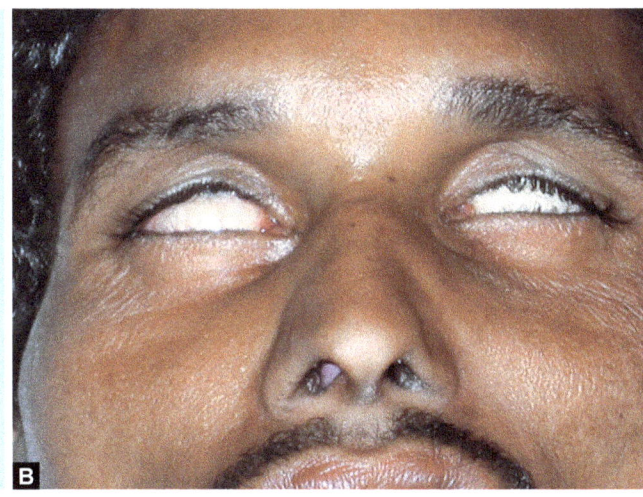

FIGS. 10A AND B: (A) Lagophthalmos of left eye due to facial nerve palsy; (B) Lagophthalmos of both eye due to bilateral facial nerve palsy.

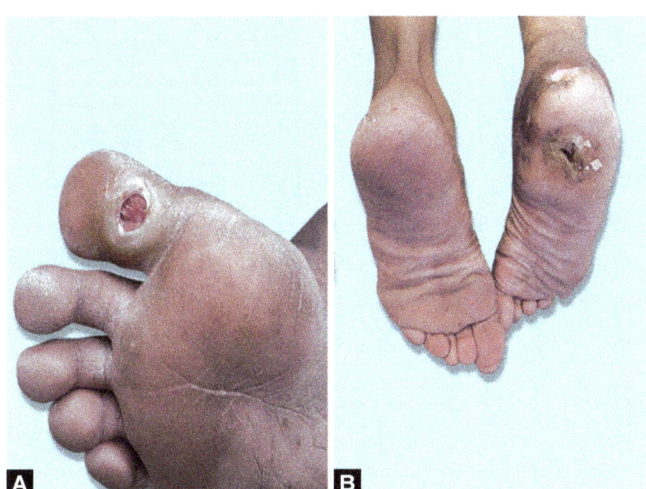

FIGS. 11A AND B: (A) Trophic ulcer over base of big toe; (B) Trophic ulcer over the heel.

Ulceration of tongue, pharynx, hard and soft palate, have been reported. Laryngeal involvement is a late phenomenon and may present as ulceration and fibrosis resulting in hoarseness of the voice.

Bones of hands, feet, and skull commonly bear the brunt of untreated disease. Repeated trauma to the anesthetic hands and feet resulting in trophic ulcers **(Figs. 11A and B)** and restricted movement of the muscles. The distal phalanges of hands undergo resorption. Metacarpals and carpals are spared. However, in the foot phalanges, metatarsals and tarsals undergo atrophy. The metatarsals become thinned out distally, a change referred to as "penciling" or a "sucked candy stick" appearance. The facial changes are the ones that carry the imprint of leprosy. Atrophy of anterior nasal spine leads to nasal collapse and that of maxillary alveolar process leading to "facies leprosa" loosening and fall of upper incisor teeth "facies leprosa."

Renal damage in leprosy is an important cause of morbidity and mortality and may be due to renal amyloidosis, glomerulonephritis, pyelonephritis, interstitial nephritis, and renal tuberculosis.

Reproductive System

Gonadal involvement in men with LL is not uncommon and manifests initially as leprous orchitis (due to acute inflammation and edema) and subsequently as testicular atrophy (due to fibrosis). Testicular atrophy can ensue in longstanding disease and as a sequelae to recurrent epididymo-orchitis during type 2 reactions (T2Rs). Sterility is followed by impotence.

There is a paucity of literature on the involvement of gonads in female leprosy patients.

Lymph Nodes

Generalized lymphadenopathy is encountered largely in MB (BL, LL) leprosy and during reactions.

Diagnosis of Leprosy

The diagnosis of leprosy is based upon three cardinal signs:
1. Hypopigmented or erythematous patch with impairment/loss of sensations
2. Enlarged peripheral nerve trunk/s **(Fig. 12)**
3. Presence of AFB in skin slit smears.

Any one of the above sign is sufficient for the diagnosis of leprosy.

- Touch, temperature, and pain sensations should be invariably tested over the lesions and over area supplied by the nerve. Power in the muscles should be assessed (voluntary muscle testing).

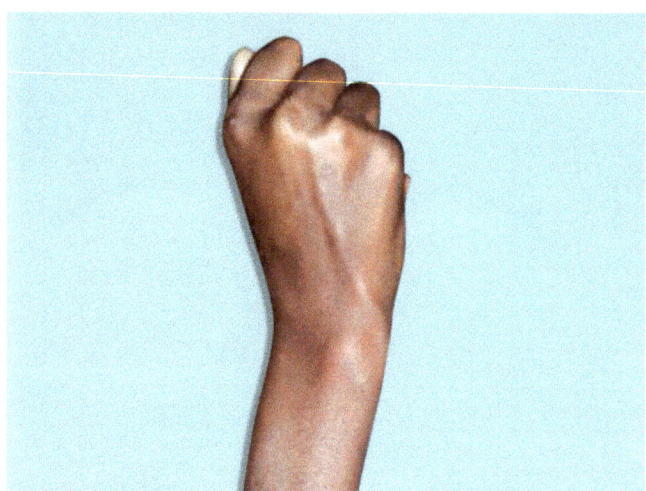

FIG. 12: Enlarged dorsal radial branch.

- *Skin biopsy*: It is performed to confirm the diagnosis and type of leprosy. AFB are demonstrable on Ziehl Neelson (ZN) or Fite-Faraco staining. As a rule, the biopsy should be taken from the most downgraded lesion.
- Histology of TT is characterized by a well-formed granuloma consisting of epithelioid cells, giant cells (Langhans type) and lymphocytes, abutting the epidermis with conspicuous absence of the nerve in the granuloma. Section is negative for AFB. On the other hand, macrophage granuloma is a distinctive feature of BL/LL leprosy. The granuloma is expansile and due to the pressure from accumulating cells the epidermis often becomes flattened with a Grenz zone **(Fig. 15)**.
- Nerve biopsy from the thickened sensory nerve may be done to confirm the diagnosis of neuritic leprosy.

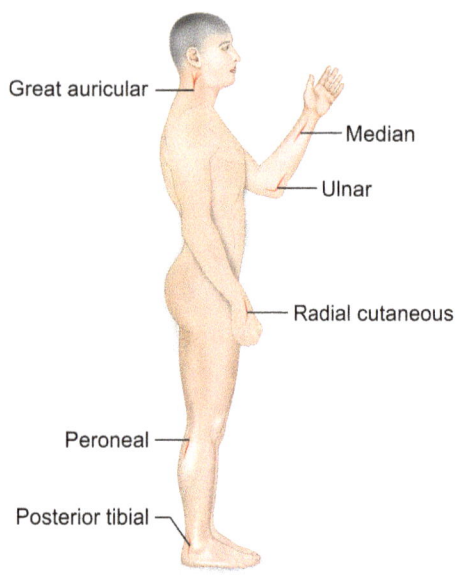

FIG. 13: Peripheral nerves commonly affected in leprosy.

- The peripheral nerves that should be palpated for thickness and tenderness include: Supraorbital, supratrochlear, greater auricular, cervical nerves, supraclavicular nerves, radial, ulnar, median, radial cutaneous, common peroneal, sural, and posterior tibial nerve **(Fig. 13)**.

Diagnosis

Laboratory Diagnosis

- *Slit-skin smear (SSS)*: SSS examination is a simple and valuable test for calculating bacteriological index (BI) and morphological index (MI). Numerous AFB are seen in MB leprosy (BL and LL) **(Fig. 14)**.

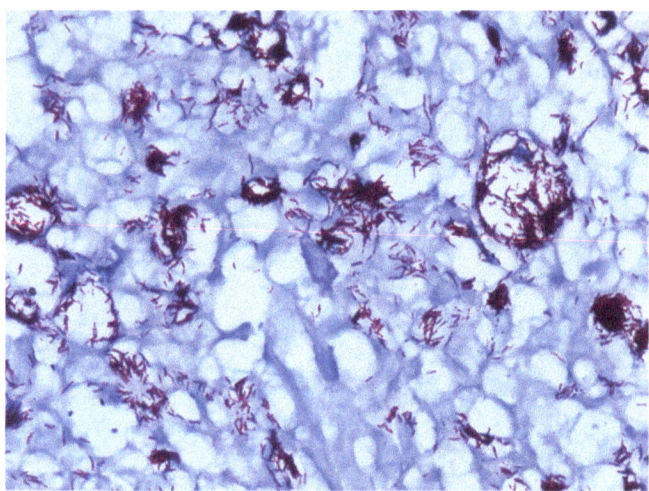

FIG. 14: Numerous acid fast bacilli (AFB) (*Mycobacterium leprae*) seen on slit-skin smear (SSS) on Ziehl–Neelsen (ZN) staining.

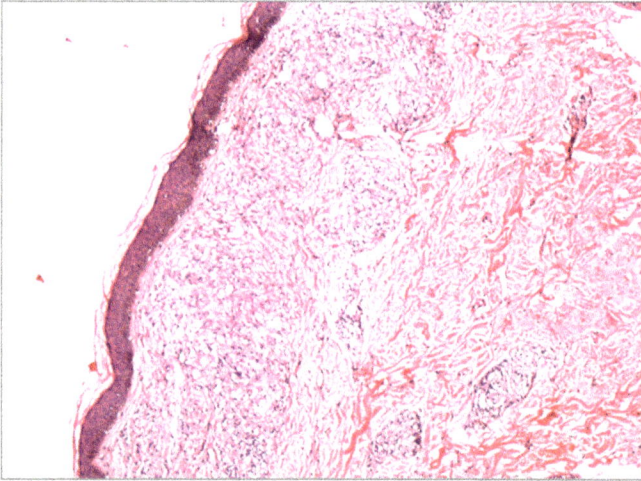

FIG. 15: Lepromatous leprosy. Note the free subepidermal zone (Grenz zone) (Hematoxylin and eosin stain, 40 × 10×).

The suitable nerves include the radial cutaneous nerve at the wrist, cutaneous nerve of the forearm and sural nerve at the back of the leg. Radial cutaneous nerve is generally chosen for ease of procedure.
- *Nerve ultrasonography*: Imaging of peripheral nerves can be done with reasonable precision with ultrasonography (USG) with broadband frequency of 10–14 MHz; color Doppler frequency of 6–13 MHz and linear array transducer. Significant correlation has been observed between clinical parameters of grade of thickening and USG abnormalities of nerve echotexture, endoneural flow, and cross-sectional area of nerves.

Indications of nerve ultrasound include an assessment of nerve involvement in leprosy, type 1 and 2 lepra reaction, and diagnosis of mononeuropathies, polyneuropathies, and peripheral nerve tumors.

Management

Multidrug therapy (MDT), i.e., simultaneous administration of two or more drugs has been the mainstay of treatment of leprosy since 1982. Rifampicin (R), dapsone (D), and/or clofazimine (C) comprises MDT.
- *MDT*: Three drugs (R, D, and C) are given in MB cases (BI positive) for at least 12 months and for PB (BI negative) cases for 6 months.

All three drugs are available in blister packs and safe in pregnancy. The dosages are modified for children **(Figs. 16 and 17)**.

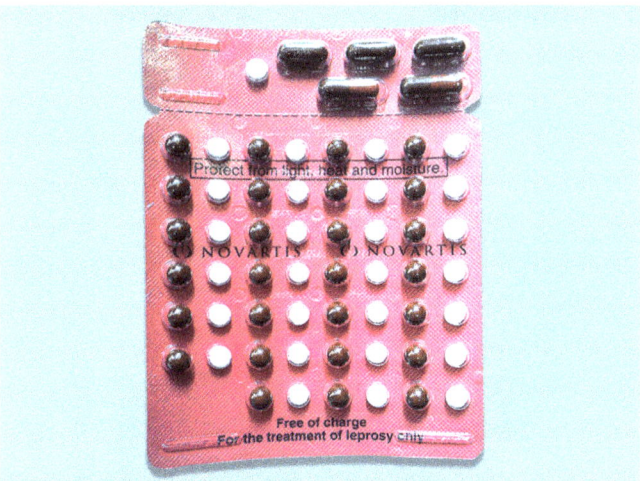

FIG. 16: Multidrug therapy (MDT) (Adult).

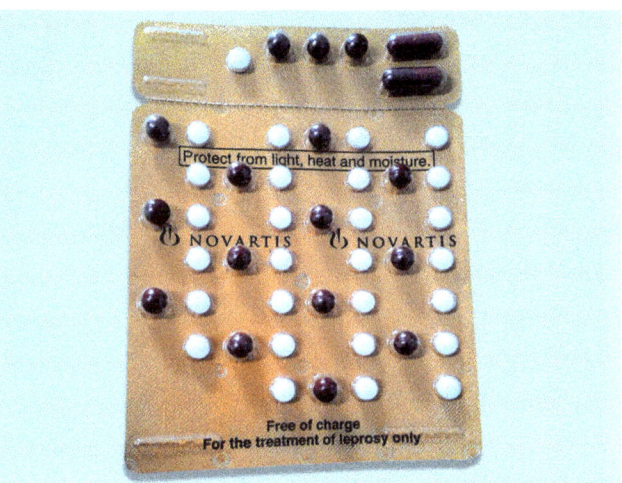

FIG. 17: Multidrug therapy (MDT) (Child: 10–14 years).

Reactions in Leprosy

Leprosy reactions are immunologically-mediated episodes of acute or subacute inflammation affecting the skin, nerves, mucous membrane, and/or other sites.
- The T1R is usually observed in the borderline spectrum (BT-BL) and is a manifestation of type 4 hypersensitivity reaction. It results in sudden shift in the patient's position in the leprosy spectrum. Some or all of the pre-existing skin patches or plaques become erythematous, edematous and tender **(Figs. 18A and B)**. Rapid swelling with severe pain or tenderness of one or more peripheral nerves is common at the site of swelling with or without nerve paresis **(Figs. 19A and B)**. In the severe form of T1R nerve abscess may be formed.
- Type 2 reaction is associated with type 3 hypersensitivity reactions (HSRs) (antigen-antibody complex mediated). It is usually observed in LL and sometimes in BL leprosy within 3–6 months of starting MBMDT. In classical T2R usually no clinical change is noticed in the original skin lesions. There is a sudden appearance of crops of evanescent (lasting for few days) pink colored tender papules, nodules or plaques, and erythema nodosum leprosum (ENL) **(Figs. 20 and 21)**. In T2R constitutional manifestations are common. Nerve damage may occur, but not as frequently as in T1R. Myositis, arthritis, iridocyclitis, glaucoma, painful dactylitis, periosteal pain (particularly in tibia), tender and swollen lymph nodes, acute epididymo-orchitis, nephritis and proteinuria, and anemia are associated features of T2R.

CHAPTER 9: Leprosy

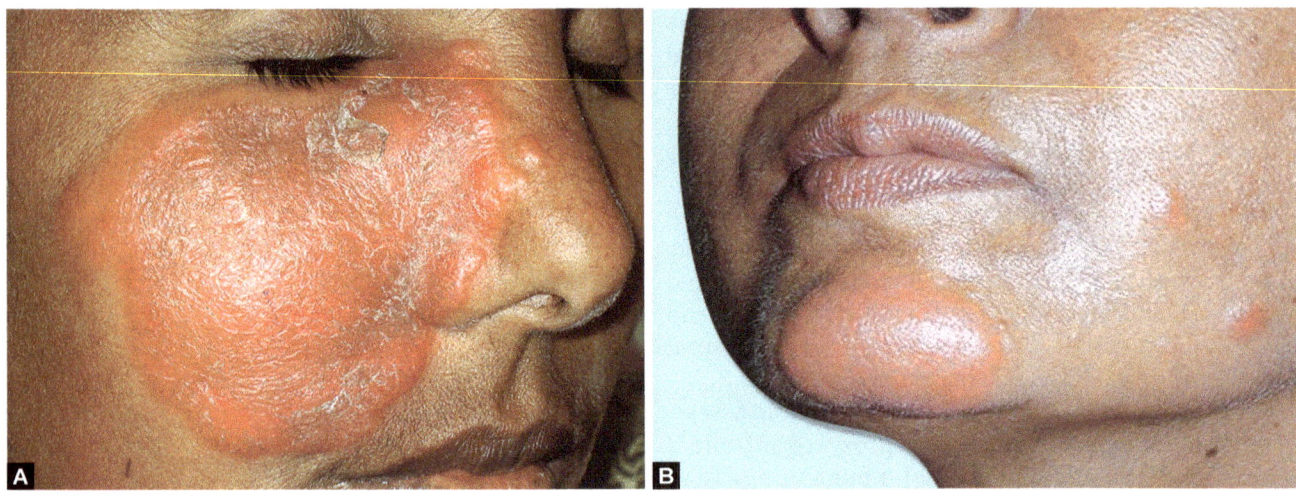

FIGS. 18A AND B: Erythematous, edematous, and tender plaque in type 1 reaction.

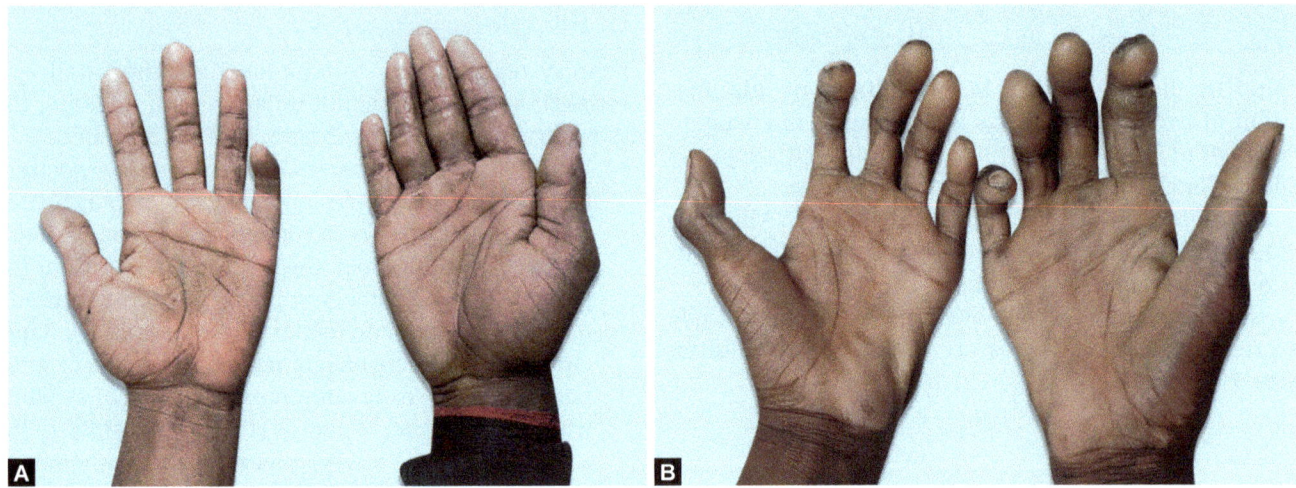

FIGS. 19A AND B: (A) Left ulnar claw hand; (B) Ulnar and median claw hands—bilateral.

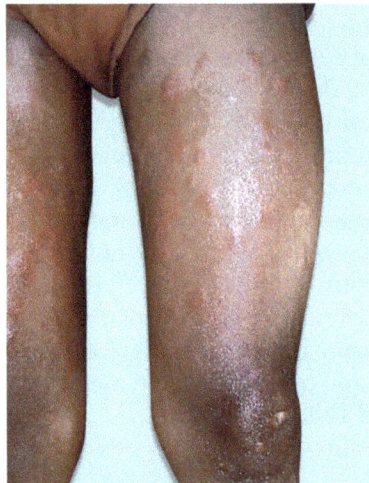

FIG. 20: Erythematous evanescent and tender nodules of erythema nodosum leprosum (ENL).

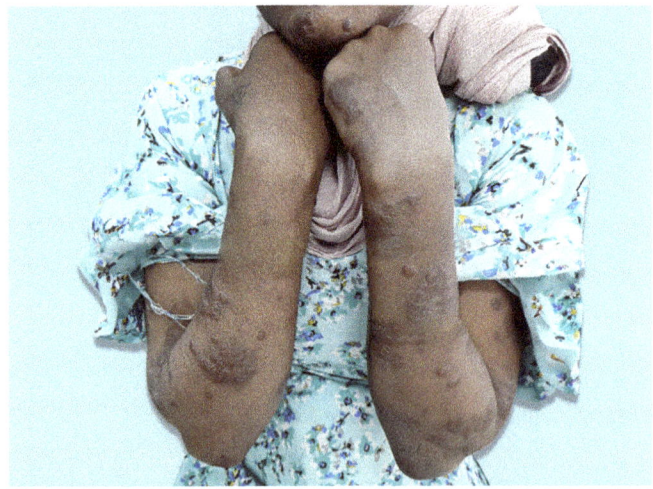

FIG. 21: Intensely erythematous and tender erythema nodosum leprosum (ENL) lesions of type 2 lepra reaction on the upper limbs and face of a young woman on multidrug therapy (MDT).

Management of Leprosy Reactions

- Mild T1R may be managed with nonsteroidal anti-inflammatory drugs (NSAIDs).
- If nerve involvement is there, oral prednisolone is given (1 mg/kg/day) and is gradually tapered when the features of T1R subside. It takes 12 weeks to even 1 year or more depending on the severity and the spectrum of disease.
- Attempts should be made to identify and treat precipitating factors of T2R such as intercurrent infections and infestations.
- In addition to NSAIDs, prednisolone (P), thalidomide (T), and clofazimine (C) are effective drugs for T2R which can be used either alone or in combination (P + C or P + T) in chronic and recurrent T2R. Thalidomide is given in 200–400 mg daily to start with, gradual tapering. It has serious teratogenic adverse reactions, therefore, contraindicated in females of reproductive age group. Clofazimine is given in 300 mg to start with followed by gradual tapering.

Newer Chemotherapeutic Agents in Leprosy

The reasons for the development of new drugs and regimens are as follows:
- The duration of treatment is long.
- Dapsone and clofazimine are weakly bactericidal.
- Administration of the daily components dapsone and clofazimine cannot be supervised.
- Patients who cannot tolerate standard ALT, need safer and effective alternative.

Fluoroquinolones (ofloxacin, pefloxacin, sparfloxacin, moxifloxacin, and sitafloxacin), tetracyclines (minocycline), macrolides (clarithromycin), ansamycins (rifabutin, rifapentine), β-lactam antibiotics (cephaloridine, cefuroxime, and co-amoxy-clavulanic acid are newer antileprosy drugs).

Prevention

- *The leprosy postexposure prophylaxis (LPEP) with single dose rifampicin (SDR)*: In this initiative, all the family contacts of the newly diagnosed index leprosy case are screened for any clinical evidence of leprosy and are given supervised SDR as a part of postexposure prophylaxis.
- Prevention primarily consists of avoiding close contact with patients with untreated disease.
- Prevention is through timely and adequate treatment of leprosy affected person as it targets the source of infection. Patients receiving long-term therapy are no longer contagious and, therefore, do not represent a risk.
- Ensure accessible and uninterrupted MDT services.
- Encouragement of self-reporting and early treatment by promoting community awareness.

CHAPTER 10

Cutaneous Tuberculosis

Introduction

Cutaneous tuberculosis (CTB) is a chronic granulomatous disease caused by *Mycobacterium tuberculosis* (MTB) and occasionally by *Mycobacterium bovis*. Commonly, CTB is divided into two major groups: true CTB and tuberculids. True CTB is a direct manifestation of infection at the site of the skin lesions. In true CTB, mycobacteria can be identified in the sites of skin involvement using tests such as smears, culture, or polymerase chain reaction (PCR). In contrast, tuberculids result from a hypersensitivity reaction to mycobacterial antigens, hence mycobacteria are not detectable on smears, histopathology, or molecular diagnostic tests.

For true CTB, based on the portal of entry into the skin (exogenous, hematogenous, lymphatic, or contiguous spread from the underlying tubercular lymph node, bone, or joint), the host's immune status, and the presence or absence of prior host sensitization to MTB, varying morphologic presentation have been described.

Tuberculous Chancre (Primary Inoculation Tuberculosis)

Clinical Features

- Tuberculous chancre occurs in individuals without previous sensitization to the bacillus; natural or artificial. Inoculation may follow trivial trauma, tattooing, ear-piercing, or ritual circumcision, or may result from exposure to unsterilized material during surgical procedures.
- Tuberculous chancre is characterized by the development of a firm, painless <1 cm sized painless, reddish brown nodule after 2–4 weeks of inoculation, at trauma prone sites such as face and extremities, which evolves into an ulcer. The ulcer is shallow with undermined bluish margins and coarse granular base **(Fig. 1)**.
- Lymphatic dissemination results in regional lymphadenopathy which may breakdown to form a discharging sinus.

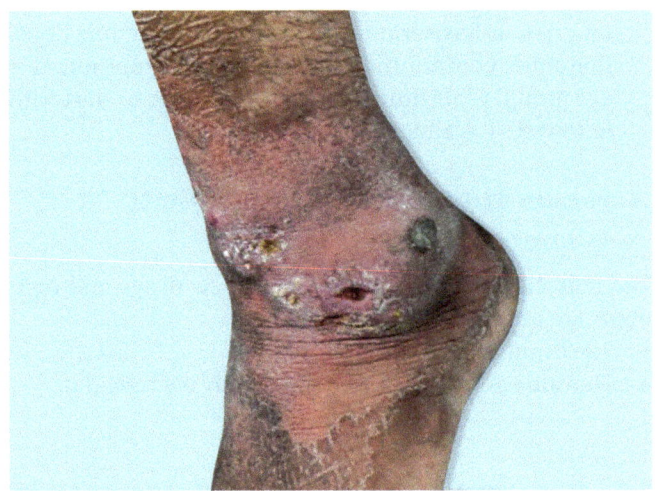

FIG. 1: Tubercular chancre following intra-articular injection with infected needle.

Diagnosis

Diagnosis is by histopathology: Early changes show acute neutrophilic inflammation. After 3–6 weeks, caseating granulomas develop and the bacilli disappear. Fine-needle aspiration cytology (FANC) from the involved lymph nodes may show epithelioid granuloma with or without acid-fast bacilli (AFB). Aspirate from fine-needle aspiration (FNA) can also be used to conduct cartridge-based nucleic acid amplification testing (CBNAAT) which is a rapid molecular diagnostic procedure to detect MTB and rifampicin (Rcin) resistance.

Differential Diagnosis
- Ulcerative lupus vulgaris
- Bacterial infection
- Scrofuloderma

Management

The chancre tends to heal spontaneously with atrophic scarring between 3 and 12 months. However, antitubercular treatment (ATT) is strongly recommended, since untreated chancre may become complicated with development of lupus vulgaris (LV) or scrofuloderma (SFD), or may disseminate resulting in acute miliary tuberculosis (TB).

Tuberculosis Verrucosa Cutis (*Synonym* "Warty Tuberculosis")

Clinical Features

- Tuberculosis verrucosa cutis (TVC) results from the primary inoculation of MTB in previously sensitized individuals who maintain moderate-to-high immunity.
- TVC presents as a solitary painless verrucous papule or plaque with serpiginous outline and central involution, over extremities and other trauma prone sites such as feet **(Figs. 2 and 3)**, hands **(Fig. 4)**, and buttocks. The surface shows fissures or clefts and often perilesional erythema is present. Sometimes, exuberant, extensive form of the disease may result in deformity of the limbs. Regional lymphadenopathy is relatively less common.

Differential Diagnosis

The TVC should be differentiated from hypertrophic LV, common warts, hypertrophic lichen planus, and subcutaneous fungal infections like chromoblastomycosis/pheohyphomycosis.

Diagnosis

Clinical diagnosis is to be confirmed on histopathology that shows striking epidermal hypertrophic changes like pseudoepitheliomatous hyperplasia, the presence of acute neutrophilic abscesses in the upper dermis and characteristic but sparse tuberculoid granulomas in the mid dermis **(Fig. 5)**.

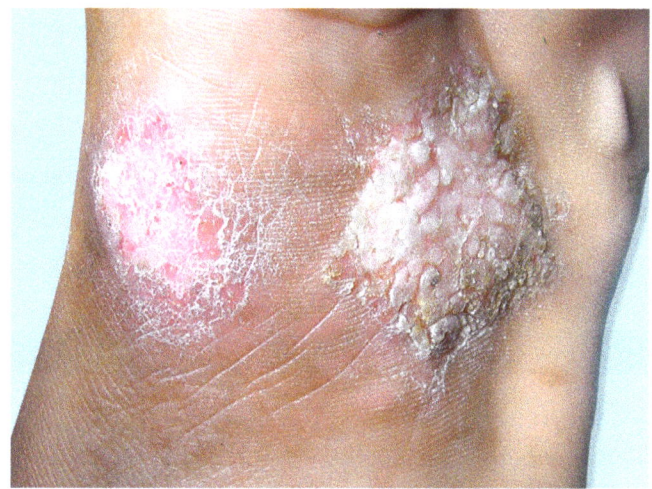

FIG. 3: Classic verrucous lesions of tuberculosis verrucosa cutis (TVC) on sole.

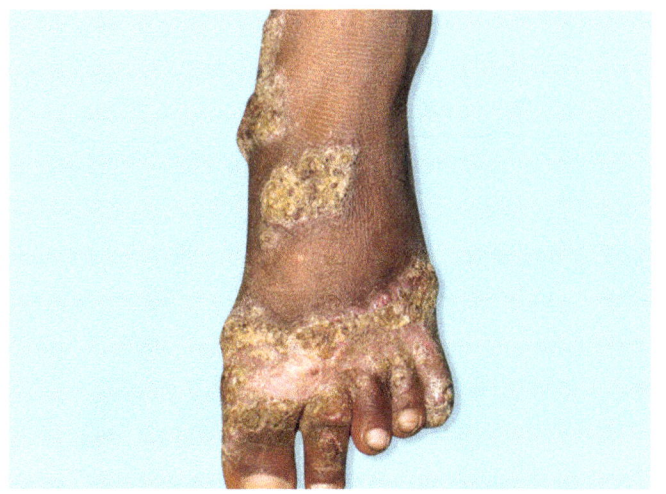

FIG. 2: Extensive, multiple tuberculosis verrucosa cutis (TVC) lesion on the left foot.

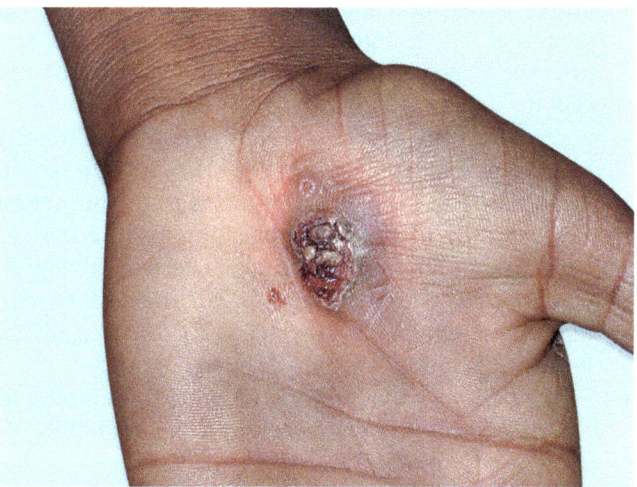

FIG. 4: Tuberculosis verrucosa cutis (TVC) lesion on the palm with fissuring and blood stained discharge.

CHAPTER 10: Cutaneous Tuberculosis

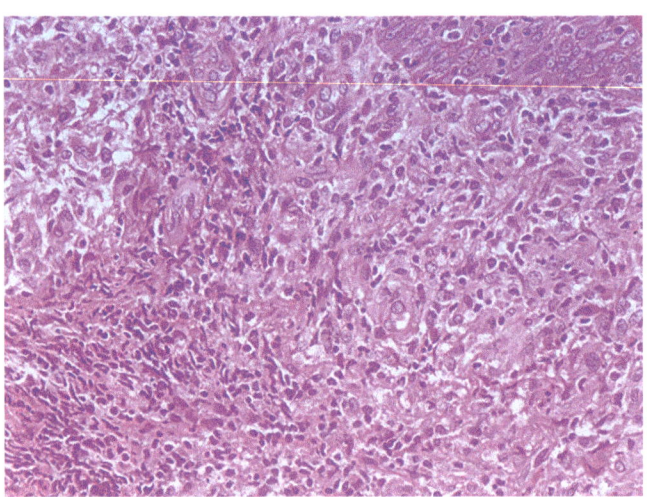

FIG. 5: Acute neutrophilic abscess formation in the upper dermis and characteristic tuberculoid epithelioid granulomas in the mid dermis (Hematoxylin and eosin staining, 400×).

Course

Without specific treatment, extension is extremely slow and the lesion tends to persist indefinitely. However, they may be complicated by secondary bacterial infection and elephantiasis.

Scrofuloderma

Clinical Features

- Scrofuloderma is the most commonly observed form of CTB in India, particularly in children and occurs as a result of contiguous spread from an underlying tubercular focus, usually lymph nodes or bone, joints and sometimes testicles.
- The cervical lymph nodes constitute the most common source of SFD lesions followed by inguinal, axillary, pre- and postauricular, occipital, and submandibular nodes.
- Scrofuloderma presents as a painless, gradually expanding cold abscesses **(Fig. 6)** overlying lymph nodes or bone/joint that ruptures with the formation of a shallow ulcer with bluish undermined edges **(Fig. 7)** that tend to heal with puckered scarring. In children and immunosuppressed, the lesions can be multiple and widespread **(Fig. 8)**. The underlying bone may show lytic lesions **(Fig. 9)**.
- Scrofuloderma is often associated with a systemic tuberculous focus such as pulmonary and abdominal TB.

Differential Diagnosis

- Bacterial abscesses
- Hideradenitis suppurativa

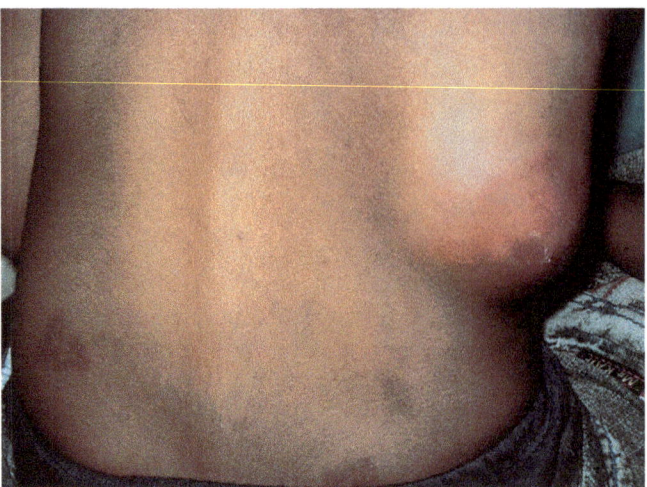

FIG. 6: Painless cold abscess just below the costal margin.

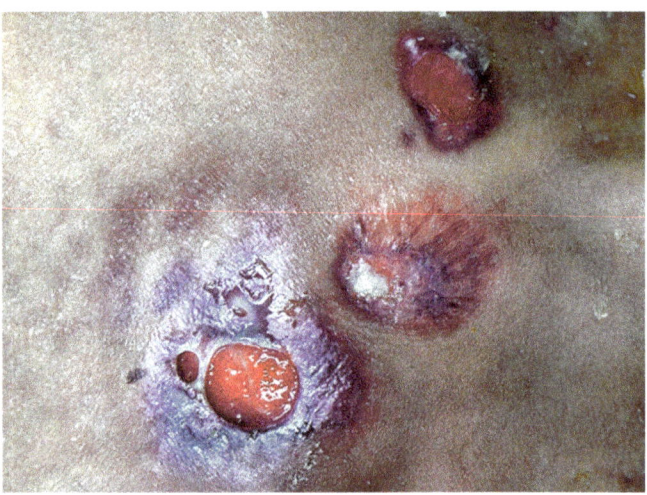

FIG. 7: Tuberculous ulcer with typical bluish undermined margins overlying sternal tuberculosis (TB) focus.

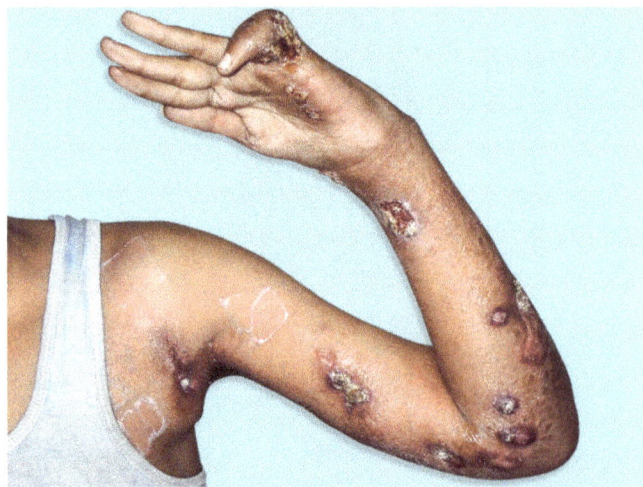

FIG. 8: Widespread lesions of scrofuloderma in a malnourished girl child.

CHAPTER 10: Cutaneous Tuberculosis

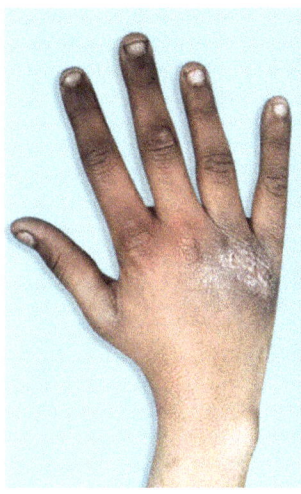
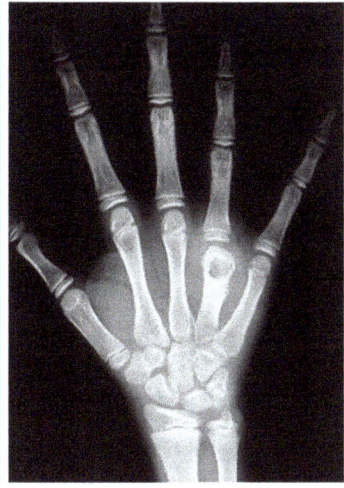

FIG. 9: Lytic lesions in the fourth metacarpal bone of right hand overlying scrofuloderma lesion.

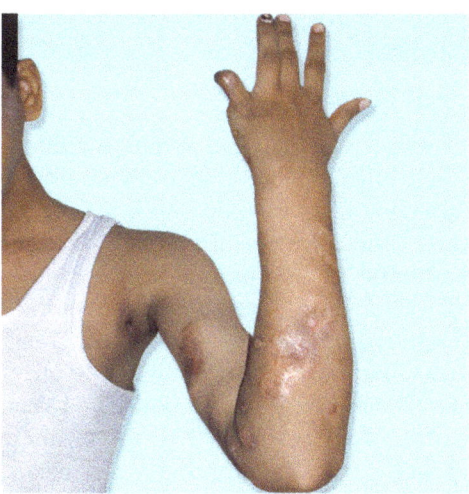

FIG. 10: Scrofuloderma lesions healing with scars following 6 months antitubercular treatment (ATT).

- Atypical mycobacterial infection (*Mycobacterium avium* and *Mycobacterium scrofulaceum*)
- Sporotrichosis
- Actinomycosis

Diagnosis

Diagnosis is mainly clinical. Cytology smears from the lymph node and biopsy from the ulcer edge show granulomas with giant cells and caseation necrosis with AFB suggestive of tubercular etiology. Mycobacterial culture on Lowenstein-Jensen medium often yields growth of *MTB*. Mantoux is strongly positive.

Course

SFD runs a very protracted course, though it may heal spontaneously over months and years with puckered scarring **(Fig. 10)**.

Orificial Tuberculosis (*Synonym* Tuberculosis Cutis Orificialis)

Clinical Features

- Orificial TB often affects the middle-aged and elderly men with impaired cell-mediated immunity. Lesions follow autoinoculation of *MTB* in to the mucosa or the skin adjoining orifices in a patient with concomitant focus of advances in intestinal or genitourinary TB. The disease is now very rare.
- Patient with orificial TB is severely ill. Lesions consist of 1–3 cm sized erythematous to yellowish, friable, and painful papules and nodules developing more commonly in or around mouth and less commonly surrounding genital or anal mucosae **(Fig. 11)**. They evolve into painful ulcers with undermined bluish edges.

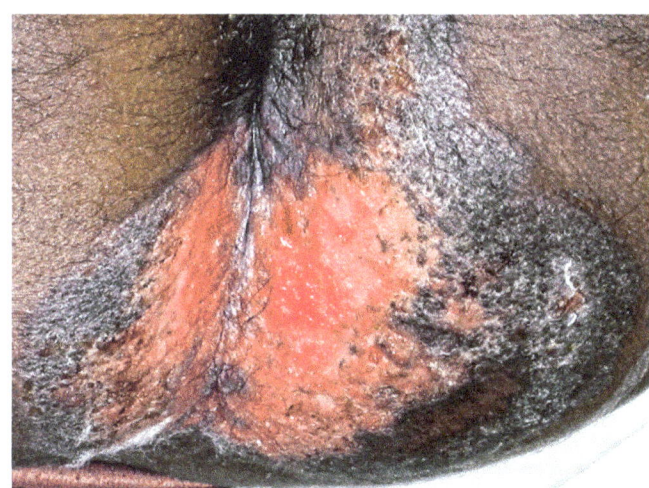

FIG. 11: Painful perianal and perineal tuberculosis ulcers.

Diagnosis

Pain is the cardinal feature and there is usually an evidence of advanced systemic TB elsewhere, generally gastrointestinal and genitourinary tract. The tuberculin test is variable and the patient is often anergic in the later stages due to profound immunosuppression.

Course

The severity of the underlying visceral disease renders a poor prognosis. In untreated cases, disease progression may result in fatality.

Lupus Vulgaris

Clinical Features

- Lupus vulgaris is the most common clinical type of CTB in adults. It occurs in individuals previously sensitized to MTB with moderate immunity.
- The most common mode of infection is hematogenous or lymphatic dissemination from an endogenous source, it may also develop from direct inoculation, at site of *Bacillus* Calmette–Guérin (BCG) vaccination **(Fig. 12)**. The most common sites of involvement are the head, neck, and gluteal region **(Fig. 13)** and lower extremities and face **(Fig. 14)**. Involvement of the upper limbs, trunk, and multiple sites has also been reported **(Fig. 15)**.
- Typical lesions consist of papules and well-defined, reddish-brown plaques that expand peripherally, with serpiginous or verrucous borders and central atrophy **(Fig. 16)**. Presence of involution in one area of the lesion and progression in another area resulting in a geographic or gyrate appearance is characteristic of LV. Diascopy of the lesion has classically been described to reveal soft reddish brown "apple jelly" nodules. Other morphological variants include hypertrophic, ulcerative, and mutilating LV. Regional lymphadenopathy is common. Systemic tubercular foci have been reported in the lymph nodes and lungs.

Differential Diagnosis

- Sarcoidosis
- Hansen's disease
- Lupus erythematosus

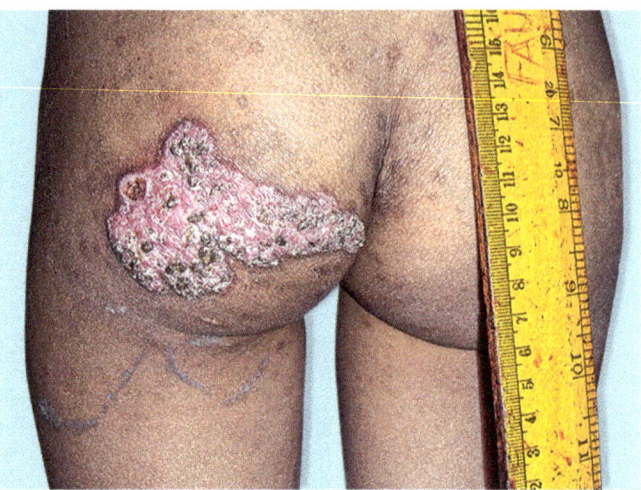

FIG. 13: Lupus vulgaris lesion on the buttock at previous injection site.

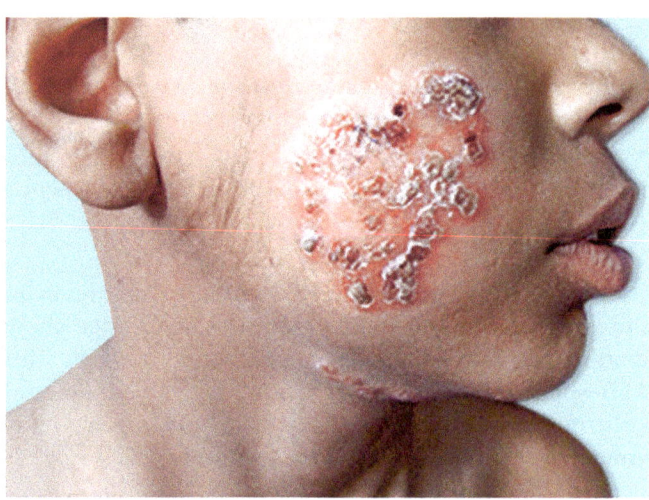

FIG. 14: Well-defined erythematous crusted plaque of lupus vulgaris on face of a child.

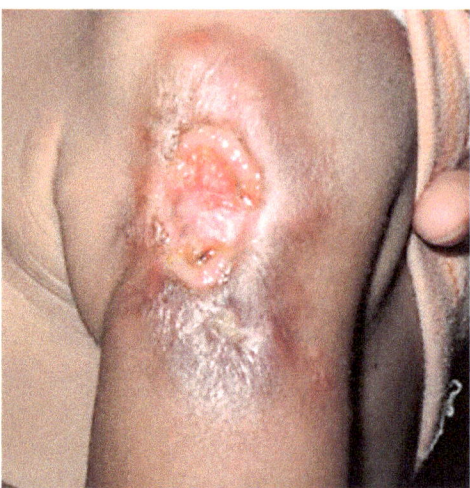

FIG. 12: Lupus vulgaris (LV) developing at the site of *Bacillus* Calmette–Guérin vaccination in a child.

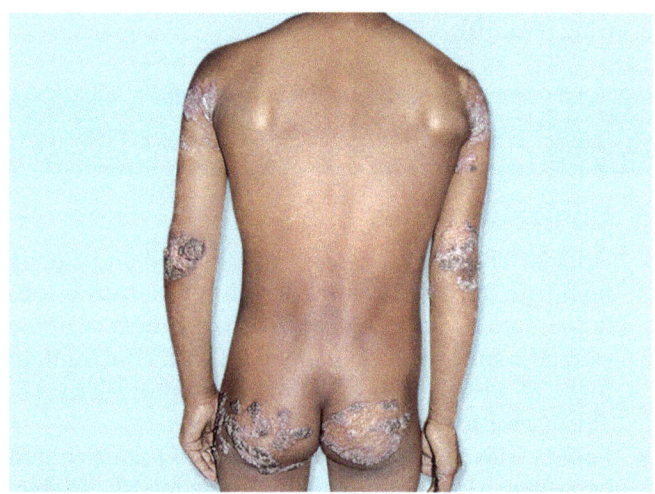

FIG. 15: Classical, multifocal lesion of lupus vulgaris in an immunocompetent boy.

CHAPTER 10: Cutaneous Tuberculosis

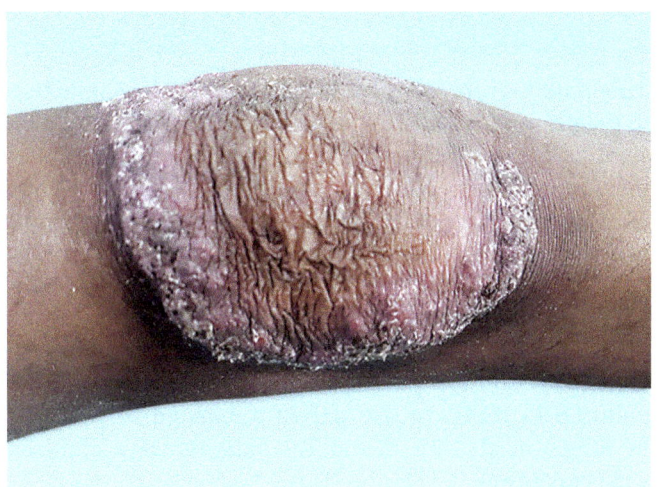

FIG. 16: Lupus vulgaris lesion with serpiginous, expanding plaque, and central clearing.

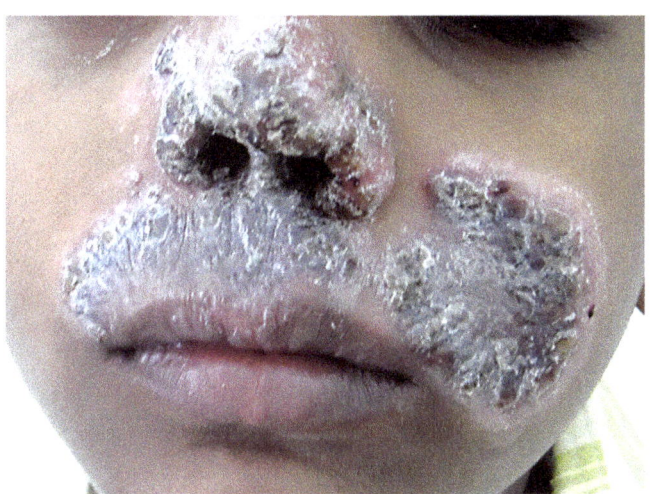

FIG. 18: Lesion of lupus vulgaris of nose leading to destruction of nasal septum.

Course

Untreated LV lesions may grow to become gigantic and often lead to tissue destruction with contractures involving the knee, elbow, and wrist, and destruction of ear and nose **(Fig. 18)**. Malignant transformation into squamous cell carcinoma of untreated LV lesions has ranged from 0.5 to 10.5%.

Tuberculous Gumma (*Synonym* Metastatic Tuberculous Abscess)

Clinical Features

- Tuberculous gumma, results from hematogenous dissemination of TB infection during periods of lowered immunity resulting in single or multiple lesions not related to the lymph nodes or joints.
- Lesions involve both trunk and extremities and are characterized by fluctuant nontender subcutaneous nodules that may later break down to form sinuses or undermined ulcers **(Fig. 19)**. Regional lymphadenopathy is usually not present.

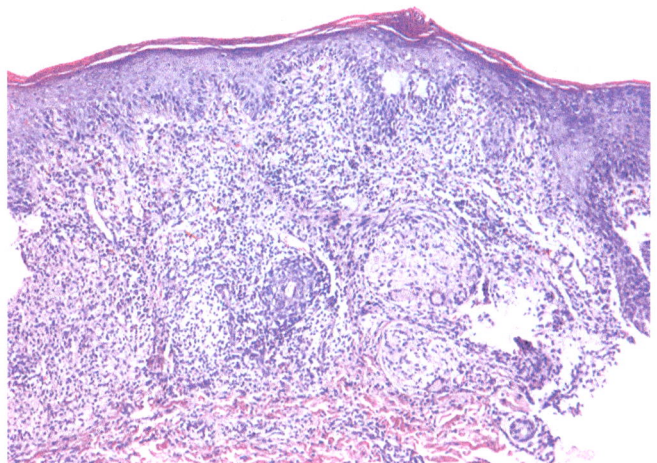

FIG. 17: Epithelioid granuloma with abundant lymphocytes and Langhans giant cell in upper dermis (Hematoxylin and eosin staining, 40 × 10×).

- Granuloma faciale
- Leishmaniasis
- Squamous cell carcinoma

Diagnosis

Histopathology of LV lesions reveals typical epithelioid granulomas in the upper dermis, with lymphocytes and Langhans giant cells in majority **(Fig. 17)**. Necrosis is absent and fibrosis is evident in areas of healing and scarring. AFB are scant and difficult to detect by staining methods or mycobacterial culture; thus LV is considered a paucibacillary form of CTB.

Diagnosis

Presence of tubercles with widespread caseous necrosis and copious amounts of AFB is seen on the FANC smears and histopathology.

Treatment

In immunocompetent individuals, abscesses may persist for years without treatment followed by spontaneous

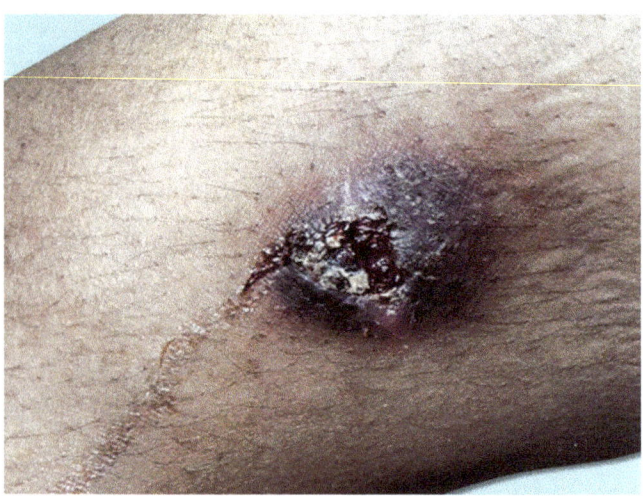

FIG. 19: Tuberculous gumma involving the right thigh in a patient with tubercular pulmonary effusion.

resolution with scarring. Patients with compromised immunity tend to have a poor prognosis.

Miliary Tuberculosis

Miliary TB of skin develops in association with generalized miliary TB due to hematogenous dissemination of mycobacteria into the skin. It is a rare and severe form of TB that affects children with poor immune status like in human immunodeficiency virus/acquired immunodeficiency syndrome (HIV/AIDS).

Clinical Features

Widespread erythematous to purplish papules, pustules, or vesicles develop that subsequently breakdown resulting in umbilication and crust formation. Lesions tend to regress in 1–4 weeks with scars. Affected patients are seriously ill with marked constitutional symptoms such as fever, anorexia, and weight loss. Tuberculin skin test is almost always negative.

Differential Diagnosis

Varicella, enteroviral exanthemata, and pityriasis lichenoides et varioliformis acuta (PLEVA).

Diagnosis

Histopathology shows acute inflammatory cells with numerous microabscesses. Being a multibacillary form of CTB, AFB are easily demonstrable.

Course

The overall prognosis is poor, but may respond to ATT.

Tuberculides

Tuberculides represent cutaneous immunologic reaction to the presence of MTB or their products in a patient with significant immunity. Diagnostic features of tuberculides include tuberculoid histology on skin biopsy, absence of AFB in smears, negative mycobacterial culture, evidence of active or healed tubercular focus elsewhere in the body, positive tuberculin test, and swift resolution of the lesions with ATT.

Lichen scrofulosorum (LS) has emerged as one of the most common presentations of CTB, especially in children in India. In the largest published series of LS by Singal et al., 70% of the 221 patients were children <15 years of age.

Lichen Scrofulosorum

Clinical Features

- It is characterized by grouped, 1–5 mm sized, asymptomatic, skin-colored to erythematous, follicular or perifollicular, flat-topped to spinous papules, most commonly over the trunk **(Fig. 20)** but may involve proximal limbs **(Fig. 21)**. LS confined to the vulva; genital tuberculid **(Fig. 22)**, associated with cervical and inguinal lymphadenitis, has been reported.
- A systemic focus of TB is detected in a majority of LS cases, the most common being involvement of lymph nodes and pulmonary TB followed by other forms of CTBs such as SFD, LV, and erythema induratum of Bazin (EIB) and with papulonecrotic tuberculid (PNT).

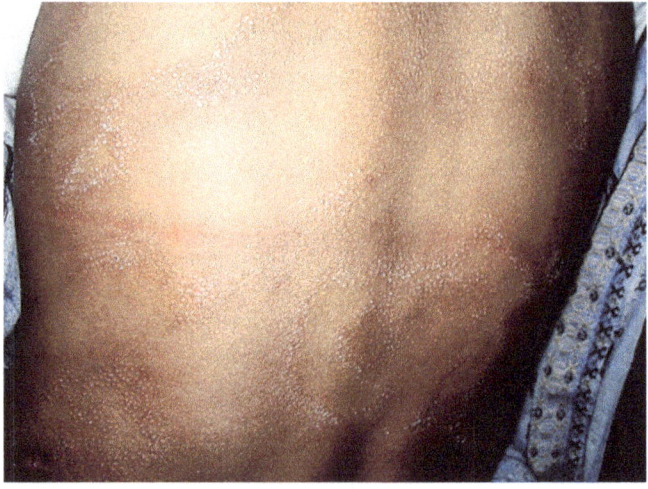

FIG. 20: Skin colored to erythematous grouped follicular papules of lichen scrofulosorum over trunk.

CHAPTER 10: Cutaneous Tuberculosis

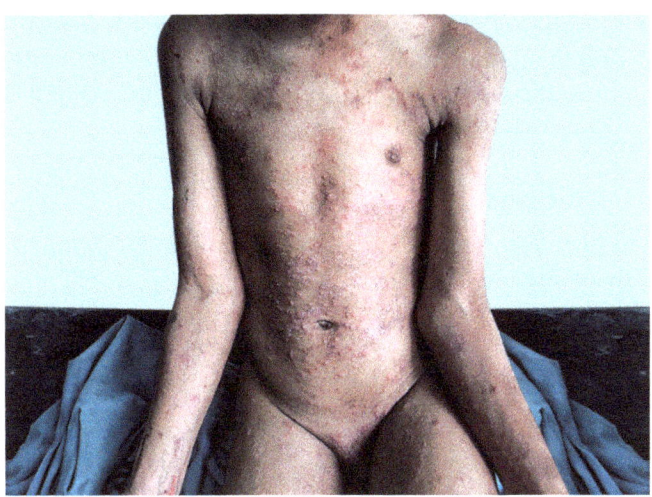

FIG. 21: Generalized lichen scrofulosorum lesions in a patient with pulmonary tuberculosis.

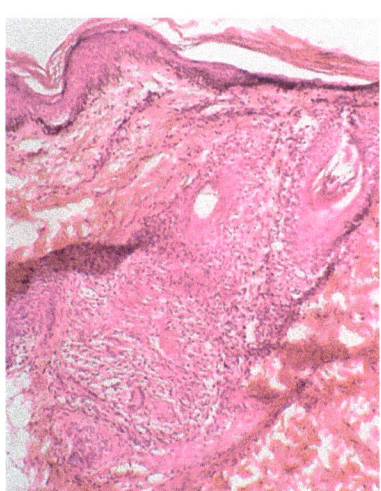

FIG. 23: Dense, perifollicular epithelioid cell infiltrate with Langhans giant cell in lichen scrofulosorum (Hematoxylin and eosin, 40 × 10×).

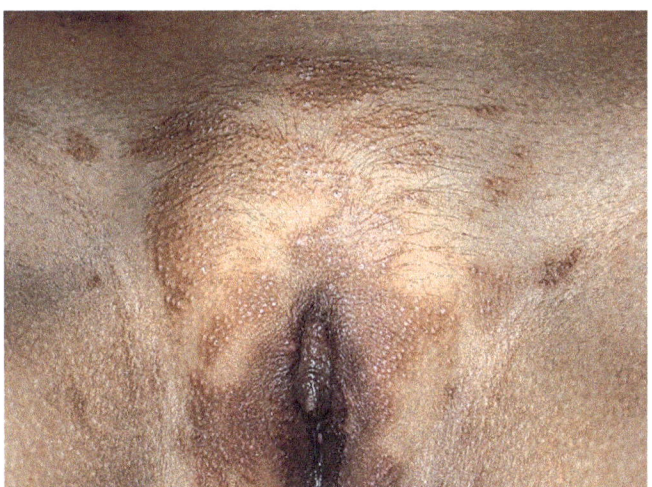

FIG. 22: Lesions of lichen scrofulosorum (LS) confined to external genitalia in a young girl (genital tuberculid).

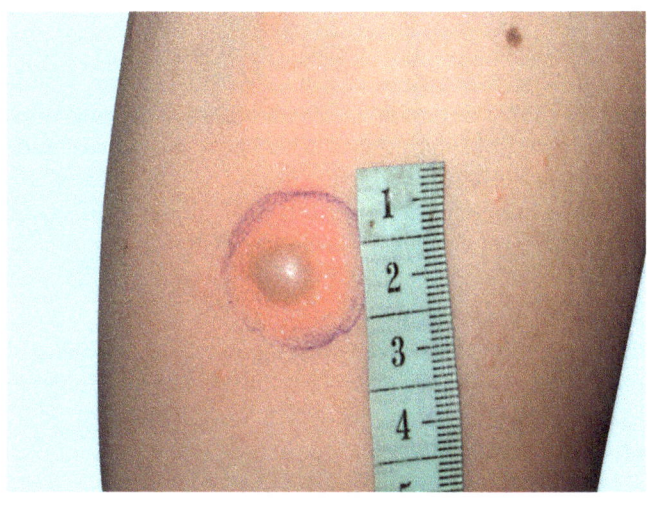

FIG. 24: Indurated erythematous plaque (>10 mm) with vesiculation at Mantoux site in lichen scrofulosorum (LS).

Differential Diagnosis

Keratosis pilaris, lichen spinulosa, pityriasis rubra pilaris (PRP), lichen nitidus, and phrynoderma.

Diagnosis

The clinical diagnosis of LS is corroborated on histology that shows perifollicular epithelioid granulomas without any caseation **(Fig. 23)**. Expectedly, AFBs are not detected and mycobacterial cultures and PCR are negative from lesional biopsies. Tuberculin test is strongly positive, with development of vesicular/vesicobullous lesions and frequent occurrence of ulceration at the test site **(Fig. 24)**.

Papulonecrotic Tuberculid

Clinical Features

Papulonecrotic tuberculid is less commonly encountered in India. It is characterized by presence of symmetrically distributed firm, dusky red necrotizing papules and pustules, mostly over the extremities **(Fig. 25)**, though, face, ears, trunk, and buttocks may also be affected. Lymphadenopathy and associated pulmonary TB may be present. PNT has also been reported after BCG vaccination. Tuberculin test is positive.

Differential Diagnosis

Varicella and pityriasis lichenoid et varioliform acuta.

CHAPTER 10: Cutaneous Tuberculosis

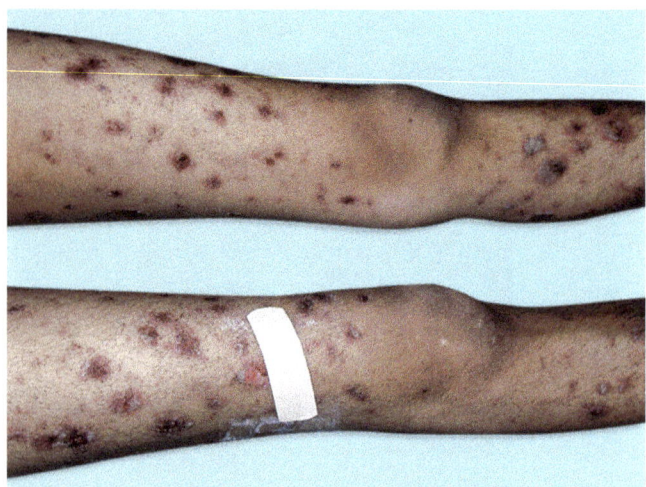

FIG. 25: Lesions of papulonecrotic tuberculid in crops on lower limbs.

▪ Diagnosis

Diagnosis is made clinically. Histopathology shows wedge-shaped necrosis of the epidermis, upper dermis with perifollicular epithelioid cell granulomas, and non-specific perivascular infiltrate. Leukocytoclastic vasculitis is a characteristic histological feature of PNT. Although, AFB are not demonstrable but *MTB* deoxyribonucleic acid (DNA) is frequently detected by PCR.

▪ Course

Eruption tends to resolve spontaneously after weeks to months, resulting in formation of depressed varioliform scars, pathognomonic of PNT. In absence of ATT, recurrences are common.

Erythema Induratum of Bazin

▪ Clinical Features

- Erythema induratum of Bazin (EIB) is a granulomatous lobular panniculitis, which affects the lower limbs of young and middle-aged adults, typically women. Children are rarely affected.
- Lesions appear as slightly painful erythematous to violaceous indurated plaques and nodules that may rupture to form deep ulcers and crusts, preferentially affecting the posterior and anterolateral aspects of the lower legs and thighs **(Fig. 26)**. EIB is frequently associated with pulmonary TB. Tuberculin test is strongly positive in patients with EIB.

▪ Differential Diagnosis

- Erythema nodosum (EN), cutaneous polyarteritis nodosa (PAN), lupus profundus, and subcutaneous sarcoid.

- Erythema nodosum also presents with painful erythematous plaques and nodules, predominantly over the extensor aspects of lower extremities **(Fig. 27)** and seldom ulcerate.

▪ Diagnosis

On histology, there is lobular or septolobular panniculitis in EIB. *MTB* DNA is detected by PCR in >50% of the cases.

▪ Course

Lesions may regress, even without treatment, after weeks to months, leaving depressed postinflammatory scarring and hyperpigmentation.

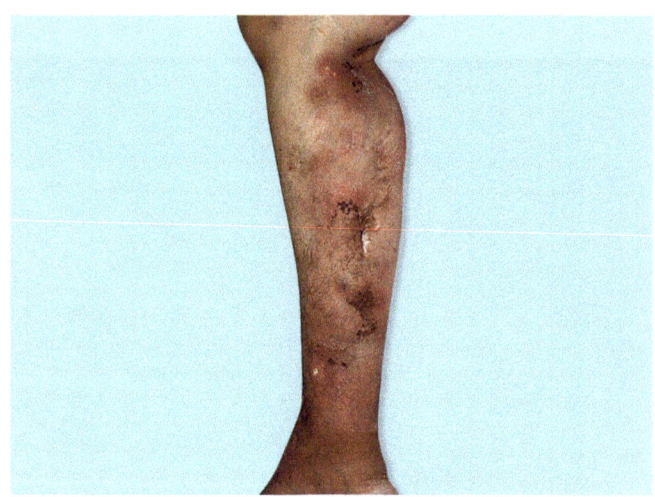

FIG. 26: Healed ulcerative lesions of erythema induratum of Bazin on the flexor aspect of leg.

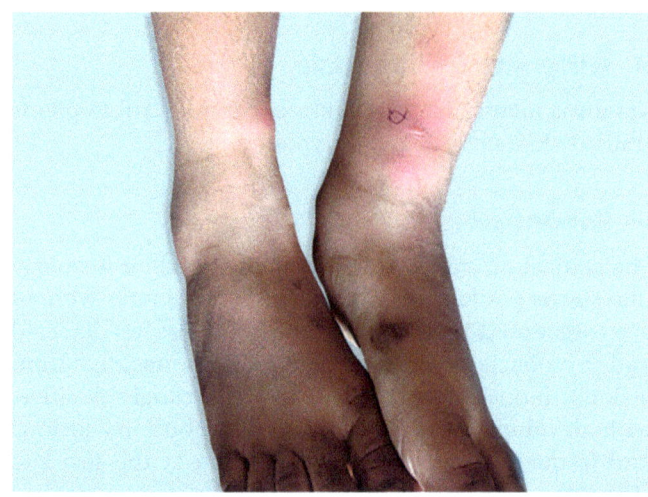

FIG. 27: Erythematous tender nodules of erythema nodosum around ankle and shins.

CHAPTER 10: Cutaneous Tuberculosis

Management

Systemic screening for tubercular focus.
- Coexistent systemic focus of TB has been observed in about 40–50% of all patients with cutaneous lesions. Associated TB focus elsewhere in the body is a guide to the duration of ATT.
- A clinical assessment of lymph nodes, pulmonary and gastrointestinal system, nervous system, eyes, and musculoskeletal system should be performed.
- Fine-needle aspiration cytology should be performed from the enlarged lymph nodes, and a part of the aspirate should be used for the culture of *MTB and CBNAAT*.
- Roentgenogram of chest and computed tomography (CT) scan (if required).
- Sputum should be sent for AFB and mycobacterial culture.
- Ultrasonography should be performed to screen for abdominal and pelvic TB.
- X-rays of the joints and bones suspected with tubercular osteomyelitis or arthritis.
- In cases with paravertebral cold abscesses, magnetic resonance imaging (MRI) spine is required.

Treatment

Antitubercular Treatment (Table 1)

Category I regimen is more suitable to provide better infection control in patients with CTB. Revised National Tuberculosis Control Program (RNTCP) Category I regimen consists of initial 2 months intensive phase of daily isoniazid (H, 6 mg/kg), rifampicin (R, 10 mg/kg), pyrazinamide (Z, 25 mg/kg), and ethambutol (E, 15 mg/kg) followed by a 4 month continuation phase with isoniazid, rifampicin, and ethambutol (2HRZE + 4HRE).

Prevention

- BCG vaccination, an essential component of Universal Immunization Program in India has doubtful efficacy in the prevention of CTB. However, its role in the containment of disseminated pulmonary and extrapulmonary disease including CTB is proven.
- Early identification and treatment of pulmonary TB in household contacts is important to prevent transmission of *MTB* through minor injuries and skin abrasions.
- Use of pasteurized and boiled milk should be encouraged.
- Promoting the use of sterilized single use disposable needles for injections, ear/nose piercings and other cultural rituals.
- Improving the overall standard of living with better hygiene and nutrition.

Clinical Pearls

- CTB has reemerged worldwide. HIV pandemic has significantly contributed to the increasing incidence in the last few decades.
- There is no gender predilection and the disease is reported in both adults and children.
- Given the plethora of cutaneous manifestations of TB, a high index of suspicion is of utmost importance in making the correct diagnosis.
- Scrofuloderma and LV are most common variants. However, tuberculides, especially, LS lesions are increasingly being recognized particularly in children.
- The clinical diagnosis of CTB should be supported by histology/cytology, culture, or PCR. Whenever possible, lymph node or lesional aspirate should be sent for CBNAAT to confirm the diagnosis and check

TABLE 1: Recommended dosage for drugs used in the treatment of cutaneous tuberculosis.				
Drug	Daily treatment adult (mg)	Daily treatment child (mg/kg)	DOTS adult (mg)	DOTS child (mg/kg)
H (Isoniazid)	300	6	600	10
R (Rifampicin)	450	10	450	10
Z (Pyrizinamide)	1,500	25	1,500	25
E (Ethambutol)	800	15	1,200	25

- for multidrug therapy resistance (MDR) (Rcin) which is becoming increasingly common.
- A diligent search to look for the systemic focus of TB should be made as concurrent TB is seen in about one-third cases.
- Response to short course ATT is generally good.
- It is important to be aware of the existence of MDR and extensively drug-resistant cutaneous tuberculosis (XDR-CTB) to prevent the transmission of primary drug resistant CTB.

CHAPTER 11

Nontuberculous Mycobacteria

Introduction

Cutaneous infections with nontuberculous mycobacteria (NTM), previously known as "atypical mycobacteria" or "mycobacteria other than *Mycobacterium tuberculosis* (MOTT)", include species other than the *M. tuberculosis* complex. NTM infections, which used to be considered unusual, are becoming frequent nowadays, particularly in immunocompromised individuals. Based on the growth rate of these organisms in culture, these are classified into slow-growing (*Mycobacterium marinum* and *Mycobacterium ulcerans*) and rapidly-growing mycobacteria (*Mycobacterium fortuitum*, *Mycobacterium chelonae*, and *Mycobacterium abscessus*). Rapid-growing mycobacteria are responsible for >90% of cutaneous infections.

Nontuberculous mycobacteria are found in water, wet soil, house dust, dairy products, vegetation, and human feces. The organism is transmitted by inhalation, ingestion, or percutaneous penetration resulting in pulmonary, lymph node, or skin disease.

Three types of cutaneous lesions caused by NTM are recognized:
1. A solitary granulomatous verrucous papule that may occasionally ulcerate and show purulent discharge.
2. Ascending lymphatic sporotrichoid lesions.
3. Rare cutaneous disseminated lesions, which occur frequently in immunosuppressed patients.

Slow-growing Mycobacteria

The mycobacteria require >7 days to reach mature growth with or without the requirement of nutritional supplementation of routine media. Cultivation of this species is difficult, as it requires up to several months to grow.

Mycobacterium marinum

Mycobacterium marinum causes an infection historically recognized as a "swimming pool" or "fish tank" granuloma, which has an incubation period of 2–3 weeks. Occupational or recreational exposure to salt or freshwater occurs in the majority of cases. Swimming pools seem to be a risk only when nonchlorinated.

Clinical Features

Most often, there is a single small violaceous papule, which may be painful in some. It usually involves the upper extremity and may progress to shallow, crusty, and ulcerative lesions. When there are multiple lesions, a "sporotrichoid" pattern can be seen **(Figs. 1A to D)**. Regional lymph nodes are generally not involved and systemic symptoms are unusual. The infection resolves spontaneously in some cases; although, complete resolution may take up to 2 years.

Differential Diagnosis

- *Solitary verrucous/ulcerated lesion*: Verruca vulgaris, sporotrichosis, blastomycosis, erysipeloid, tuberculosis verrucosa cutis, nocardiosis, leishmaniasis, syphilis, iododerma, and malignant skin tumors.
- *Sporotrichoid lesion*: Staphylococcal or group A streptococcal lymphangitis, sporotrichosis, leishmaniasis, nocardiosis, actinomycosis, and anthrax.

Diagnosis

- A history of contact with water, fish tanks, aquariums, etc., combined with granulomatous histology is suggestive of the diagnosis
- *Acid–fast bacilli (AFB)* can be demonstrated in some cases on direct microscopy of pus.
- *Skin biopsy*: For older lesions more typical tuberculoid architecture is developed with epithelioid cells

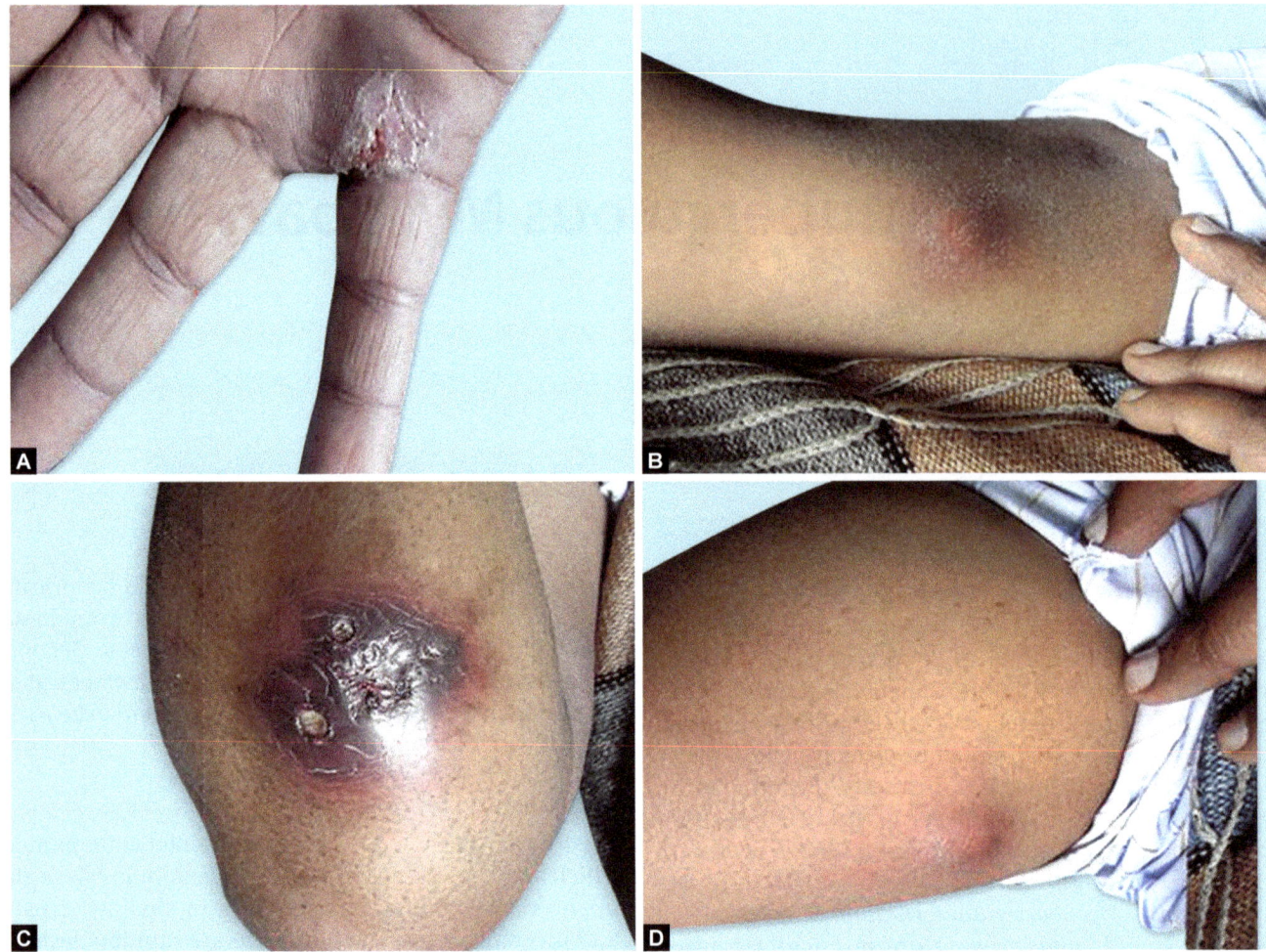

FIGS. 1A TO D: Multiple lesions of *Mycobacterium marinum* infection arranged in an ascending fashion on the right upper limb.

and Langhans giant cells. Intracellular AFB, longer and broader than *M. tuberculosis* are detectable in approximately 10% of cases.
- *Culture*: Positive in 70–80% of cases. *M. marinum* grows at 32°C in 2–4 weeks. Early lesions yield numerous colonies.
- *Serology*: Species-specific monoclonal antibody against 56-kDa *M. marinum* antigens has been identified using polymerase chain reaction (PCR)-reverse cross-blot hybridization assay with species-specific gene probes.

Treatment
- Clarithromycin is the drug of choice and can be used in combination with rifampicin and continued for 1–2 months after resolution of symptoms, typically at least 3–6 months in total.
- Minocycline > doxycycline, ethambutol, and trimethoprim–sulfamethoxazole have also been used with variable success.

Mycobacterium ulcerans (Buruli Ulcer)

It is believed to be the third most common mycobacterial infection after tuberculosis and leprosy. The major virulence factor is a lipid toxin, mycolactone, which causes necrosis of fat and subcutaneous tissue. This is usually seen in wetlands in tropical countries and northern areas of Australia. Exposure to riverine areas (swamps, lakes, slow-flowing rivers, etc.) with humid hot climates is thought to play a role; although, the exact mode of transmission is not known.

Clinical Features
About 70% of patients are children below 15 years of age. The lesions usually begin as single, asymptomatic, firm, mobile subcutaneous nodules commonly involving extremities (lower > upper), which become fluctuant and ulcerate **(Fig. 2)** after 1 or 2 months. The floor of the ulcer is formed of necrotic fat, and there may be a clear mucoid discharge. Ulcers may heal spontaneously with

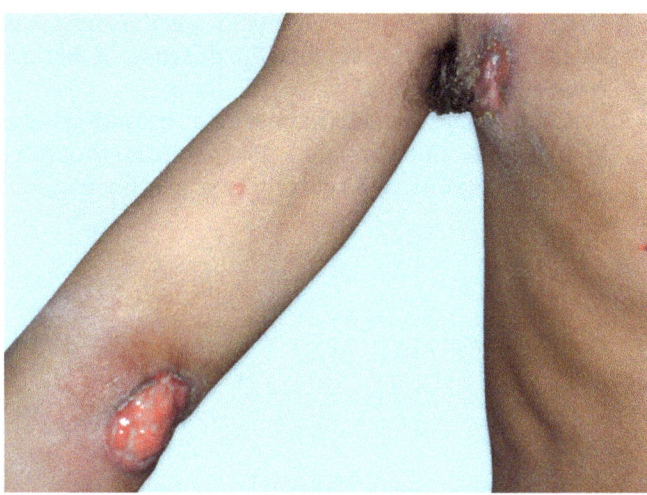

FIG. 2: Subcutaneous ulcerated nodular lesion caused by *Mycobacterium ulcerans*.

scarring or may spread to involve large areas of skin or even underlying soft tissue and bone.

Differential Diagnosis
- *Initial phase*: Panniculitis, nodular fasciitis, cysts, foreign body granuloma, and other granulomatous diseases.
- *Ulcerative phase*: Fungal infections, pyoderma gangrenosum, and suppurative panniculitis.

Diagnosis
- Ziehl–Neelsen-stained smears of exudate or pus reveal clumps of AFB.
- *Culture*: Visible growth often requires 6–8 weeks of incubation at 32°C optimally on routine mycobacteriological media.
- *Histopathology*: Characteristically, there is an extensive involvement of the subcutaneous fat as septal panniculitis. There is poor inflammatory response despite clusters of extracellular bacilli. Ulceration is surrounded by granulation tissue with giant cells but no caseation necrosis or tubercles. AFBs are always demonstrable.
- *PCR*: IS2404 PCR, which can be performed directly from ulcer swabs, approaches 100% sensitivity and specificity.

Treatment
- Recent studies suggest that clarithromycin is highly active *in vitro* against *M. ulcerans*. Treatment with oral rifampicin (10 mg/kg daily) plus clarithromycin (7.5 mg/kg twice daily) for 8–12 weeks is now recommended as first-line treatment by the World Health Organization (WHO).
- Trimethoprim–sulfamethoxazole 80/400 mg BD, quinolones (ciprofloxacin and moxifloxacin), and nitrogen oxide-releasing topical creams may also be used.
- Surgical excision is the traditional treatment with or without skin graft.
- Local continuous heat (40°C) and hyperbaric oxygen are other therapeutic options.

Mycobacterium fortuitum and *Mycobacterium chelonae*

These organisms are widely distributed in the environment in soil, dust, and tap water and may also be commensal organisms of human skin. Infection typically occurs following trauma, surgery, contact with contaminated medical instruments, implants, tattooing, and post-injection.

These organisms are commonly isolated from municipal tap water. *M. chelonae* was found as a contaminant in a gentian violet solution. Pseudo-outbreaks have been most commonly related to contaminated bronchoscopes, endoscopic cleaning machines, and contaminated hospital water supplies.

Mycobacterium chelonae infections are seen primarily in patients who are immunosuppressed, especially on long-term corticosteroids. The *M. fortuitum* group accounts for 60% of community-acquired, localized cutaneous infections caused by rapidly growing mycobacteria (RGM). *M. fortuitum*, localized cutaneous and subcutaneous infections, usually have no predisposing immunosuppression.

Clinical Features
The most common presentation is multiple erythematous subcutaneous nodules, in a sporotrichoid pattern on the distal limbs. Other forms of cutaneous involvement range from cellulitis, abscesses, and papulopustules to sinuses and ulcers.

Differential Diagnosis
- Foreign body reaction
- Subcutaneous mycoses
- Osteomyelitis

Diagnosis
- *Histopathology*: A biopsy from the margin of the abscess is more likely to yield the organism than aspirated pus. The presence of both neutrophilic microabscesses and granuloma formation with foreign body-type giant cells is characteristic. Necrosis may occur.

- *Culture*: The organisms grow on routine bacterial culture media, such as 5% sheep blood agar and chocolate agar, within 7 days producing visible colonies between 5 and 7 days at temperatures ranging between 22 and 45°C.
- *Treatment*: The *M. fortuitum* group is much less drug-resistant than the *M. chelonae*. Macrolides such as clarithromycin and azithromycin are the only oral agents reliably active *in vitro*. The duration of therapy is usually 4–6 months.
- In addition, surgical debridement may be undertaken. Minocycline, ciprofloxacin, ofloxacin, trimethoprim-sulfamethoxazole, and cefoxitin have also been used.

CHAPTER 12

Human Helminthic Infections (Nematodes, Cestodes, and Trematodes)

Introduction

Helminths are a group of parasites that infect humans, either as definitive hosts or as intermediate hosts. The helminths causing cutaneous disease primarily belong to two phyla:
- *Nemathelminthes*: These cause common and disabling diseases among people living in poor and unhygienic conditions including lymphatic filariasis and river blindness.
- *Platyhelminthes*: Cestodes (tapeworms) and trematodes (flukes) are common parasites endemic in Africa, causing skin disease by allergic response or ectopic deposition of their eggs or adult worms.

Lymphatic Filariasis

- It is a disabling parasitic disease caused by human nematodes, spread from person to person by the bite of infected mosquitoes.
- It is prevalent in the tropics and subtropics of Asia, Africa, the Western Pacific, and parts of the Caribbean and South America, affecting over 120 million people worldwide.
- Bihar, Karnataka, Maharashtra, Odisha, Dadra and Nagar Haveli are some of the high endemic zones in India.
- Causative organisms include *Wuchereria bancrofti* (most common), *Brugia malayi*, and *Brugia timori*.
- The life cycle of *W. bancrofti* has been depicted in **Figure 1**.

Clinical Features

- Acute dermato-adeno-lymphangitis (ADLA) is the hallmark of this disease, which causes lymphedema of the legs **(Fig. 2)**.
- Recurrent attacks of fever and painful swelling of lymph nodes of the affected limb are common, leading to progressive lymphatic damage and elephantiasis.
- In bancroftian filariasis, acute epididymo-orchitis (funiculitis) is characterized by severe pain, tenderness, and swelling of the scrotum, usually with fever and rigor. The testes, epididymis, or the spermatic cord may become swollen and extremely tender.
- Hydrocele and tropical pulmonary eosinophilia are other common presentations.
- In endemic areas, a substantial number of patients may be asymptomatic, having microfilariae in their peripheral blood without overt clinical manifestation.
- Lymphedema of extremities is the most common chronic manifestation. In advanced stages, skin is thickened and thrown into folds **(Fig. 2)**, pigmented, warty, with intertrigo in toe webs **(Fig. 3)** and chronic nonhealing ulcers.
- Stemmer's sign involves tenting (pinching) the skin on the upper surface of the toes. Stemmer's sign positive is considered grade 3 of lymphedema. This sign is determined by skinfold thickness over the second toe.
- The most dreaded complication of lymphedema is cellulitis.
- ADLA episodes responsible for the progression of lymphedema continue to occur with even greater frequency in higher grades of edema.

Diagnosis

The diagnosis of lymphedema is mostly clinical.
- In the early asymptomatic phase, night blood samples are helpful to establish the diagnosis with detection of microfilariae in peripheral smear. A definite diagnosis depends solely on microscopic examination of a thick blood smear (20–60 µL) obtained by finger prick, air dried, dehemoglobinized, and stained with Leishman's or Giemsa stain. This helps to identify the

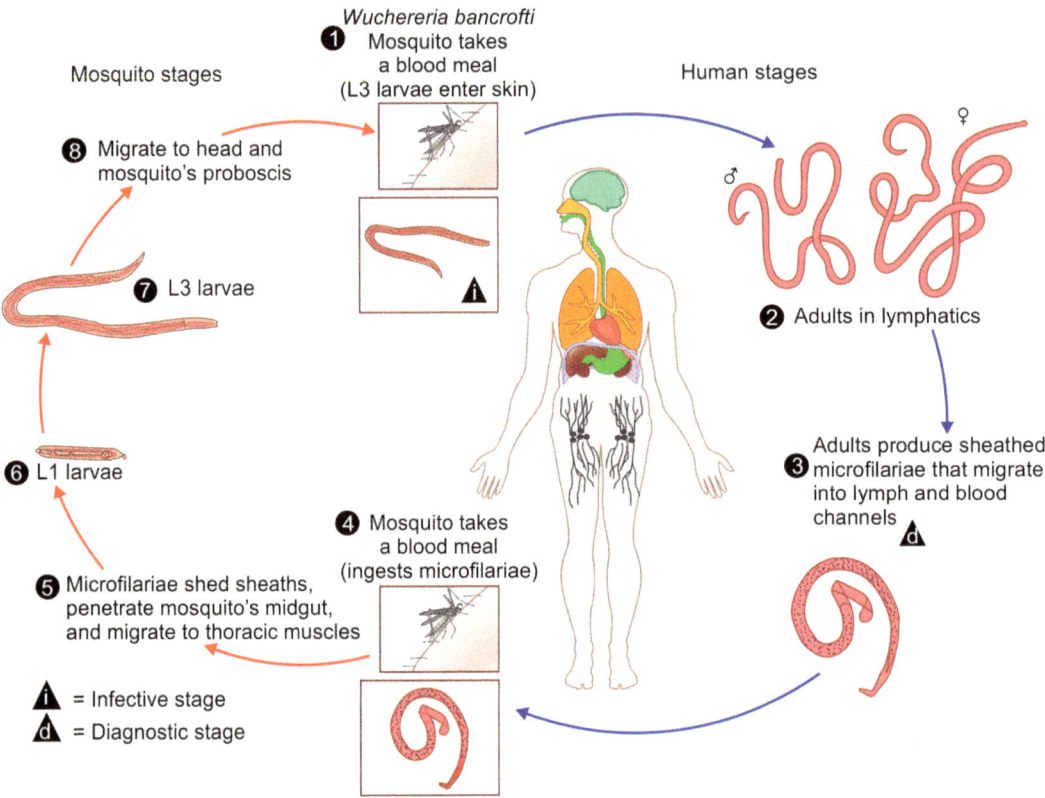

FIG. 1: Life cycle of *Wuchereria bancrofti* showing the infective as well as diseased state. Note the predilection of the worms to localize to the lymph and blood channels, in contrast to *Onchocerca* which localizes to the subcutaneous tissue.
Source: Courtesy of the Centers for Disease Control and Prevention (CDC) [https://www.cdc.gov/dpdx/lymphaticfilariasis/index.html.]

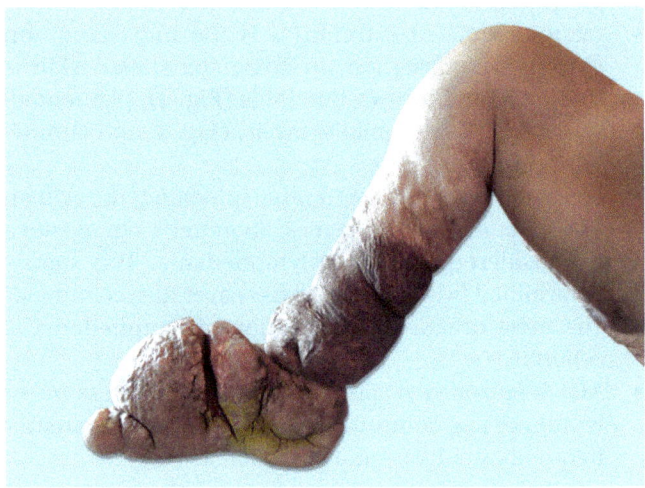

FIG. 2: Elephantiasis of the leg is associated with warty thickening, vesiculation, and pigmentation.

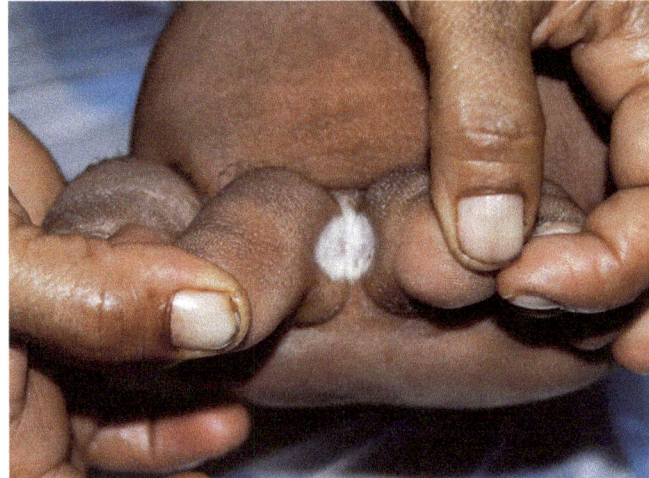

FIG. 3: Fungal intertrigo is a common bacterial entry lesion and must be treated in all patients to prevent attacks of cellulitis.

microfilariae and their species. Microfilariae are rarely seen in the peripheral blood once lymphedema sets in.
- In the majority of cases, etiological diagnosis is by exclusion or is presumptive.
- Antibody determination is considered sufficient as corroborative evidence.

- Filarial antigen detection assays are available as card tests and enzyme-linked immunosorbent assay (ELISA)-based formats. The tests are highly sensitive and specific.
- Immunochromatographic card test (ICT) can be performed on blood samples drawn by finger prick

CHAPTER 12: Human Helminthic Infections (Nematodes, Cestodes, and Trematodes)

at any time of the day. It is positive in the early stages, becoming negative once the worms are dead.
- Ultrasonography with a 7.5–10 MHz probe can locate clusters of living adult filarial worms in the scrotal lymphatics, with their characteristic constant thrashing movement in their "nests", described as the "filarial dance". It is generally not useful in patients with filarial lymphedema, as living adult worms are generally not present at this stage.
- Lymphoscintigraphy can also be useful.

Treatment

For filariasis:
- Diethylcarbamazine citrate (DEC) at 6 mg/kg/day, in three divided doses, for 14 days is the drug of choice as it is both microfilaricidal as well as active against adult worms. In patients with microfilaremia, it is advisable to start with low doses and then scale up like in treatment of onchocerciasis. Concomitant glucocorticoids and/or antihistamines may be required to deal with allergic reactions induced by disintegrating microfilariae.
- Single dose of albendazole 400 mg either with ivermectin 200 µg/kg or DEC 6 mg/kg is effective in reducing *W. bancrofti* microfilaremia.
- Oral doxycycline 100 mg daily for 6 weeks is found to suppress the microfilaremia. It is essential in the prevention of transmission of the disease.

For peripheral lymphedema:
- The late phase of chronic disease is not affected by chemotherapy. Treatment consists of conservative (nonoperative) and operative techniques. The cornerstone for success of virtually all treatment approaches includes meticulous skin hygiene, cleansing care, application of low-pH lotions, and emollients. Basic range of motion exercises of extremities, combined with external limb compression, and limb elevation are also helpful.
- Operative management could include microsurgical procedures (reconstructive methods involving the use of a lymphatic collector or an interposition vein segment or lymphatic-venous and lymph nodal-venous shunts) or surgical resection (debulking, omental transposition, enteromesenteric bridge operations, and implantation of tubes or threads to promote substitute lymphatics). Postsurgery worsening or shifting of lymphedema may also occur **(Fig. 4)**.
- An integrative treatment of lower limb lymphedema has been found effective both at medical centers and resource-poor Indian villages **(Fig. 5)**.
- This includes general measures, including limb elevation by 10–20 cm at bedtime as well as even while

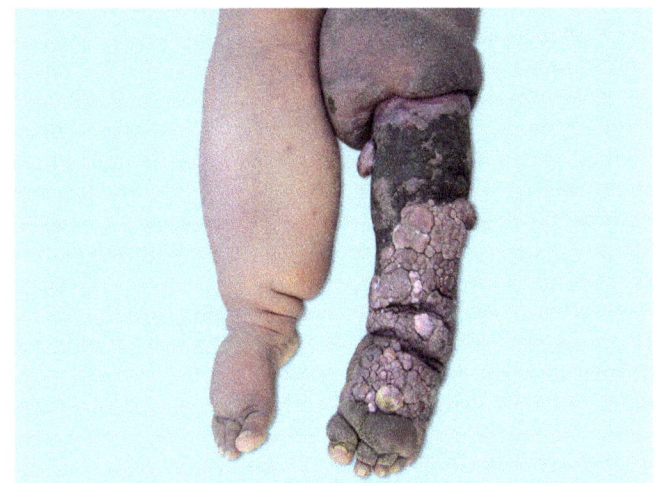

FIG. 4: Scarring following the debulking surgery on the left lower limb lymphedema. The patient subsequently developed lymphedema of the thigh above the area of scaring. Right lower limb lymphedema was not operated.

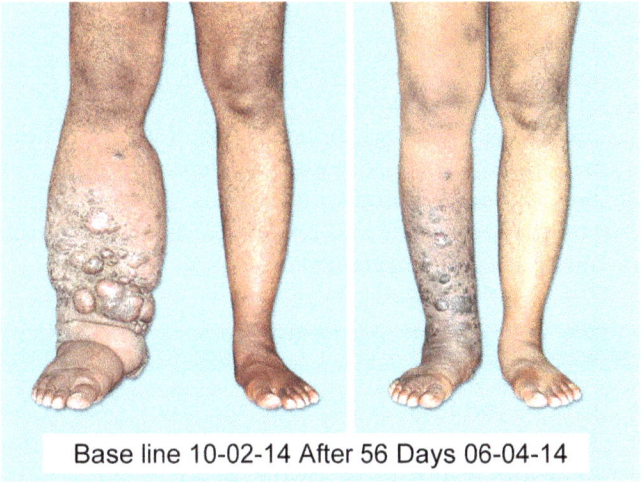

FIG. 5: Response of lower limb lymphedema to integrative treatment. Response to treatment depends on the concordance to treatment by patients back home after the initial 2 weeks of treatment. Treatment involves ayurvedic massages, yoga exercises, and compression bandaging.

sitting, counseling, skin wash, soaking the limb in herbal Phanta solution, a set of yoga exercises, manual lymph drainage, compression bandaging, and postdrainage yoga. Special care of bacterial entry points should be strictly ensured in lymphedema patients.
- Associated gravitational eczema should be treated with topical betamethasone dipropionate (0.05%) cream. Ulcers, if infected, should be treated with appropriate antibiotics. Skin care should include the regular cleaning and paring of nails and hair. Patients are strictly advised to use good, well-fitting footwear,

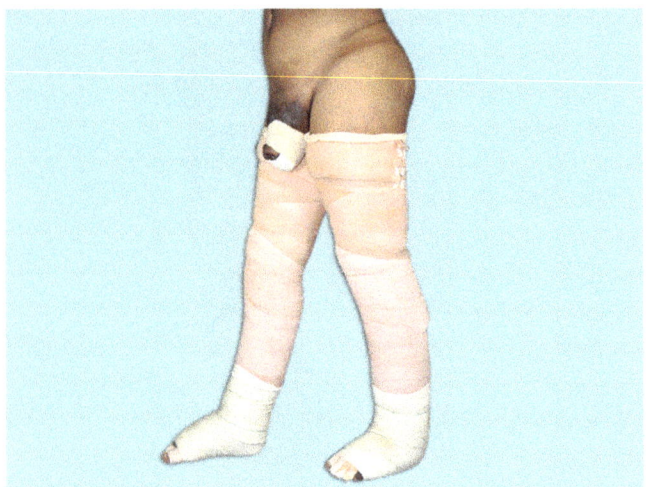

FIG. 6: Compression bandaging.

which sometimes requires customized making. Folliculitis, fissures, and paronychia should be treated properly.
- Compression therapy with long-stretch compression bandages is routinely used in lymphedema and ulcer management **(Fig. 6)**. It helps by reducing capillary filtration, increasing lymphatic resorption, stimulating lymphatic transport, improving venous pump, and breaking down fibrosclerotic tissues. The selection of compression grade and proper size is critical to the success of garment control.

Enterobiasis

- It is a common helminthic infection caused by *Enterobius vermicularis*, also known as threadworm, pinworm, seatworm, or oxyuriasis.
- It has a worldwide distribution and is the most common helminthic infection of industrialized nations.
- Children are most commonly affected.
- The causative agent is *E. vermicularis* for which humans are the only host.
- The infection is transmitted by ingestion of infected eggs **(Fig. 7)** through fecal–oral route, sexual or fomite-borne transmission. The incubation period is 2–8 weeks.

Clinical Features

- A large number of infected children are asymptomatic.
- Primary presenting complaints are nocturnal, anal, and perineal pruritus, with sleeplessness and irritability.
- Anal intertrigo, nocturia, and secondary infection may also occur.

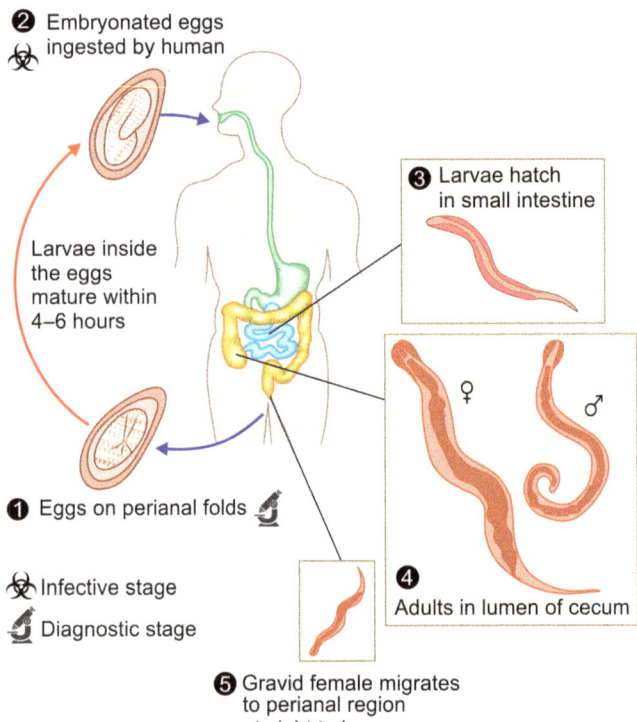

FIG. 7: Life cycle of *Enterobius vermicularis* showing infective as well as diseased state.
Source: Courtesy of the Centers for Disease Control and Prevention (CDC) [https://www.cdc.gov/dpdx/enterobiasis/index.html]

- It may lead to pruritus vulvae and from here may even migrate up into the female genital tract, leading to mucoid vaginal discharge and rarely salpingitis or peritonitis.

Diagnosis

The adult female worm may be visualized in the perianal area and perineum at night or in stools.

Microscopic visualization of the worm or eggs confirms the diagnosis, best done with a 6 cm strip of adhesive cellulose tape over the butt end of a test tube or a wooden spatula, with the sticky side outward. This is then rubbed over the perianal skin on waking. The eggs and adults stick to the adhesive which can be mounted on a slide and examined under the microscope with a drop of toluene.

Treatment

- Mebendazole is the most effective drug, acting on all stages of the worm. For mass treatment campaigns, 100 mg single dose; while for individual treatment, a dose of 100 mg twice daily for 3 days, to be repeated after 2 weeks, is used.
- Albendazole is also efficacious, and the dose needs to be repeated after 2 weeks.

CHAPTER 12: Human Helminthic Infections (Nematodes, Cestodes, and Trematodes)

- Ivermectin is less effective and may be used as an adjunct with albendazole.
- The whole family should be treated simultaneously.
- Cleanliness of hands and nails should be encouraged.

Hookworm Disease

This category includes diseases caused by *Ancylostoma duodenale* (Old World hookworm disease or ancylostomiasis) and *Necator americanus* (New World or American hookworm disease).

This disease is very common and widely distributed in the tropics and subtropics, especially in areas with poor sanitation. The definitive hosts are humans, cats, and dogs, and transmission occurs through penetration of intact skin by the larvae **(Fig. 8)**.

Clinical Features

- A transient eruption when larvae penetrate the skin is known as "ground itch", "dew itch", and "uncinarial dermatitis". It is characterized by localized erythema, edema, and papulovesicular lesions localized to the feet, lasting up to 2 weeks.
- Pulmonary symptoms include cough, wheezing, or dyspnea, 1–3 weeks after penetration by the worm. A transient respiratory illness due to eosinophilic alveolitis or pneumonitis induced by migrating larvae is known as Loeffler's pneumonia. It may be associated with peripheral eosinophilia and urticaria.
- Gastrointestinal symptoms develop after 1 month such as abdominal pain, diarrhea, and, occasionally, melena. Due to persistent blood loss, features of malnutrition, such as pallor, edema, puffy face, listlessness, and growth retardation, may be seen.

Diagnosis

- *Chest X-ray*: Loeffler's syndrome may be visualized radiographically as transient patchy pulmonary infiltrates.
- Peripheral blood eosinophilia is a nonspecific marker.
- Stool microscopic examination can show characteristic eggs in the feces. The eggs of *A. duodenale* and

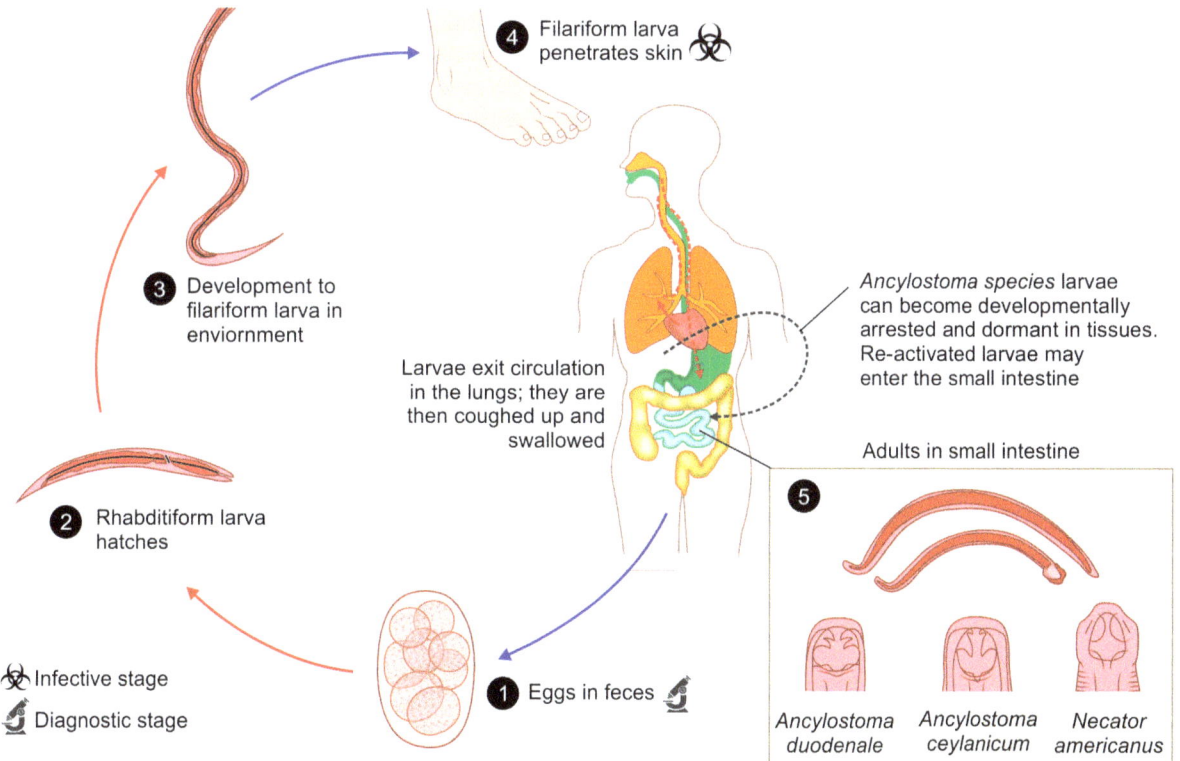

FIG. 8: Life cycle of hookworm showing the infective as well as diseased state. Humans acquire the infection primarily by walking barefoot on infected soil or grass.
Source: Courtesy of the Centers for Disease Control and Prevention (CDC) [https://www.cdc.gov/dpdx/hookworm/index.html#:~:text=Intestinal%20hookworm%20infections%20are%20commonly,occur%20especially%20in%20heavy%20infections.].

N. americanus cannot be distinguished microscopically.
- The presence of occult or frank blood in stools can point toward a diagnosis.
- The presence of iron deficiency anemia and hypoalbuminemia are suggestive diagnostic tests.

■ Treatment

- Ground itch usually responds to antipruritic creams and oral antihistamines.
- Pulmonary symptoms are self-resolving; but if severe, a short course of corticosteroids may be required.
- Specific therapy involves a 3-day course of albendazole 400 mg, mebendazole 100 mg, or pyrantel pamoate 11 mg/kg.
- Oral iron supplementation to overcome iron deficiency may be needed.

Cutaneous Larva Migrans

It is also known as creeping eruption, sandworm eruption, plumber's itch, and Duck hunter's itch. It is a common eruption in tropical and subtropical countries, especially during the warm and rainy season caused by hookworm *Strongyloides stercoralis* infection.

Cutaneous larva migrans (CLM) is a common disease in India, especially in children living in less hygienic conditions, among construction workers, and those walking barefoot on beaches.

■ Clinical Features

- Animal hookworms inhabiting the intestines of dogs and cats are responsible. The excreted ova passed in their feces that contaminate the soil, hatch into infective larvae, and penetrate the human skin of barefoot walkers. Thus, humans act as a dead-end host.
- Creeping eruption presents as intensely pruritic papules over the feet, ankle, back, buttocks, etc., whichever was in contact with contaminated sand. It is seen to begin as multiple papules, sudden in onset, and intensely pruritic.
- Within 2–3 days, the lesions are seen as "expanding" or "migrating". They present as intensely itchy, erythematous, edematous papules and/or vesicles arranged as serpiginous (snake-like) or bizarre patterns. The lesions are slightly elevated, 2–3 mm wide. They may track 3–4 cm away from the penetration site **(Fig. 9)**.
- The larvae may lie quiet for weeks or months or may immediately begin creeping activity.

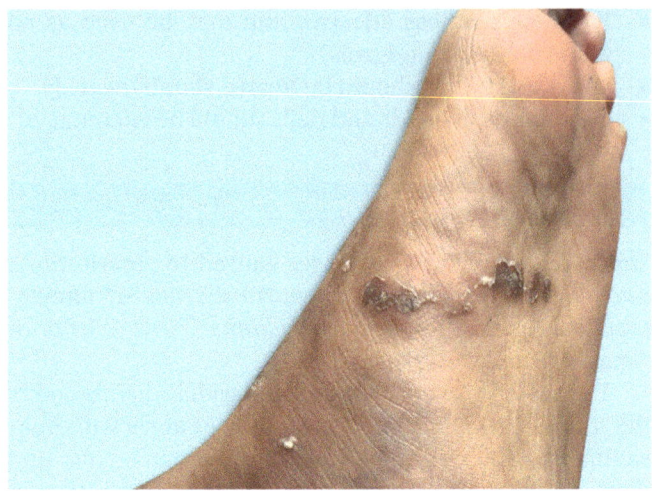

FIG. 9: Pruritic, serpiginous advancing lesion of cut larva migrans in a young man after a beach holiday.

- Dermatitic changes and bacterial infection are common due to the highly pruritic nature.
- The disease is self-limiting.

■ Treatment

- Albendazole 400 mg/day for 3 days is the recommended treatment.
- Ivermectin administered as a single dose of 200 µg/kg, to be repeated the next day, is an alternative treatment.
- Topical ivermectin and thiabendazole in 10% suspension, to be applied 4 times a week, have also been used. Oral thiabendazole is less effective and more toxic than the topical formulation.

Cysticercosis

Taeniasis and cysticercosis are two different conditions caused by the *Taenia solium* tapeworm. The patient may remain asymptomatic for years or develop a few or multiple localized cutaneous swellings. Cysticercosis is a tissue infection caused by the larval cysts of the tapeworm. If the brain is affected, the condition is called neurocysticercosis and is one of the leading causes of adult-onset seizures in developing nations. Cysticercosis has a worldwide distribution.

The causative agent is *T. solium* (pork tapeworm), and humans are the definitive hosts while pigs serve as intermediate hosts **(Fig. 10)**. Transmission of infection is a result of ingestion of contaminated food, water, or inadequately cooked pork. Adult *T. solium* lives attached to the wall of the small intestine. In comparison, cysticercosis caused by the lodging of the larval stage

CHAPTER 12: Human Helminthic Infections (Nematodes, Cestodes, and Trematodes)

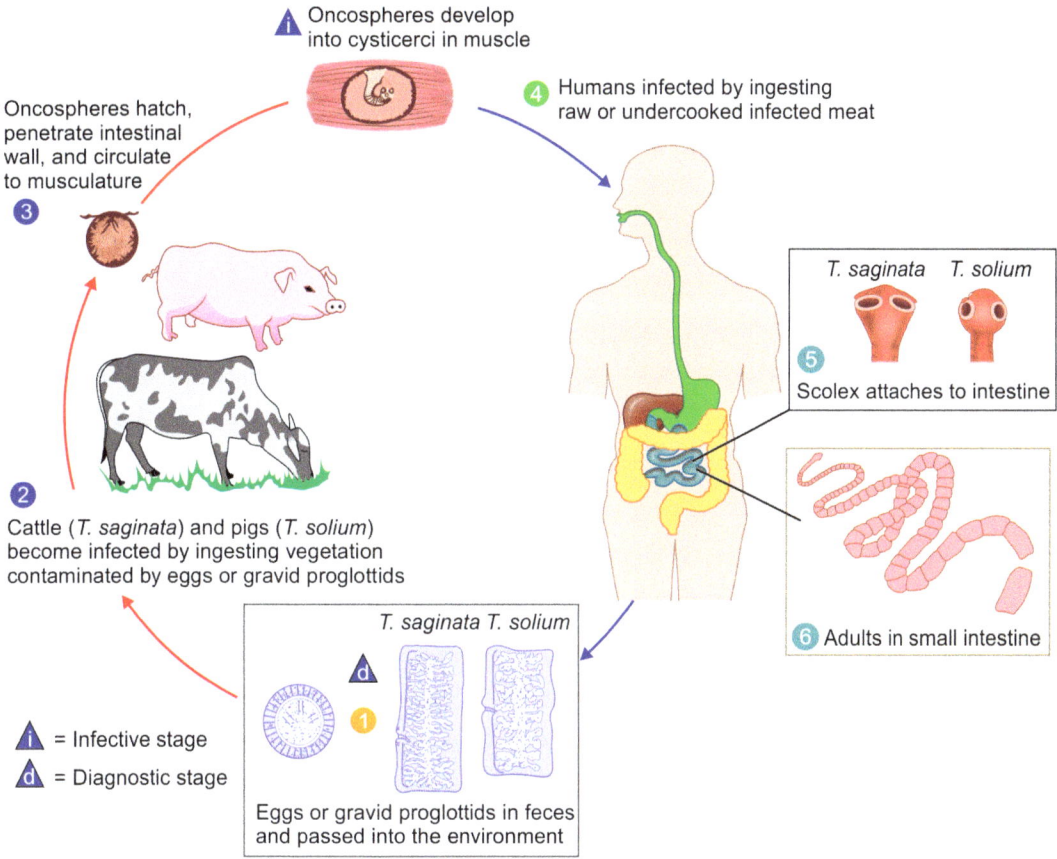

FIG. 10: Life cycle of *T. solium* and *T. saginata* showing the infective as well as diseased state.
Source: Courtesy of the Centers for Disease Control and Prevention (CDC) [https://www.cdc.gov/dpdx/taeniasis/index.html#:~:text=Taeniasis%20is%20the%20infection%20of,to%20months%20in%20the%20environment.]

(*Cysticercus cellulosae*) in numerous organs, especially effects subcutaneous tissue, muscle, brain, etc. The larvae are enclosed in a cyst.

Clinical Features
- Taeniasis is usually asymptomatic
- Cutaneous lesions are generally a part of cysticercosis cellulosae cutis, characterized by the development of multiple 1–2 cm painless, firm, and rounded subcutaneous nodules, which may persist for years.
- Other organs such as muscles, eyes, lungs, and brain may also be involved, with symptoms depending on the organ involved as well as major function hampered by the cyst.

Diagnosis
It is based on the following investigations:
- Stool microscopic examination reveals the presence of eggs in the stool.
- Histopathologic examination of an excised cyst is diagnostic. There is a central cystic cavity containing clear fluid and a white irregularly shaped membranous structure, the cysticercus larva. It is surrounded by a thick fibrous capsule covered by epithelioid cells and a few Langhans giant cells.
- Serology is helpful, but cross-reactions are known to occur.
- X-ray examination frequently shows calcific foci in muscle, although rarely such lesions may also be seen in the brain.
- Computed tomographic (CT) scan shows typical appearances in the brain and muscle.

Treatment
- Subcutaneous cysticercosis is usually harmless but serves as a pointer toward the possibility of cerebral infection, hence, all suspected cases should be screened.

- If the patient desires, individual cosmetically disfiguring lesions or subcutaneous cysts can be surgically removed.
- For cerebral disease, if the parasite is dead, treatment is confined to the control of seizures with the help of anticonvulsants.
- Antihelminthic drugs (albendazole and praziquantel) are used only in case of viable or live cysts. These should be given under the cover of steroid therapy. Albendazole is the preferred drug due to higher efficacy, given at 15 mg/kg in two divided doses for 15 days.
- Obstructive lesions of the brain require surgical relief.
- Prognosis is good for taeniasis, but with cysticercosis, serious consequences can be anticipated when vital organs are involved.

13

Leishmaniasis

Introduction

Cutaneous leishmaniasis (CL) is a protozoal disease caused by over 20 species of *Leishmania*. The disease is transmitted to humans by the bite of infected female *phlebotomine* sandflies. The disease burden remains significant with a worldwide prevalence of 12 million and an annual incidence of 1.5–2 million new cases each year. In India, outbreaks of CL have been reported chiefly in the hot and dry areas of Rajasthan (Bikaner, Ganganagar) and Gujarat, with occasional case reports from Punjab, Assam, and Haryana. Recently, Himachal Pradesh and Union Territory of Jammu and Kashmir (Chenab region) have emerged as a challenging focus of disease.

Clinical Features

There are three major clinical forms of leishmaniasis:
1. *Cutaneous type*: Most common type, restricted to the skin and often seen in the old world (*Leishmania major, Leishmania tropica, Leishmania infantum*) (Europe), or *Leishmania aethiopica* (Ethiopia and Kenya) as compared to new world (*Leishmania mexicana*).
2. *Mucocutaneous type*: Affects both the skin and mucosal surfaces, and occurs almost exclusively in the new world (*Leishmania braziliensis*).
3. *Visceral type*: Also known as kala-azar, it is fatal in 95% cases if left untreated. Affects the organs of the mononuclear phagocyte system, e.g., liver, spleen (*Leishmania donovani* complex, i.e., *Leishmania donovani, Leishmania infantum*, and *Leishmania chagasi*) and is followed by the sequel of post-kala-azar dermal leishmaniasis (PKDL).

Cutaneous Leishmaniasis

The lesions are ulcers/nodulo-ulcers, often solitary but may be multiple that are present on the exposed body parts, face being the most commonly affected site. The majority of acute cutaneous infections resolve spontaneously with scarring in about a year.

Old World Cutaneous Leishmaniasis (Oriental Sore/Baghdad Boil/Delhi Boil)

The clinical morphological spectrum is wide. Lesions generally start as a small, well-circumscribed, erythematous papule at the inoculation site. These enlarge over few weeks to form nodules/plaques, which often ulcerate and become crusted **(Fig. 1)**. The volcanic,

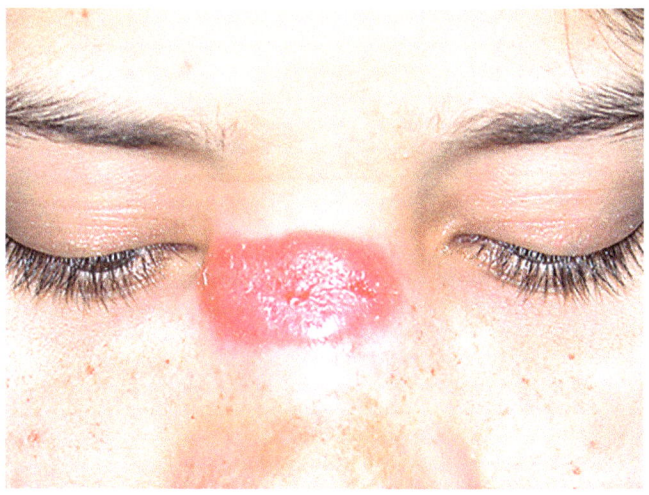

FIG. 1: Erythematous indurated plaque of cutaneous leishmaniasis with scale crust and ulceration over the bridge of the nose.

nodulo-ulcerative morphology is characteristic and consists of a painless crateriform ulcer with a rolled out margin and a necrotic base, which tends to be covered with an adherent crust **(Fig. 2)**. Other presentations include iceberg nodules, eczematoid, psoriasiform, erysipeloid, zosteriform, paronychia, chancriform, annular, palmoplantar, verrucous, and keloidal lesions. Satellite lesions, regional lymphadenopathy, and sporotrichoid spread along lymphatics, **(Fig. 3)** have also been described. Secondary bacterial infection in these lesions is common.

- Pure cutaneous disease is very similar to old world CL and isolated ulcers are the most common presentation.
- Various reported complications of CL include scarring, disfigurement, social stigma, and evolution into diffuse cutaneous, chronic cutaneous, and mucocutaneous (new world) forms.

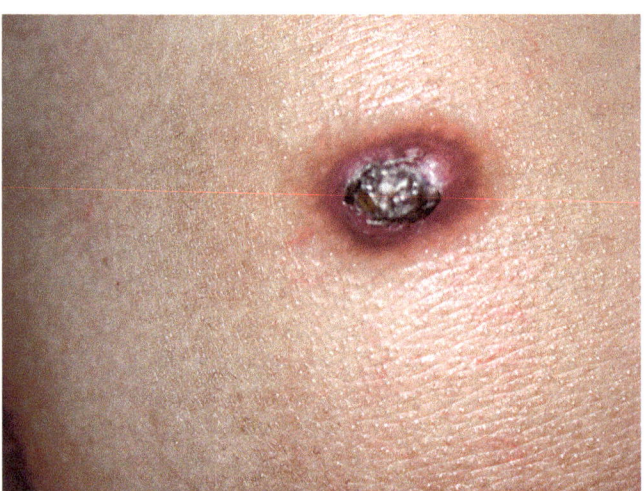

FIG. 2: Volcanic nodule of cutaneous leishmaniasis.

Diffuse Cutaneous Leishmaniasis

Diffuse cutaneous leishmaniasis (DCL) is characterized by the presence of multiple (>10) pleomorphic lesions involving two or more noncontiguous areas of the body. This is seen in the setting of deficient cell-mediated immunity and can mimic lepromatous leprosy clinically and histologically. Parasite-laden, nonulcerative nodules start disseminating from the initial site of infection, gradually with a predilection for various exposed areas such as extremities or face, where lesions may coalesce to form leonine facies. DCL is caused by *L. aethiopica* (in Africa) and the mexicana complex (*Leishmania amazonensis*), in the Americas. DCL variant is difficult to treat.

Mucosal/Mucocutaneous Leishmaniasis

After few months to many years, some patients go on to develop mucocutaneous disease. In most endemic areas, 1–10% of localized CL infections result in mucosal leishmaniasis, 1–5 years after the localized lesions has healed. Mucocutaneous leishmaniasis (MCL) is often caused by *L. braziliensis* and *Leishmania panamensis* in Central and South America. In the old world, similar mucosal lesions caused by *L. aethiopica* may be seen but carry an overall better prognosis. MCL results from a direct spread/hematogenous/lymphatic spread to the upper respiratory tract, and rarely to ocular and genital mucosa. Mucosal lesions range from a simple edema of the lips and nose **(Fig. 4)**, to perforation of the nasal cartilage (tapir nose, parrot beak) and laryngeal cartilage as well as the palate. Infiltration and/

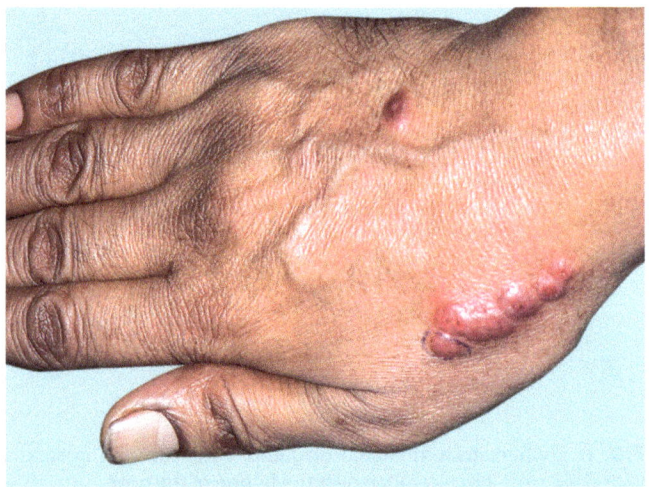

FIG. 3: Nodules of cutaneous leishmaniasis showing sporotrichoid pattern over the hand.

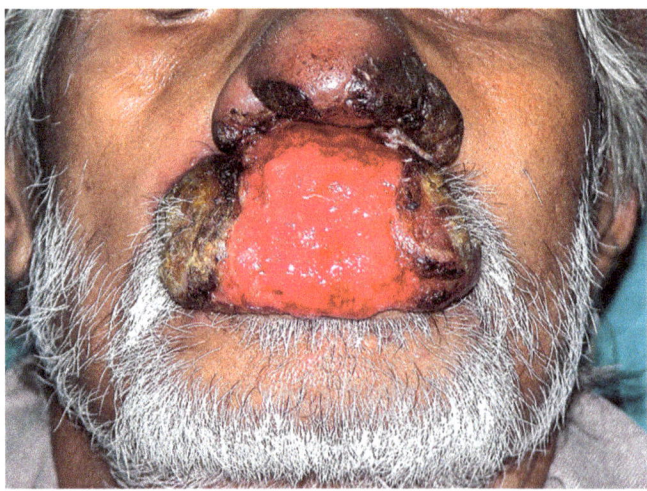

FIG. 4: Ulcerated and crusted plaque of mucocutaneous leishmaniasis over the upper lip and nose.

or ulceration of the nasal mucosa, buccal mucosa, lips, and oropharynx is its characteristic. In some patients, there is extensive nasopharyngeal mutilating ulceration (espundia), as well as an alteration in phonation because of the destruction of the vocal cords. Bone involvement usually does not occur. Mucosal leishmaniasis does not heal spontaneously and is very difficult to treat, secondary bacterial infection is common, and is potentially fatal.

Chronic Cutaneous Leishmaniasis

In this form, the lesions evolve from papules to chronic disfiguring nodules/plaques that are larger than average lesions. These may exhibit variable degree of scaling, ulceration, verrucosity, and scarring. Erythematous scaly papules, often with apple jelly appearance over the borders of a completely/partially healed lesion are its characteristics. The disease is mostly caused by *L. tropica* in the old world and *L. braziliensis* in the new world.

Post-kala-azar Dermal Leishmaniasis

Post-kala-azar dermal leishmaniasis is the most common cutaneous manifestation of leishmaniasis in India and is prevalent in areas where *L. donovani* is endemic. It is a sequel of visceral leishmaniasis (VL) in majority. PKDL is extremely rare in the new world and is mostly seen in Sudan and India. In contrast to Sudan variant, spontaneous resolution is rare in Indian patients. PKDL develops in about 12% of patients treated with sodium stibogluconate (SSG) monotherapy for VL. In contrast to patients with VL, patients with PKDL are constitutionally well.

Three grades of severity of PKDL are described:
1. *Grade 1:* Scattered maculopapular or nodular rash on the face (predilection for the area around the chin and mouth), with or without lesions on the upper chest or arms **(Fig. 5)**.
2. *Grade 2:* Dense maculopapular or nodular rash covering most of the face and extending to the chest, back, upper arms and legs, with only scattered lesions on the forearms and legs **(Fig. 6)**.
3. *Grade 3:* Dense maculopapular or nodular rash covering most parts of the body, including the hands and feet; the mucosa of the lip and palate may be involved **(Figs. 7 and 8)**.

Lesions tend to be quite symmetrical in distribution and are not itchy. At times, only hypopigmented macules are present **(Fig. 9)**. The papules may further increase in size, evolving into nodules or plaques, or a combination of these, i.e., polymorphic form **(Figs. 10A and B)**.

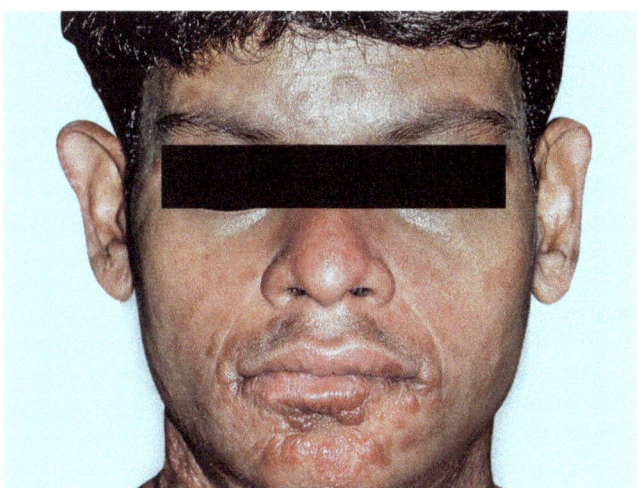

FIG. 5: Skin colored papules and plaques of post-kala-azar dermal leishmaniasis (PKDL) in the perioral area and the face resembling lepromatous leprosy.

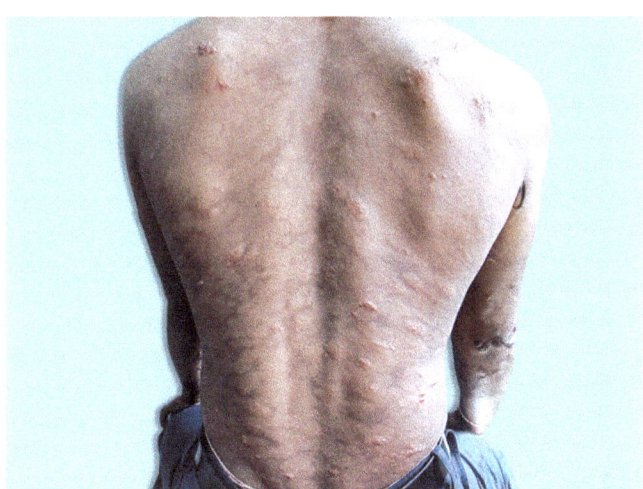

FIG. 6: Extensive involvement over the back with hypopigmented macules and prominent papulonodular lesions.

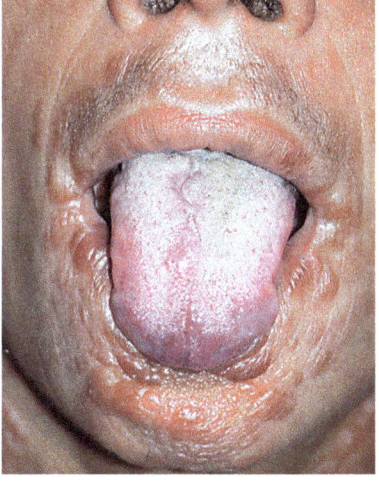

FIG. 7: Nodular lesions of post-kala-azar dermal leishmaniasis (PKDL) over the tongue and inner lips.

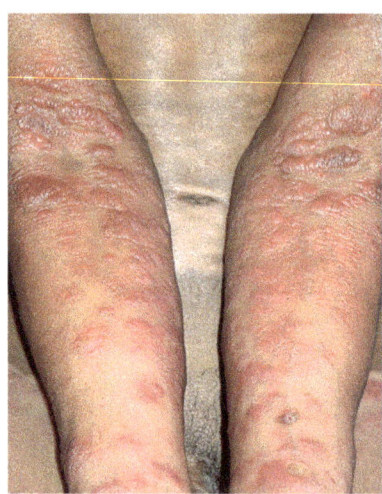

FIG. 8: Lesions of post-kala-azar dermal leishmaniasis (PKDL) involving the forearms.

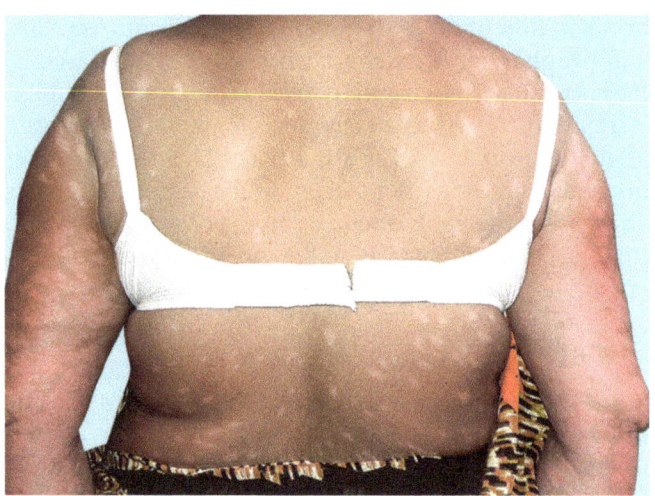

FIG. 9: Hypopigmented macules of post-kala-azar dermal leishmaniasis (PKDL) discrete over the trunk and confluent over the upper limbs.

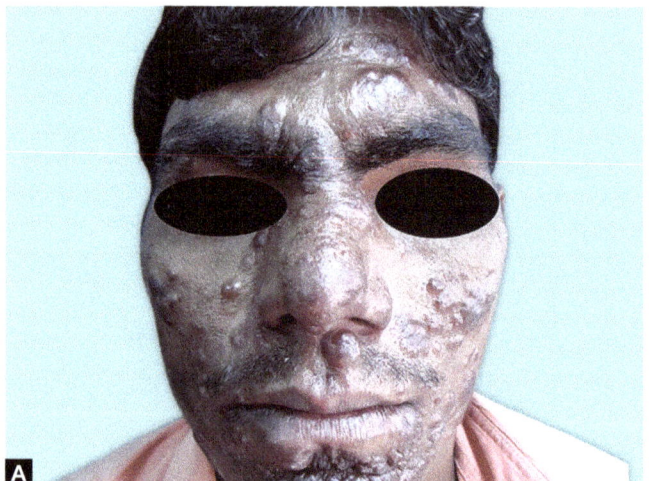
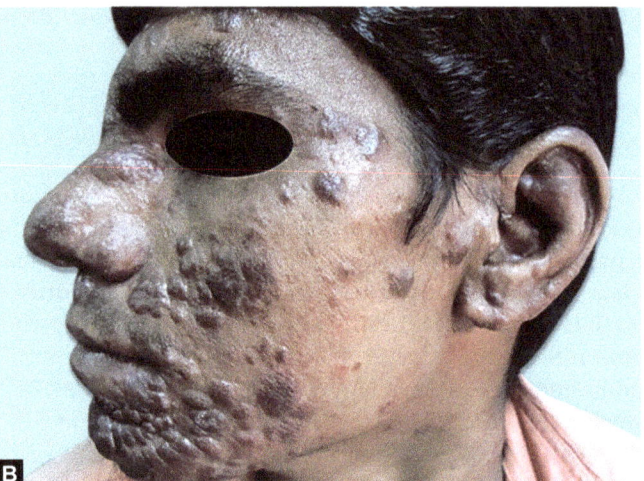

FIGS. 10A AND B: Extensive infiltration with nodules and plaques in a patient with long-standing disease.

Diagnosis

Characteristic single, indurated, and nodulo-ulcerative lesion on the face (nose, cheeks) in a patient coming from high endemic area should raise a suspicion on clinical examination.

Various diagnostic techniques can be utilized for confirming the diagnosis of different forms of leishmaniasis, depending on the clinical type as well as the stage of disease.

Direct Demonstration of Organisms

Parasitological diagnosis remains the reference standard in the diagnosis of CL because of its high specificity. It is advised that a full thickness scalpel biopsy should be taken from the infiltrated margin of the lesion/ulcer and divided into three parts to prepare an impression smear, for histological examination as well as for culture on Novy–MacNeal–Nicolle (NNN) media. The smears can then be stained with Giemsa and examined for the presence of amastigotes. Culture is the gold standard for diagnosis, with a sensitivity of 50%.

Direct Smears

The sensitivity of direct slit skin smear has been reported to vary from 30 to 80% on Giemsa-stained sections in various studies. Fine needle aspirates from the ulcer margin using an aseptic technique, stained with Hematoxylin and eosin (H&E) stain or Giemsa stain can be performed.

Crush Smear

The harvested tissue is crushed between two slides, fixed, stained, and then examined.

Leishman–Donovan bodies **(Fig. 11)** are visualized as round to oval structures (amastigote form) measuring only 2–5 microns; surrounded by a plasma membrane and containing large, deeply basophilic, nucleus, and a smaller, deeply staining, rod-shaped kinetoplast.

Histopathology (Fig. 12)

In early lesions, dermal infiltrate is composed of predominantly histiocytes, lymphocytes, and plasma cells with scattered multinucleate giant cells. The hallmark of the disease is the presence of parasitized macrophages (Wright cells) which contain Leishman–Donovan bodies. These can be observed in around 70% of cases. The overlying epidermis becomes hyperkeratotic and subsequently breaks down to form an ulcer.

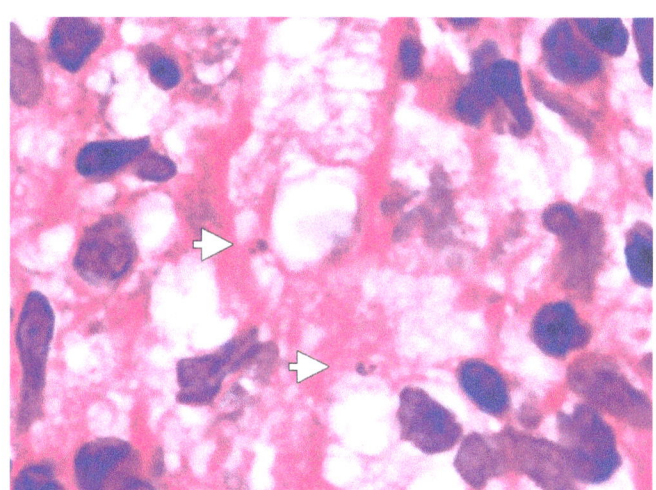

FIG. 11: Leishman–Donovan bodies seen on tissue smear.

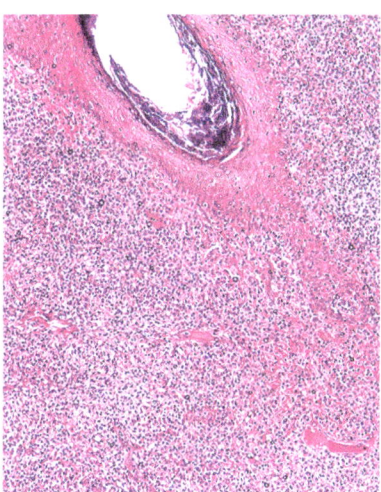

FIG. 12: Dense pandermal infiltrate composed of predominantly epithelioid cells, foamy histiocytes admixed with a few lymphocytes, and plasma cells.

PKDL shows a diffuse dermal infiltrate of macrophages, lymphocytes, and plasma cells. The histopathology in PKDL has sensitivity varying from 7 to 33% in macules, 34–67% in papules, and 67–100% in nodules.

Serological Tests

Serology alone may not be useful due to its low sensitivity and specificity. However, the antibodies may be present in high titers in cases with VL and PKDL. The commonly used antigens are rK39 and rK16 which can be detected with the help of immunochromatography.

Molecular Techniques

Species-specific polymerase chain reaction (PCR) has been shown to amplify deoxyribonucleic acid (DNA) using kinetoplast DNA, heat shock protein 70 (hsp70), or glycoprotein 63 (gp63). This may be used on skin biopsy samples or slit skin specimens in well-equipped laboratories and has a sensitivity of 90–100%.

Differential Diagnosis

Many disorders can be confused with CL. Few are mentioned in the following text:
- *Cutaneous leishmaniasis*: Cutaneous tuberculosis, infected insect bites, foreign body granuloma, tropical ulcers, fungal infections, traumatic ulcers, pyoderma, etc.
- *Mucocutaneous leishmaniasis*: Paracoccidioidomycosis, tertiary syphilis, Wegener's granulomatosis, or angiocentric natural killer (NK)/T-cell lymphoma.
- *Diffuse cutaneous leishmaniasis*: Lepromatous leprosy; however, the former spares the eyebrows and the lesions are usually not as infiltrative as those of lepromatous leprosy.

Treatment

The treatment approach depends in part on the *Leishmania* species and natural history of infection, geographical region, risk for mucosal dissemination, drug susceptibilities, and the number, size, location, and evolution of skin lesions. It is generally seen that old World CL is often self-limiting, whereas infections due to *L. braziliensis* can progress to mucocutaneous disease and therefore require systemic treatment. Various antileishmanial medications available include:
- *Pentavalent antimonials:* For localized disease, an intralesional pentavalent antimonial, SSG, can be administered at a dose of 0.5 mL/cm^2 (100 mg/mL solution) three times weekly until cure is achieved, or for a maximum duration of 10 weeks. For larger lesions

(diameter >5 cm or a cumulative area >10 cm^2) and for PKDL, the SSG is administered once daily, intravenously or intramuscularly slowly over 5–10 minutes, at a dose of 20 mg/kg/day (maximum 800 mg/day) for 3 weeks with continuous cardiac monitoring. With this regimen, the outcome is generally favorable **(Figs. 13A and B)**.

A prolongation of a corrected Q-T interval (>0.5 seconds) signals the likely onset of serious and fatal cardiac arrhythmia. Other side effects include an elevation of pancreatic enzymes but clinical pancreatitis is uncommon. Elevated liver enzyme, leukopenia, anemia, and thrombopenia have been reported. The presence of serious side effects in the form of hepato- or cardiotoxicity signals that the drug should be changed.

- *Azoles medicines:* For limited cutaneous lesions, azole drugs such as itraconazole, ketoconazole, fluconazole, are now been increasingly recommended due to their easy availability, safety profile, and efficacy. The success of treatment depends upon the type and severity of the infection.
- *Liposomal Amphotericin B deoxycholate*: For localized cutaneous lesions, weekly intralesional injection of 2.5–5 mg/mL of liposomal amphotericin-B for 8 weeks has been recommended as efficacious and safe drug. For extensive disease, administration is in the form of an intravenous infusion over 2 hours. Mild infusion reactions (fever, chills, and rigor) and back pain may occur in some patients. Transient nephrotoxicity or thrombocytopenia can also be occasionally seen.

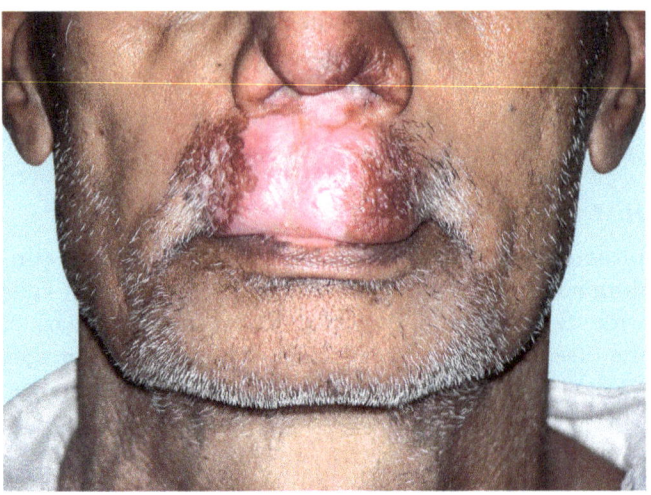

FIG. 14: Resolution of mucocutaneous leishmaniasis lesions with 12 weeks of miltefosine therapy (patient in **Fig. 4**).

- *Miltefosine*: Miltefosine has effective antileishmanial activity in doses of 50 mg twice daily (or 100 mg OD) in adults used mainly for PKDL **(Fig. 14)**. Miltefosine commonly induces gastrointestinal side effects; anorexia, nausea, vomiting (38%), and diarrhea (20%). Most episodes are brief and resolve as treatment is continued. An extensive skin rash, elevated hepatic transaminases and renal insufficiency may rarely be observed. Miltefosine should be taken after meals. It is potentially teratogenic and should not be used by pregnant women or women with childbearing potential for whom adequate contraception cannot be assured for the duration of treatment and 3 months, thereafter.

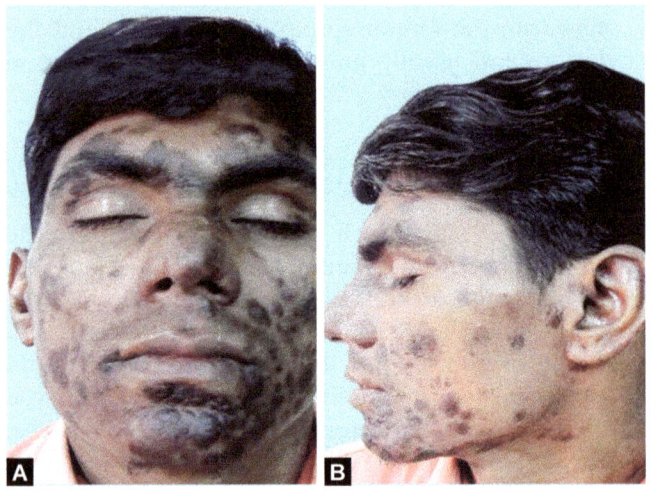

FIGS. 13A AND B: Resolution of PKDL lesions with 4 weeks of sodium stibogluconate infusion therapy (patient in Figs. 10A and B).

Approach to Therapy

In general, the initial approach to treatment of uncomplicated CL involves local therapy.

Systemic therapy is warranted for treatment of complicated CL. This category would include:
- Infection with species associated with MCL.
- More than four lesions and individual lesions being 5 cm or more in size.
- Presence of subcutaneous nodules and regional lymphadenopathy >1 cm size.
- Lesions present on face, fingers, or toes.
- Immunosuppressed host
- Clinical failure of local therapy even after 2–3 months of appropriate treatment.

Definitions of Cure

- *Clinical cure*: Demonstrated by clinical cure of papular and nodular lesions, and complete resolution of macular lesion or repigmentation of macular lesions at 12 months follow-up visit.
- *Parasitological cure:* At the end of treatment and at subsequent follow-up visits, parasites should no longer be present.

Prevention

Prevention should be directed toward the elimination of reservoirs or reduction of human-vector contact. Sandflies are highly susceptible to insecticides such as dichloro-diphenyl-trichloroethane (DDT), organophosphates, pyrethroids, and carbamates. Use of bed nets should be encouraged in endemic areas.

CHAPTER 14: Infestations

Introduction

Infestation is a state of being invaded or inhabited by a pest or parasite. Epidermal parasitic skin diseases (EPSD) are a heterogeneous category of infestations wherein the parasite-host interactions are confined to stratum corneum. This includes scabies, pediculosis, and demodicidosis as the common infestations seen in Indian population.

Scabies

- Human scabies is a contagious infestation caused by the mite, *Sarcoptes scabiei* var. *hominis*, an ovoid, 8-legged, obligate human ectoparasite **(Fig. 1)**.
- Transmission is predominantly via direct skin-to-skin contact and also by fomite. The mite takes less than 30 minutes to penetrate the skin. Transmission of mites requires intensive skin-to-skin contact of at least 5–10 minutes' duration, as occurs, e.g., in the breastfeeding or cuddling of an infant, sexual intercourse, or even sitting with an infested individual. In common scabies patients, only 10–15 adult mites are present on the skin surface, because the mites can be washed and scratched away. The cell-mediated immune response begins 3–6 weeks after the infestation resulting in symptoms. The mites can survive outside the human body and remain infectious for 24–36 hours at normal room temperature (21°C) in relatively humid air (40–80%) and can survive much longer at lower temperatures and higher humidity.

Clinical Features

- Patient presents with a severe generalized pruritic rash that is worse at night.
- The host immunity toward the mite and its feces results in erythematous, discrete, excoriated papules, and papulovesicles, symmetrically distributed in the intertriginous areas, finger-web spaces **(Fig. 2)**, flexor

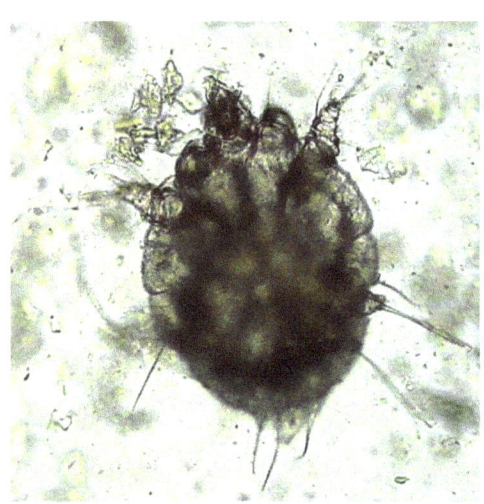

FIG. 1: Scabies mite.

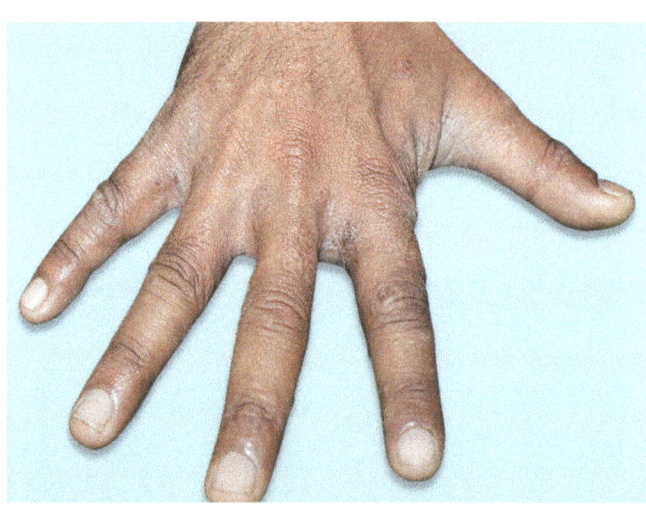

FIG. 2: Classical scabies affecting the web spaces.

aspect of the wrists, anterior axillary folds, breasts in females, periumbilical region, waist, penis, and scrotum. An imaginary circle formed by these sites of predilection is called the "Circle of Hebra" **(Fig. 3)**.
- Head, face, neck, palms, and soles in adults are typically spared but can be affected in infants.
- "S"-shaped burrows may be seen in web spaces of fingers and on male genitalia **(Fig. 4)**.

Clinical Variants of Scabies

- **Scabies in infants/children:** Lesions may involve the face, scalp, palms, and soles **(Fig. 5)**.
- **Nodular scabies:** Severely pruritic nodular lesions are seen on the genitals **(Fig. 6)**, thighs, axilla, or periareolar region. They may persist for weeks even after eradication of the mite and are extremely pruritic.
- **Crusted scabies (Norwegian scabies)** is a severe variant of scabies, extremely contagious and tends to occur in old, immunocompromised, mentally retarded, Parkinson's disease, Down's syndrome patients, and in patients with poor sensory perception. Clinical presentation includes generalized erythematous scaling rash **(Fig. 7)** with hyperkeratotic crusted lesions on the hands, feet, and under nails **(Fig. 7)** and scalp **(Fig. 8)**. Pruritus is mild or absent.

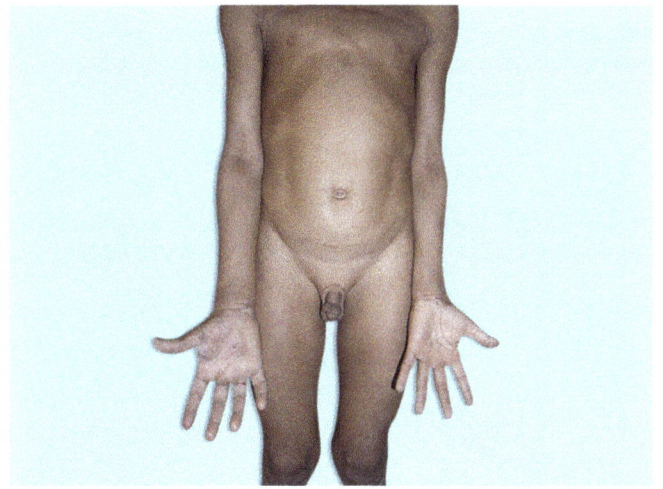

FIG. 3: Classical lesions of scabies seen involving the Circle of Hebra.

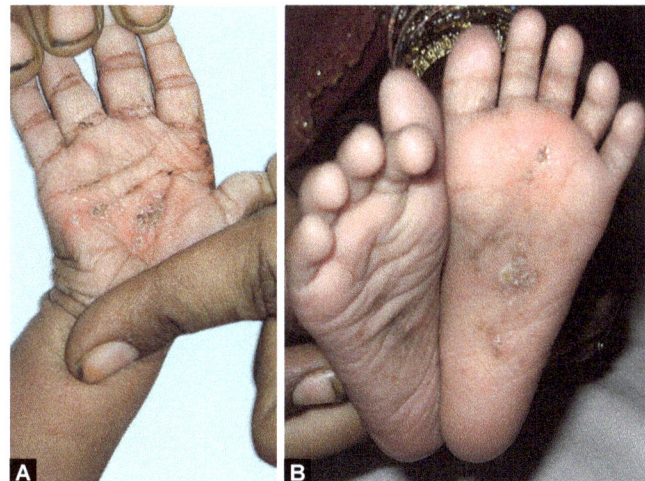

FIGS. 5A AND B: Involvement of palms and soles in a young child.

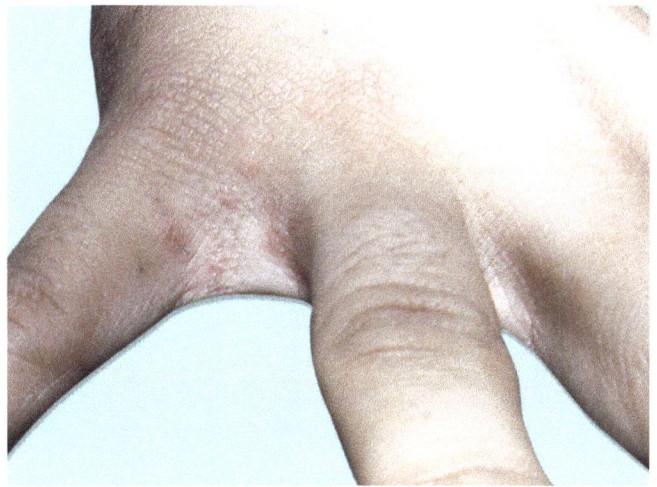

FIG. 4: Characteristic S-shaped burrows of scabies.

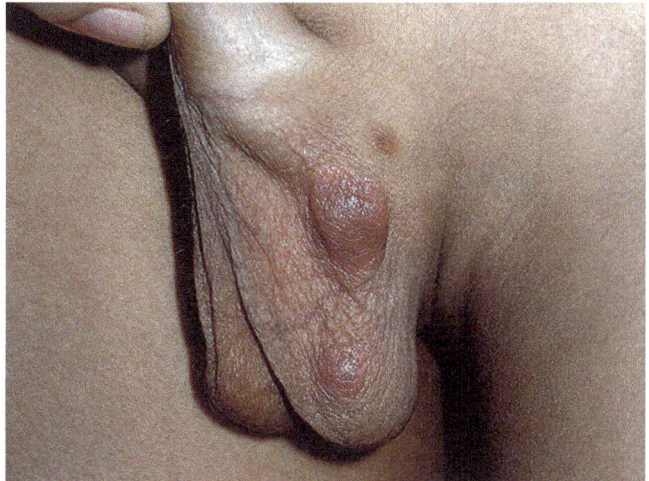

FIG. 6: Nodular scabies involving the scrotum.

CHAPTER 14: Infestations

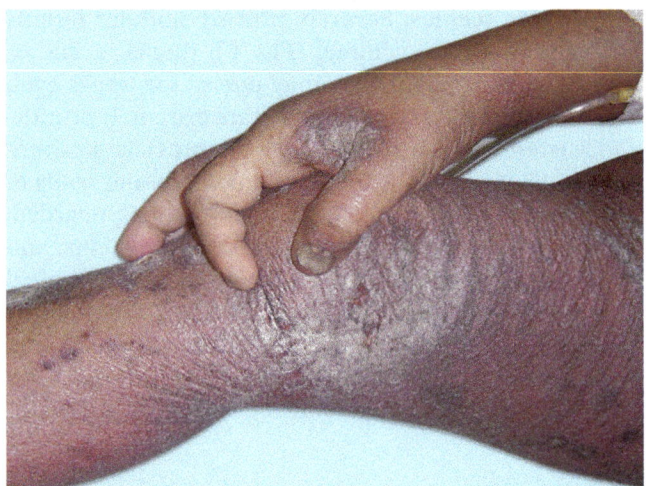

FIG. 7: Subungual involvement in a case of Norwegian scabies.

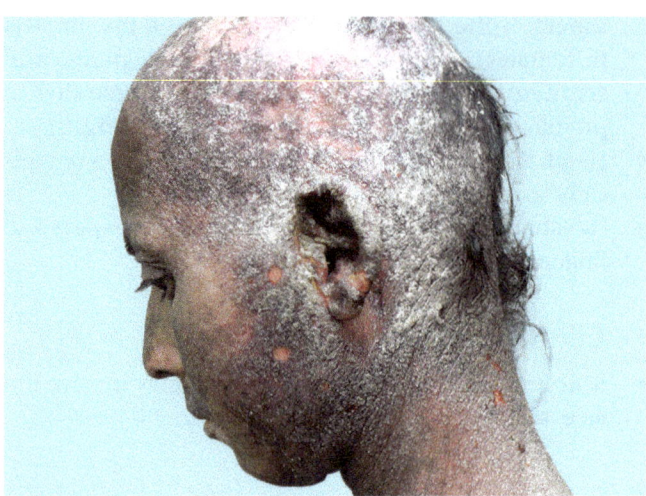

FIG. 8: Norwegian scabies with marked scalp involvement in a patient of systemic lupus erythematosus on systemic steroids.

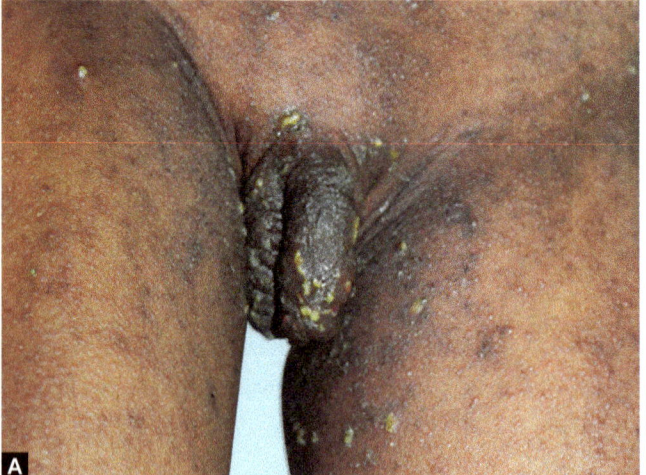

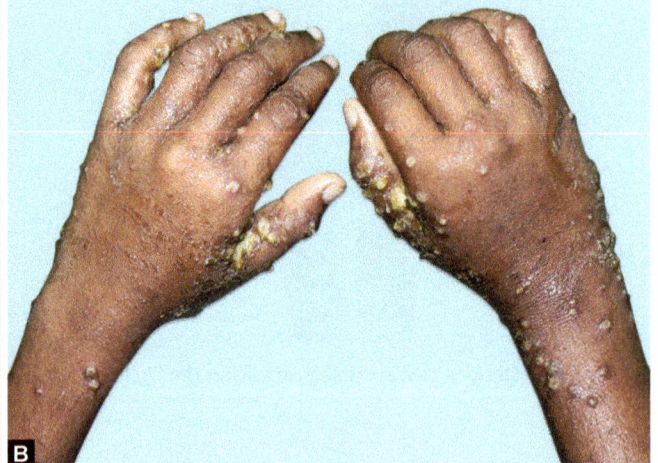

FIGS. 9 A AND B: Scabies with extensive secondary infection in the (A) genital location and (B) on hands.

Complications

Secondary bacterial infection manifesting as impetigo, cellulitis, and abscess **(Figs. 9A and B)** and eczematization may complicate scabies.

Diagnosis

- Diagnosis is mostly clinical. Pruritus that is worse at night, rash in the typical distribution, and positive family history should raise a high index of suspicion.
- Skin scrapings in 10–20% potassium permanganate (KOH) from papules, burrows, or subungual debris may reveal mites, eggs, or its fecal pellets **(Fig. 10)**. Dermatoscopic visualization of the mite in its burrow shows a characteristic "jet with contrail" appearance.

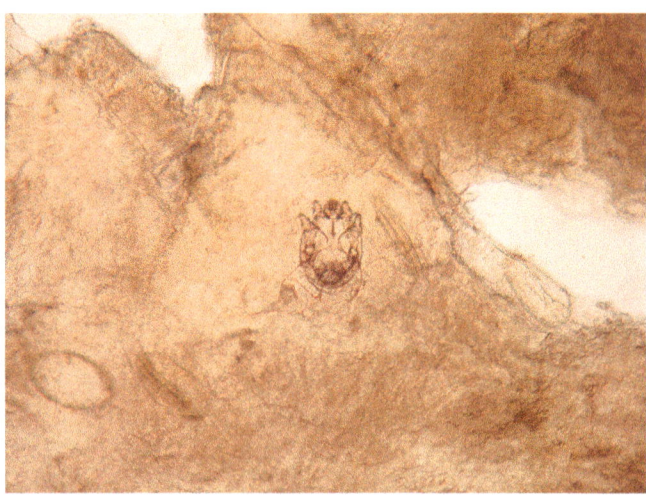

FIG. 10: Skin scraping showing the mite, with eggs as well as fecal pellets.

Differential Diagnosis

- Atopic dermatitis
- Insect bites
- Papular urticaria
- Dermatitis herpetiformis
- Dyshidrotic eczema
- Adverse drug reaction
- Psoriasis

Treatment

- Counseling regarding isolation, proper application of scabicidal drugs, and simultaneous treatment of all family members and close contacts
- Topical permethrin 5% lotion/cream (~30 g) should be applied over the entire body excluding the head and scalp with special attention to areas such as web spaces, nails, folds, and external genitalia for 6–8 hours followed by a thorough bath. A second application is sometimes required after 1–2 weeks.
- Topical permethrin is safe in infants, pregnant, and lactating women.
- Other topical creams include crotamiton cream 1%.
- The nails should be trimmed very short.
- Oral ivermectin (200 µg/kg) in a single dose that may be repeated after 2 weeks.
- A combination of permethrin and ivermectin is used to treat otherwise intractable cases and is generally indicated for the treatment of crusted scabies.
- *Crusted scabies*: Patient isolation and daily application of permethrin for 5–7 days along with keratolytic agents such as urea. All the people who have come in even brief contact with should be treated.
- *Nodular scabies*: After topical and/or systemic treatment, topical steroids may be applied on the nodular lesions. Rarely, intralesional steroids may be needed to resolve the recalcitrant nodular lesions
- Secondary infection and eczematization need to be treated prior to topical antiscabetic application with antibiotics and a topical steroid.
- Sedating antihistamines are needed to control the itch of scabies, as patients may continue to complain of itch for 2–6 weeks even after adequate antiscabetic treatment.
- *General measures*: Patients are advised to disinfect or machine wash all recently used textiles (underwear, pyjamas, bed linen, towels) at a temperature of at least 50°C for at least 35 minutes. A simple approach is to iron all the garments and linen after washing.

Treatment failure: It is common in scabies and the common causes include:
- Faulty application of topical antiscabies drugs
- Poor compliance
- Failure to treat contact/family members simultaneously and the lack of repeated treatment
- Inadequate decontamination of the fomites

Pediculosis

- Infestation by *Pediculus humanus* var. *capitis* (head louse; **Fig. 11**), var. *corporis* (body louse) and *Pthirus pubis* (pubic louse), is termed pediculosis.
- The prevalence of pediculosis in India in children ranges from 16.5% to 48%, with head lice being more prevalent in girls compared to boys.
- The most common mode of transmission of head lice is head-to-head contact, but fomites such as head brush, comb, headgear, and towels could be a causative factor.
- Body louse is seen more commonly in hygiene-poor situations, e.g., in homeless individuals, postnatural calamities, and those living in extremely crowded conditions.
- Pubic louse infests the hair in the pubic area and rarely the eyebrows and eyelashes. Transmission is by close physical contact and, therefore, it is listed as a sexually transmitted disease.
- The organism is a small (1–4 mm in size), six-legged, wingless insect **(Fig. 12)**. Body and head lice appear similar, with three pairs of short legs arising

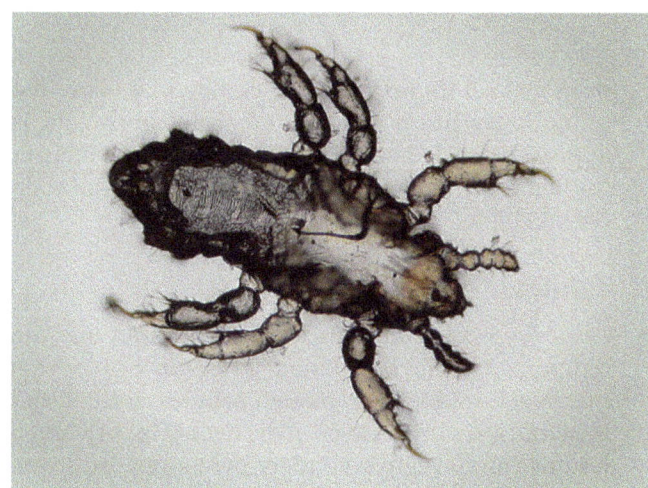

FIG. 11: Head louse.

CHAPTER 14: Infestations

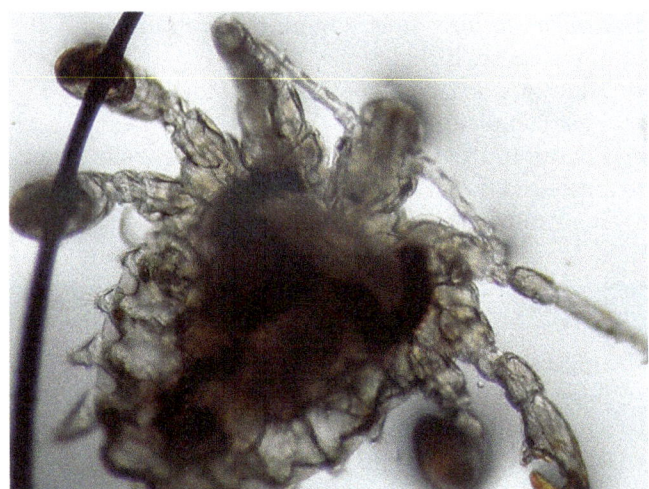

FIG. 12: Pubic louse.

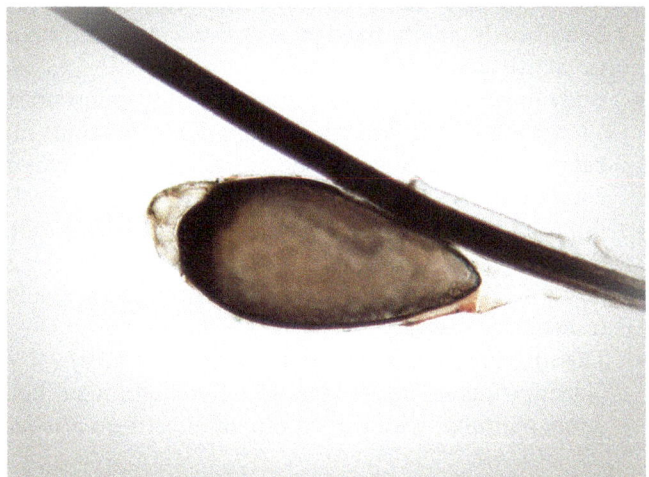

FIG. 13: Nit with chitinous covering, cemented to the hair shaft.

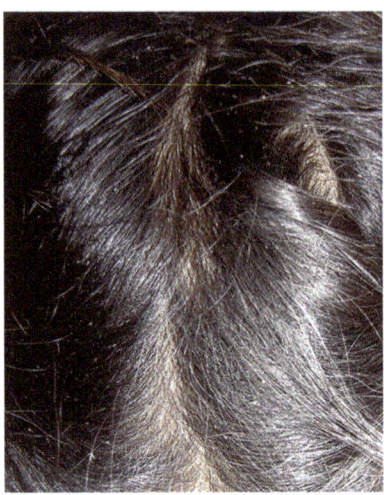

FIG. 14: Nits and lice in the occipital area of a young girl.

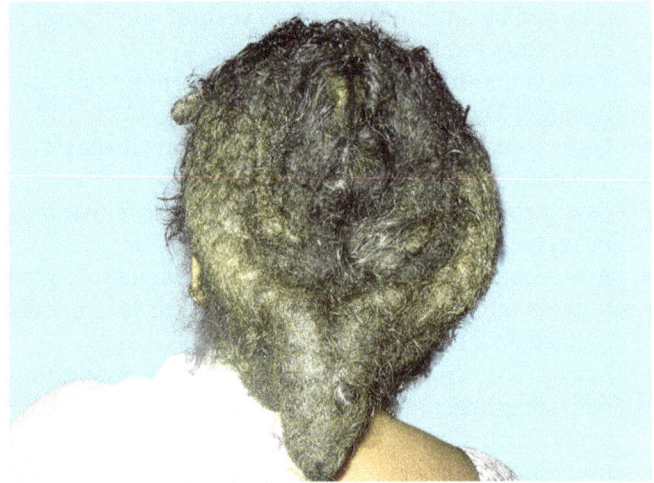

FIG. 15: Plica polonica.

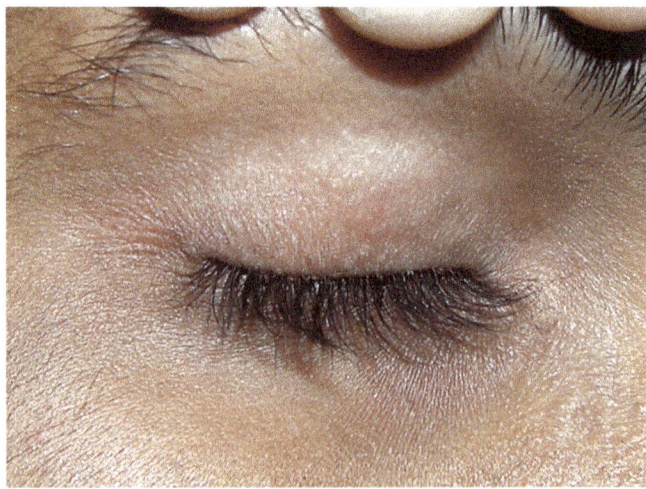

FIG. 16: Nits cemented at the base of eyelashes.

from a small thorax, each leg ending in a claw. The pubic louse has a shorter and wider body and is approximately 1-2 mm in size **(Fig. 13)**. Nits adhere to the hair ensheathing the hair shaft away from the scalp **(Fig. 14)**.

Clinical Features

- *Head louse*: Lice and nits favor the occiput and the temporal region. The patient presents with severe pruritus, resulting in excoriated papules, scaling, and lichenification on the nape of the neck **(Fig. 14)**. These lesions can develop secondary pyoderma. In severe neglected infections, the hair can get matted due to the exudates and pus secretion. This is called plica polonica **(Fig. 15)**. Occasionally, eyelashes may also be involved with a head louse **(Fig. 16)**.

- *Body louse*: The patient presents with pruritus with scaling and eczematization, especially on the back, neck, shoulders, and waist. Most lesions are excoriated and sometimes impetiginized with areas showing postinflammatory hyperpigmentation **(Fig. 17)**. This presentation is also known as Vagabond's disease.
- *Pubic louse*: Pruritus in the pubic area is the most common presentation. In many cases, they appear as hemorrhagic crusts that move on touch and shift position **(Fig. 18)**. On the eyelashes, the lesions may appear as scales similar to squamous blepharitis. It may also appear as mascara, which is the fecal accumulation of lice. In chronic infestation, bluish-gray ill-defined macules may be seen on the thighs, buttocks, and trunk, called macula cerulea.

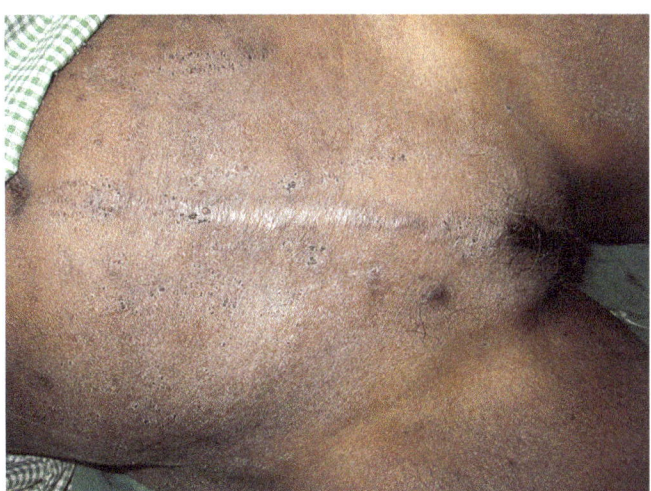

FIG. 17: Vagabond's disease. Note the extensive hyperpigmentation, excoriations, and crusting.

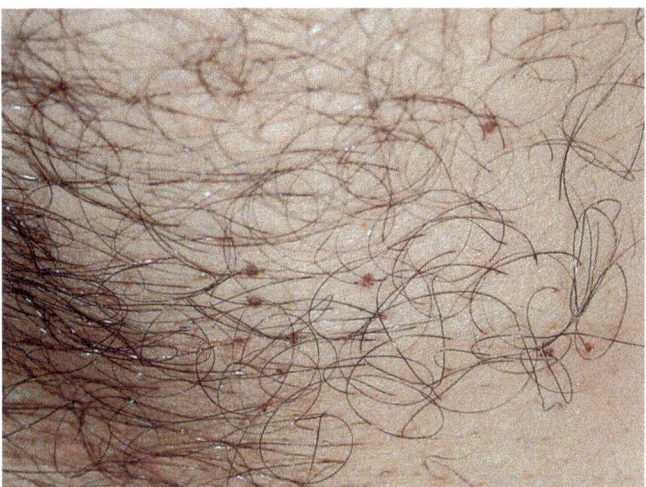

FIG. 18: Infestation of the pubic area with crab louse.

Diagnosis

Mainly clinical, by finding the nits and adult lice on scalp hair. A simple bedside investigational tool is contactless dermatoscopy, called entomodermoscopy when applied to the insect world.

Differential Diagnosis

Pediculosis capitis and corporis:
- Seborrheic dermatitis
- Psoriasis vulgaris
- Hair casts
- Dried hair products such as sprays and gels
- Piedra
- Trichorrhexis nodosa

Pubic louse:
- Scabies
- Other arthropods
- White piedra
- Trichomycosis pubis or axillaris

Treatment

- *Basic care and preventive measures*: Care of hygiene, clothes, and environment, evaluation of family members and playmates, nit removal, instruction for parents and school/teachers. Wet hair combing with a fine light-colored nit comb slows down the movement of the lice and allows easy removal. It is repeated every 2–3 days and continued for several weeks.
- *Topical pediculicides*: Permethrin cream rinse/lotion 1% applied along the length of the hair for 30–45 minutes before washing and combing the wet hair with a fine-toothed comb.
- Other alternative topical preparations include gamma benzene hexachloride 1%, malathion, and spinosad.
- Occlusive petroleum jelly massaged on the scalp and hair overnight with a shower cap is believed to be effective in head louse infestation
- *Oral pediculicides*: Cotrimoxazole, albendazole, and ivermectin
- *Body louse infestation*: Laundering and heat treatment (ironing) of such clothing in the seam help in killing the lice and nits.
- *Pubic louse*: Avoid contact with the partner until both have been treated and when the absence of infection is confirmed on follow-up. Additionally, all bedsheets, towels, and clothing should be washed and ironed. Shaving pubic hair might help.

Demodicosis

- *Demodex* mite (*Demodex folliculorum* and *Demodex brevis*) is an obligate human ectoparasite found in or near the pilosebaceous units on the face. *Demodex* infestation usually remains asymptomatic but may be pathogenic in high density. The density of more than 5 mites per follicle has been considered a pathogenic criterion.
- Cutaneous diseases caused or associated with *Demodex* mites are named as demodicosis or demodicidosis. The prevalence of infestation is highest in the 20–30 years age group, when the sebum secretion rate is at its highest, and is low in infants and children. Sebaceous hyperplasia with oily or mixed skin favored *Demodex* proliferation. *Demodex* is associated with rosacea, steroid-induced dermatitis, seborrheic dermatitis, nonspecific facial dermatitis, and acne vulgaris.
- *Sites of involvement*: *Demodex* is commonly found on the face and is also present on the neck, ears, and bald scalp.

Clinical Features

It is unclear whether these conditions are caused by *Demodex* or the increase in mite density contributing to the inflammation. They include *Demodex* rosacea, steroid-induced rosacea, nonspecific facial dermatitis, lupus miliaris disseminatus faciei (LMDF), perioral dermatitis, androgenic alopecia, madarosis, blepharoconjunctivitis and dissecting folliculitis **(Fig. 19)**. Rosacea-like demodicidosis is characterized by dryness, follicular scaling, superficial vesicles, and pustules **(Fig. 20)**.

Diagnosis

Demodex mites are identified microscopically on KOH preparation of skin scrapings, biopsy, or by using the skin surface biopsy technique. A count of more than 5 mites/cm^2 from lesions is diagnostic. Dermatoscopy can be a useful aid for diagnosis, the two distinct dermoscopic findings are *Demodex* tails and follicular openings.

Treatment

- Topical crotamiton 1% and permethrin 5% have been used. Topical azelaic acid 10–20% or topical metronidazole 0.75–2% for weeks to months may be beneficial due to their anti-inflammatory effects.
- Oral ivermectin (200 μg/kg/dose, 2 doses 1 week apart) may be used in severe cases.
- Systemic metronidazole [250 mg three times a day (TID) for 2–8 weeks], doxycycline (50 mg daily for 2–8 weeks), tetracyclines, and ivermectin have also been used.
- A combination of oral and topical treatment may also be used.

Prevention

Prevention of the proliferation of mites can be achieved by regular facial cleansing and avoidance of oil-based cleansers and greasy cosmetics.

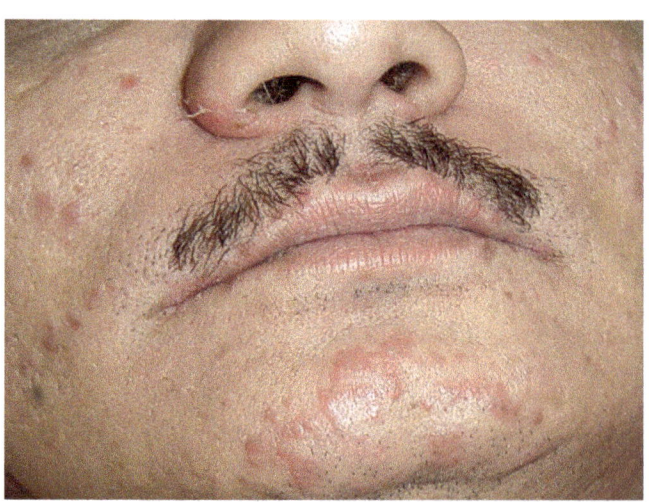

FIG. 19: Nonspecific facial dermatitis associated with demodicidosis.

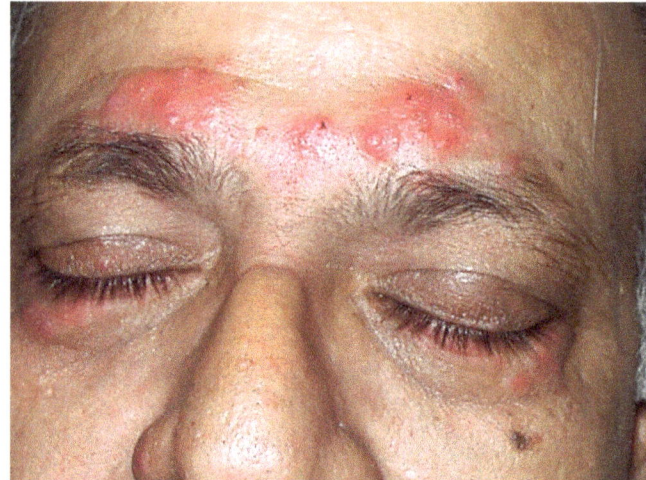

FIG. 20: Rosacea-like presentation of demodicidosis.

15. Bites and Stings

Introduction

A "bite" describes the process of toxins injected via structures associated with the mouth, such as fangs and mandible, while a "sting" connotes the injection of venom via a tapered structure most accurately called a sting (noun). Persons in tropical climates with fewer clothes are more prone to get bites or stings especially on the exposed parts. Occupations carrying increased risk include forest workers, dock workers, people handling foodstuff, and humans working with animals.

Arthropod Bites and Stings

These are a common occurrence worldwide. Mostly, it results in minor temporary cutaneous changes; though, rarely fatal anaphylactic reactions may occur. Clinical type and distribution of skin lesions vary for different arthropods. Most often observed lesion is papular urticaria **(Fig. 1)**.

Clinical Features

- Local irritation is a very common symptom of arthropod bites, and rubbing and scratching may lead to eczematization.
- Constitutional symptoms such as fever and malaise may also occur.
  Complications include secondary infection, impetigo, folliculitis, cellulitis, and lymphangitis.

Management

Management includes cleansing using soap and water in order to prevent secondary infection. Topical steroids

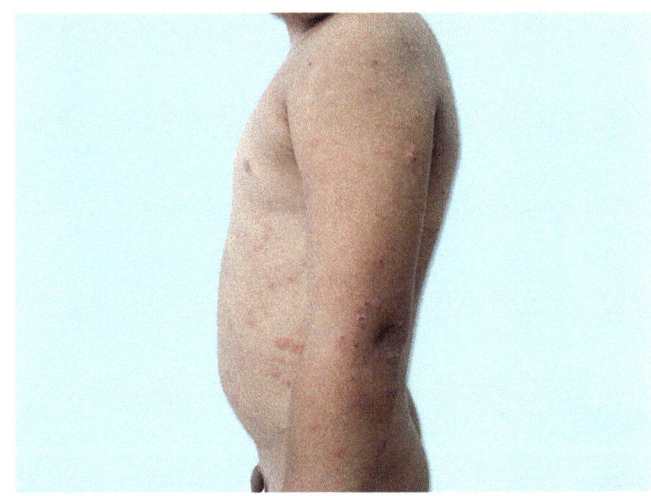

FIG. 1: Arms and trunk of a young child showing papular urticaria.

and oral antihistamines can be given for a short period. Aggressive treatment is only required for severe allergic reactions, which are rare and will include injectable steroids such as hydrocortisone and dexamethasone.

Bedbug Bites (Cimicosis)

The species of bedbugs commonly found in India are the common bedbug (*Cimex lectularius*) and tropical bedbug. In recent years, there has been an increase in the population as well as incidence of bites with bedbugs. These are nocturnal feeders which stay in groups, hidden in the crevices of the furniture, wall, picture frames, etc. Poor sanitation, overcrowding and trade in second-hand furniture facilitate infestation.

CHAPTER 15: Bites and Stings

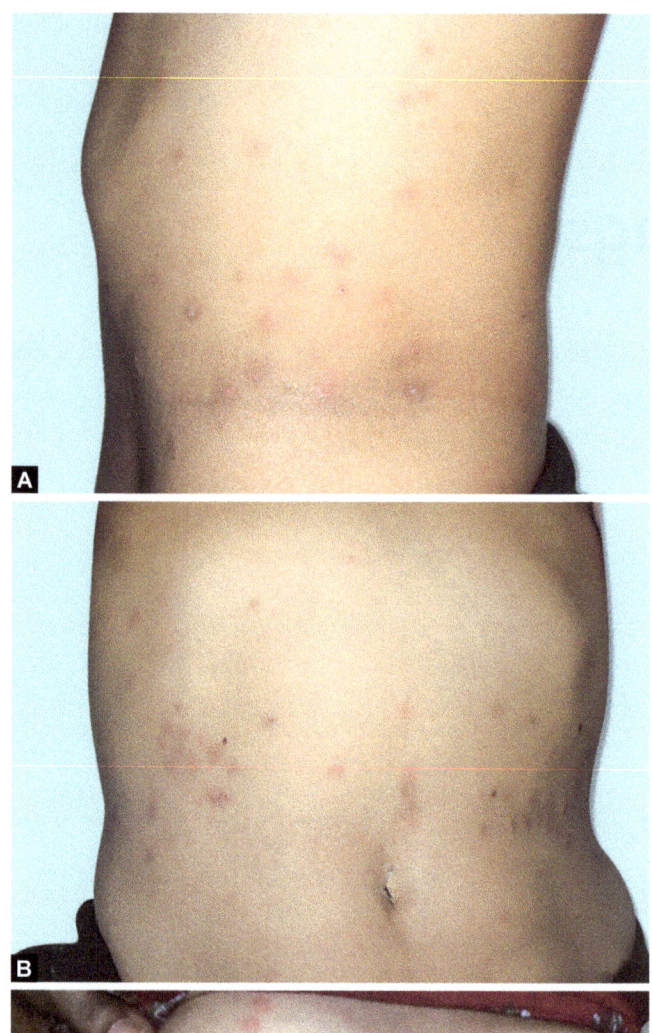

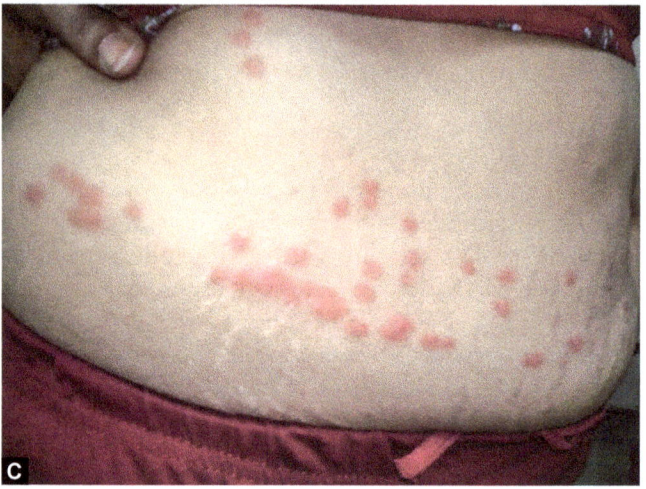

FIGS. 2A TO C: Bedbug bites with characteristic distribution.

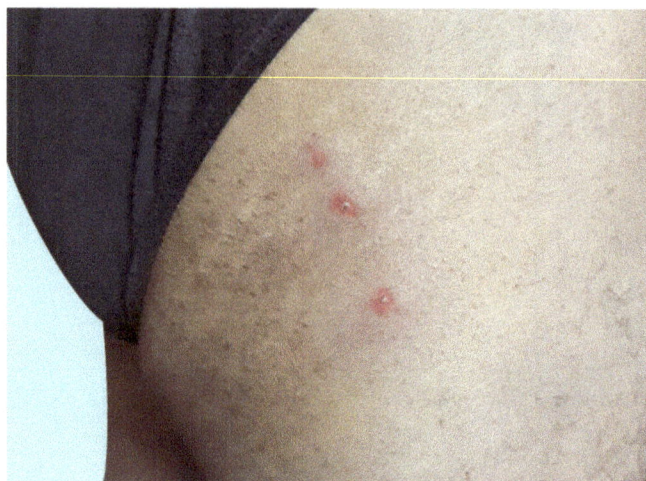

FIG. 3: "Breakfast, lunch, and dinner sign" in an adult.

irregular manner (**Figs. 2A to C**), with the arrangement in three rows being known as "breakfast, lunch, and dinner" sign (**Fig. 3**). The lesions are commonly present on exposed areas such as head, neck, arms, shoulders, and legs.

Treatment

Bedbug eradication is needed by removing infested furniture. The most effective insecticides are pyrethroids, dichlorvos, and malathion. Resistance of bedbugs to insecticides is known.

Blister Beetle Dermatoses (*Paederus* Dermatitis)

It is a seasonal vesicobullous disorder caused mainly by vesicant beetles belonging to the genus *Paederus* which have nocturnal habits, can fly, and are attracted to artificial lights. The vesicant action is caused by "pederin" which is a powerful crystalline caustic amide, acting on deoxyribonucleic acid (DNA) to block mitosis. This leads to erythema and smaller vesicles which converge to form blisters. Normally, the beetles do not bite or sting. The clinical manifestations are a result of the secretions of the beetle getting rubbed into the skin, after the insect has been crushed in an attempt to ward it off. The exposed areas of the body, such as face, neck, and limbs, are most commonly affected. The lesions heal in a week's time leaving behind erythematous or hyperchromic macules. The lesions are linear or elongated in configuration as the insect is rubbed against the skin (**Figs. 4A to C**).

Bites manifest as delayed hypersensitivity reaction with pruritus; painless, erythematous macules, papules, or nodules. Bites tend to be arranged in a linear or

CHAPTER 15: Bites and Stings

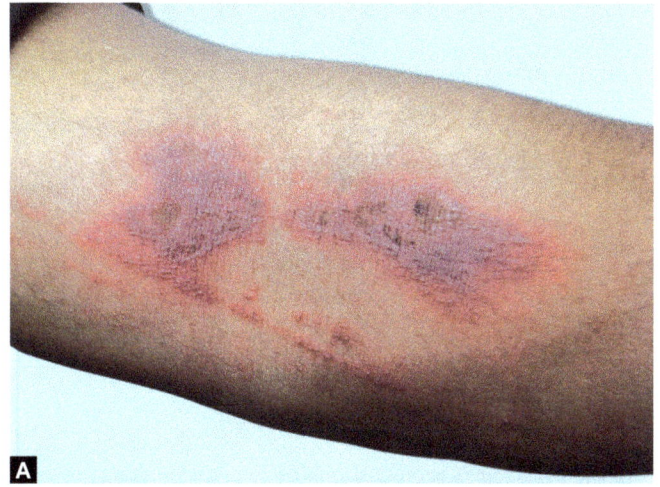
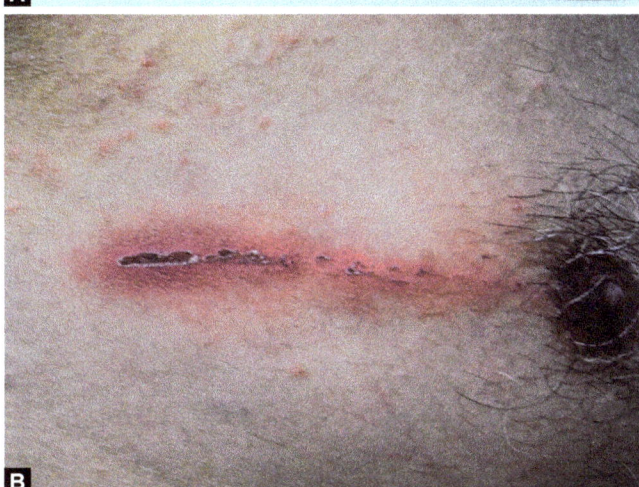
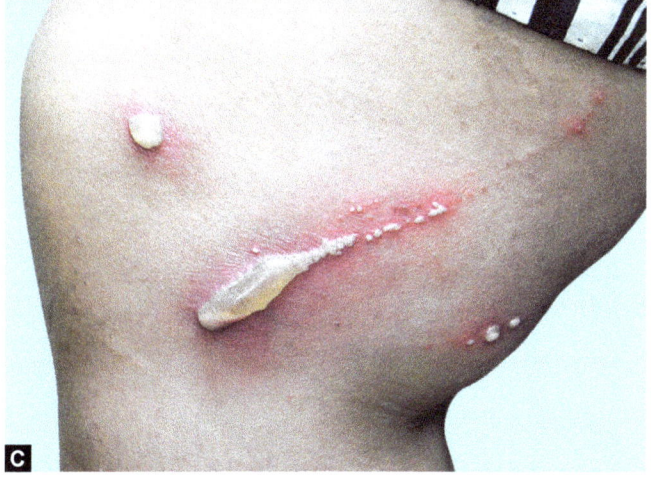

FIGS. 4A TO C: (A) Extensive dermatitis in a linear fashion on the arm. (B) There is vesiculation with subsequent eschar formation. (C) This case had presented with large bullae with hypopyon formation. The linear distribution and surrounding erythema reveals the etiology.

Tick Bites

Ticks act as vectors for infections such as Rocky Mountain spotted fever, Colorado tick fever, tularemia, tick paralysis, babesiosis, tickborne relapsing fever, ehrlichiosis, and Lyme disease.

They get attracted to the smell of sweat, white color, and body heat and their bites could produce characteristic skin lesions. Upon attaching to the host, the tick feeds on it for 2 hours to 7 days.

Tick bites are normally painless, but can sometimes cause a foreign body reaction, hypersensitivity reaction, or rarely a delayed hypersensitivity reaction with fever, pruritus, and urticaria. Retained mouthparts of the tick can also result in granulomatous foreign body reaction.

The tick *Ixodes scapularis* can cause Lyme's disease (erythema migrans) **(Fig. 5)**.

Prevention

Prevention of tick bites is critical for controlling the spread of tickborne diseases. Permethrin applied directly to the clothes is the most effective tick repellent. N, N-diethyl-m-toluamide (DEET) can also be applied on exposed skin surface. Thin tipped tweezers or forceps are used to grasp the tick as close to the skin surface as possible. The tick is to be pulled straight upward with even pressure so that mouthparts are not left behind.

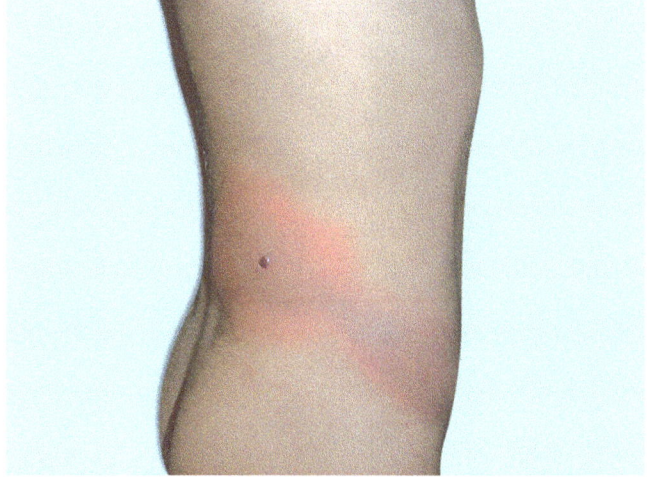

FIG. 5: Cutaneous manifestation of Lyme disease (erythema migrans).

Leech

Leeches are classified in the phylum *Annelida* (segmented worms). They attach themselves to the host skin using their powerful jaws, and feed on blood till they are engorged, after which they release their grip and drop to the ground. Their saliva possesses fibrinolytic, anticoagulant, vasodilator, and anesthetic properties. During this process, substances introduced in the host can be antigenic. If sensitization occurs, the bite reaction may be urticarial or bullous **(Fig. 6)**.

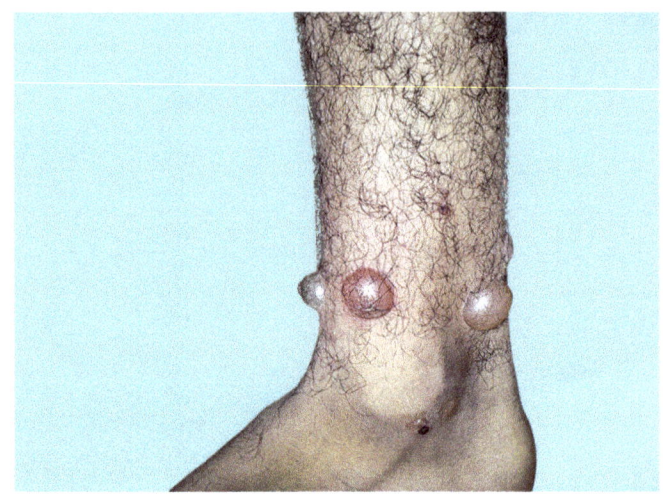

FIG. 6: Bullous lesions due to leech bite.

CHAPTER 16

Sexually Transmitted Infections

Introduction

Sexually transmitted infections (STIs) are the ones transmitted predominantly through sexual contact including vaginal intercourse, anal, or oral sex. They were earlier referred to as STDs or venereal diseases (VD); however, the term STI is now preferred in view of a broader meaning including infections that can exist without any disease manifestation.

STIs are broadly divided into genital discharge disease (GDD) and genital ulcer disease (GUD).
- *Genital discharge disease*: *Neisseria gonorrhoeae*, *Chlamydia trachomatis,* and organisms such as Ureaplasma or mycoplasma are the major causative agents responsible for genital discharge disease.
- *GUD*: This chapter includes chancroid, syphilis, and lymphogranuloma venereum (LGV), with genital herpes being included in the chapter on herpes viral infections.

Common risk factors for acquiring STIs include high-risk sexual behavior, age younger than 25 years, inconsistent use of contraception, substance abuse, history of STIs, promiscuity, or multiple sexual partners.

Gonorrhea

It is one of the oldest known human infections, a common human STI. It is caused by *N. gonorrhoeae*, which is an exclusively human pathogen, transmitted sexually or rarely, and perinatantly to newborns. Men with gonorrhea are usually symptomatic (asymptomatic/mild urethral infection in 10–15% of cases), while the majority of women with gonorrhea have no symptoms. Untreated, gonorrhea can be a serious health hazard, particularly in women, leading to tubal scarring, infertility, and increased risk of contracting and transmitting human immunodeficiency virus (HIV).

Neisseria gonorrhoeae (gonococci), the causative agent of gonorrhea, is a gram-negative, nonmotile, and nonsporing diplococcus that is seen in pairs with adjacent sides flattened. It is a fastidious organism with complex growth requirements. It infects only mucosae lined by columnar or cuboidal noncornified epithelial cells. Thus, it can infect the male urethra, paraurethral glands and ducts, cervix, Bartholin's ducts, rectum, and conjunctiva. Female urethra escapes infection because of only a few scattered areas of columnar epithelium. Gonococcal vulvovaginitis in prepubertal girls is due to infection of the stratified squamous epithelium of the vagina.

Clinical Features

The mean incubation period after contact is 2–5 days (range: 1–14 days) and the clinical spectrum varies from asymptomatic infection to systemic dissemination.
- Asymptomatic infection involves the urethra, endocervix, rectum, and pharynx, accounting for 15% of cases in males and 50% of cases in females.
- Anterior urethritis is the most common manifestation in men. It starts with scanty mucoid or mucopurulent discharge, progressing to profuse thick purulent discharge per urethra within 24 hours **(Fig. 1)**. It can be associated with dysuria, frequency, urgency, perimeatal erythema, and edema. Gonococcal balanoposthitis may develop due to direct contact with the discharge **(Fig. 2)**.
- Cervicitis in females can be gonococcal in etiology. The endocervical canal is the primary site of infection **(Fig. 3)** and is usually associated with urethral colonization. Dysuria, frequency, urgency, and scanty discharge is seen. Involvement of periurethral gland or Bartholin's gland ducts can occur.
- Primary rectal infection can occur in men who have sex with men (MSM) while in women, rectal gonorrhea

CHAPTER 16: Sexually Transmitted Infections

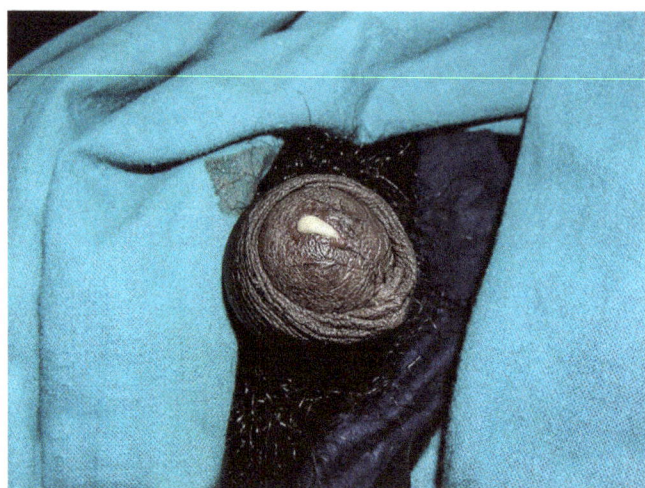

FIG. 1: Acute gonococcal urethritis with thick profuse discharge.

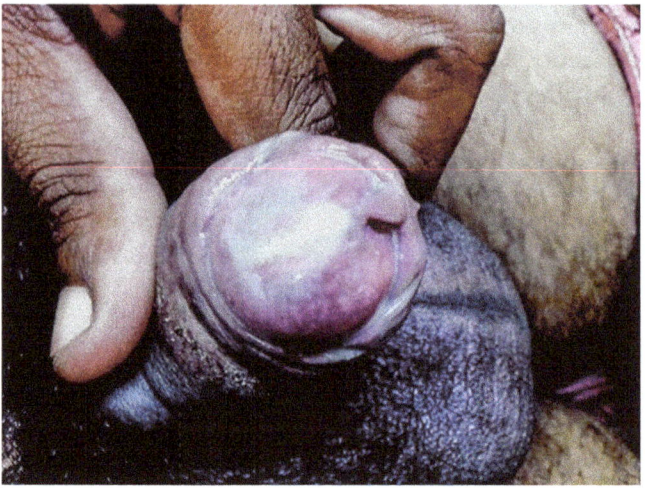

FIG. 2: Acute gonococcal urethritis with surrounding balanoposthitis.

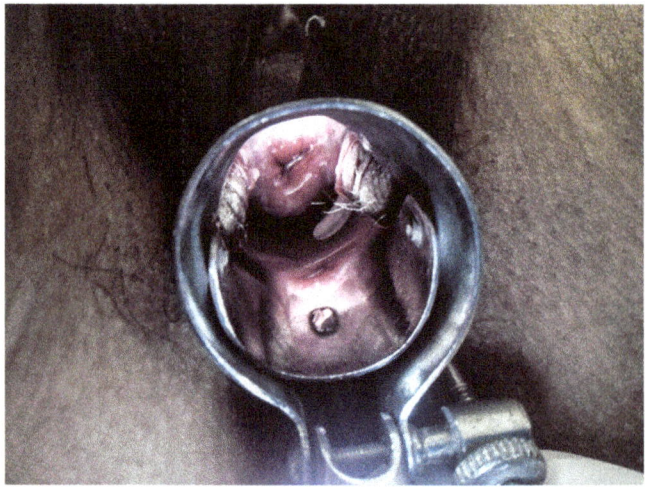

FIG. 3: Acute gonococcal cervicitis.

is secondary to perineal contamination from infected cervical discharge. It may vary from asymptomatic infection to mild discharge, bleeding, or overt proctitis.
- Pharyngitis is more commonly seen in MSM, where 90% of cases are asymptomatic. Others may have acute pharyngitis or tonsillitis.
- Gonococcal conjunctivitis can occur due to inoculation. Rare cutaneous infection can be localized ulcer of the genitals, perineum, upper thighs, or finger.
- Infection in infants is primary gonococcal conjunctivitis (5–15% of conjunctivitis in newborns), due to exposure to infected cervical exudate at birth. It is an acute illness that manifests 2–5 days after birth. Manifestations include ophthalmia neonatorum and sepsis (including arthritis and meningitis), rhinitis, vaginitis, urethritis, and reinfection at sites of fetal monitoring.

Complications

Complications associated with gonorrhea are summarized in **Table 1**.

Diagnosis

Diagnosis is based on the microscopic identification of *N. gonorrhoeae* from infected sites, culture, and the serological tests.
- *Specimen collection*: Urethral swab is obtained by passing a small sterile wool cotton swab or loop into the urethra. If no discharge, milking of urethra is performed. A 15–30 mL of first voided urine after 6–8 hours of urine holding can also be used as a specimen. For specimen collection in females, the cervix is cleaned; a swab is inserted 1–2 cm into

TABLE 1: Complications of gonorrhea.

	Local		Systemic
In men		**In women**	**DGI**
Epididymitis		Acute salpingitis	Endocarditis
Posterior urethritis		Pelvic inflammatory disease	Meningitis
Urethral strictures		Infertility	Arthritis
Cowper's gland inflammation		Ectopic pregnancy	
Tyson's gland inflammation		Chronic pelvic pain	
Seminal vesiculitis		Hydrosalpinx	
Penile lymphangitis		Pyosalpinx	
Periurethral abscess		Tubo-ovarian abscess	

(DGI: disseminated gonococcal infection)

the endocervical canal and rotated gently for up to 10 seconds. If per speculum is not possible, blind vaginal specimen can also be obtained. Extragenital specimens may be used for nucleic acid amplification techniques (NAAT). Anorectal specimens are collected by swabs passed 2–3 cm into the anal canal, avoiding gross fecal contamination. Pharyngeal specimens are collected by swabbing the posterior pharynx including the tonsillar areas and faucial pillars.

- *Direct microscopy*: Swab specimen is homogeneously spread on a clean slide, dried and heat fixed, stained with Gram's stain, and examined under oil immersion objective. Gonococci are identified as gram-negative diplococci within or in close association with polymorphonuclear cells **(Fig. 4)**. Smears from the rectum or endocervical canal are less sensitive and less specific than urethral smears.
- *Bacterial culture*: It is the most specific investigation. As gonococci are fastidious organisms, antibiotic-containing selective media such as modified Thayer–Martin medium (MTM), Chacko Nair medium, Martin Lewis, and New York City (NYC) medium are used. Stuart's medium or Amies medium is used as transport media when prompt incubation of the specimen is not possible. The diagnostic sensitivity of selective media depends on the anatomic site being cultured as well as on the time gap between the collection of the specimen and its incubation. Culture methods provide the additional advantage of monitoring gonococcal antibiotic susceptibility.
- *Nonculture tests*: Nonamplified DNA probe tests, NAAT, polymerase chain reaction (PCR) based assays, enzyme-linked immunosorbent assay (ELISA), DNA hybridization, etc. have become popular in recent years. With these tests, a single specimen can be used for simultaneously testing *C. trachomatis*.
- *Serology*: Antibody detection by complement fixation, latex agglutination, immunofluorescence, hemagglutination, immunoprecipitation, ELISA, radioimmunoassay, immunoblotting, bacterial lysis, etc. has low diagnostic sensitivity and specificity, hence, not useful for screening and diagnostic purpose.

Based on the diagnostic tests, *case classification* (effective January 1, 2014) has been proposed:

- *Probable gonorrhea*: Demonstration of gram-negative intracellular diplococci in a urethral smear obtained from a male or an endocervical smear obtained from a female.
- *Confirmed gonorrhea*: Laboratory isolation of typical gram-negative, oxidase-positive diplococci by culture (presumptive *N. gonorrhoeae*) from a clinical specimen or demonstration of *N. gonorrhoeae* in a clinical specimen by detection of antigen or detection of nucleic acid via nucleic acid amplification (e.g., PCR) or hybridization with a nucleic acid probe.

Treatment Recommendations

These treatment recommendations are based on "Sexually Transmitted Infections Treatment Guidelines, 2021" (published July 2021 by CDC).

Uncomplicated gonococcal infections of the cervix, urethra, and rectum:

- Recommended regimen is ceftriaxone 500 mg intramuscular (IM), a single dose for weight <150 kg (if weight is more than that, then the dose is 1 g).
- If chlamydial infection has not been excluded, treat for chlamydia with doxycycline 100 mg orally 2 times/day for 7 days.
- If ceftriaxone is not available, use gentamicin 240 mg IM + azithromycin 2 g orally as a single dose or cefixime 800 mg orally as a single dose.

Uncomplicated gonococcal infections of the pharynx:

- Recommended regimen is ceftriaxone 500 mg IM, a single dose for weight <150 Kg (if weight is more than that, then the dose is 1 g).
- If chlamydial infection has not been excluded, treat for chlamydia with doxycycline 100 mg orally 2 times/day for 7 days.
- No reliable alternative regimens available

To maximize adherence with recommended therapies:

- Medication should be provided on-site and directly observed.

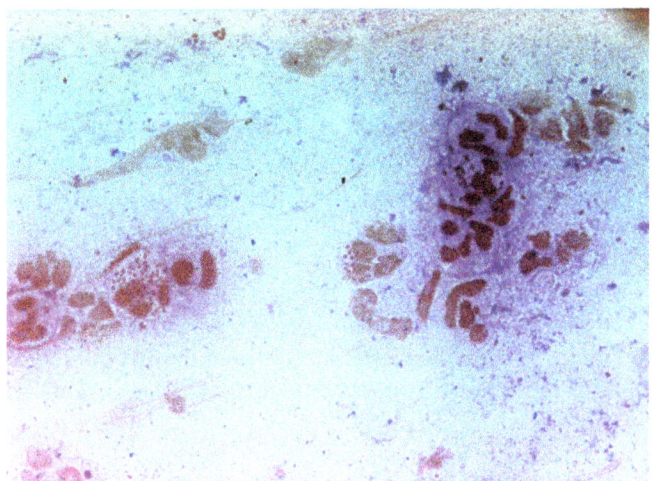

FIG. 4: Gram-negative intracellular diplococci in urethral smear full of polymorphonuclear cells (Gram's stain 1,000×).

- If medications are unavailable, linkage to an STI treatment facility should be provided for same-day treatment.
- To minimize disease transmission, persons treated for gonorrhea should be instructed to abstain from sexual activity for 7 days after treatment and until all sex partners are treated (7 days after receiving treatment and resolution of symptoms, if present).
- All persons who receive a diagnosis of gonorrhea should be tested for other STIs, including chlamydia, syphilis, and HIV.
- Those persons whose HIV test results are negative should be offered HIV pre-exposure prophylaxis (PrEP).
- Test of cure at 7 days is unnecessary for those treated with these regimens.
- *Pregnancy*: Do not use quinolones or tetracyclines. Only a recommended or alternate cephalosporin is to be given. Women who cannot tolerate cephalosporin should be administered a single 2 g dose of azithromycin.
- *HIV infection*: Same treatment regimen as of those who are HIV negative

Gonococcal conjunctivitis in adolescents and adults:
- Recommended regimen is ceftriaxone 1 g IM, single dose.
- Consider the lavage of the infected eye with saline solution once.

Disseminated gonococcal infection (arthritis and arthritis-dermatitis syndrome):
- Recommended regimen is ceftriaxone 1 g IM or intravenously (IV) every 24 hours.
- If chlamydial infection has not been excluded, treat for chlamydia with doxycycline 100 mg orally 2 times/day for 7 days.
- Alternative regimens are cefotaxime 1 g IV every 8 hours, or ceftizoxime 1 g IV every 8 hours.
- These should be continued for 24-48 hours after improvement begins then switched to cefixime 400 mg orally twice daily to complete at least 1 week.

Gonococcal meningitis and endocarditis:
- Recommended regimen ceftriaxone 1-2 g IV every 12 hours
- Therapy for meningitis continued for 10-14 days while for endocarditis continued for at least 4 weeks.
- If chlamydial infection has not been excluded, treat for chlamydia with doxycycline 100 mg orally 2 times/day for 7 days.

Ophthalmia neonatorum (by N. gonorrhoeae):
- *Prophylaxis*: Erythromycin 0.5% ophthalmic ointment in each eye in a single application at birth
- Recommended regimen is ceftriaxone 25-50 mg/kg IV or IM, single dose, not to exceed 250 mg.

Disseminated gonococcal infection in neonates:
- Ceftriaxone 25-50 mg/kg/day IV or IM, single daily dose for 7 days. Duration 10-14 days if meningitis is documented.
- Cefotaxime 25 mg/kg/day IV or IM every 12 hours for 7 days. Duration 10-14 days if meningitis is documented.

Prophylactic treatment for infants with mothers having gonococcal infection:
- Recommended regimen in the absence of signs of gonococcal infection is ceftriaxone 25-50 mg/kg IV or IM, in a single dose, not to exceed 250 mg.

Children (<45 kg) with uncomplicated gonococcal vulvovaginitis, cervicitis, urethritis, pharyngitis, or proctitis:
- Recommended regimen is ceftriaxone 25-50 mg/kg IV or IM, in a single dose, not to exceed 250 mg.
- For children >45 kg, treat as adults.

Children with bacteremia and arthritis:
- Children weighing <45 kg, ceftriaxone 50 mg/kg IV or IM, not to exceed 2 g in a single dose daily, every 24 hours for 7 days
- Children weighing >45 kg, ceftriaxone 1 g IV or IM, in a single dose daily, every 24 hours for 7 days

Management of sex partners:
- Patients should be instructed to refer their sex partners for evaluation and treatment.
- All sex partners within 60 days before the onset of symptoms or diagnosis should be evaluated and treated for *N. gonorrhoeae* and *C. trachomatis* infections.
- Advised to avoid sexual intercourse until therapy is completed and until they and their sex partners no longer have symptoms.

Follow-up

- Uncomplicated gonorrhea treated with any of the recommended or alternative regimens does not need a test of cure.
- Persistent symptoms after treatment should be evaluated by culture for *N. gonorrhoeae*, and gonococci isolated should be tested for antimicrobial susceptibility. It might also be caused by *C. trachomatis* or other organisms.
- Retesting is recommended approximately 3 months after treatment, or whenever on the next visit in 12 months posttreatment, regardless of the sex partner management.

Prevention

- Education of the population, identification of symptomatic and asymptomatic contacts, and effective diagnosis and treatment
- Latex condoms, to be used consistently and correctly
- Individual and group-based prevention counseling

Chlamydial Infections

- Genital infections caused by *C. trachomatis*, an obligate intracellular human pathogen, are the most common bacterial STIs worldwide.
- Clinical spectrum varies from asymptomatic urethritis or cervicitis to serious complications and infertility, quite similar to gonorrhea.
- Inflammation of the urethra, caused by organisms other than *Gonococcus*, is called nongonococcal urethritis (NGU). *C. trachomatis* is the causative agent of 35–50% of the NGU cases.
- *Chlamydiae* are obligate intracellular parasites as they lack the capacity to synthesize adenosine triphosphate (ATP) and thus are dependent on the host cells for ATP and nutrient supply.
- The unique developmental cycle of Chlamydia is shown in **Figure 5**.
- The organism infects columnar or transitional epithelium, involving the urethra, epididymis, endocervix, endometrium, salpinx, peritoneum, and rectum.

Clinical Features

Chlamydial infections are commonly asymptomatic or mild genital infections that occur after an incubation period of 1–3 weeks or longer.

Infection in men:
- *Urethritis*: This is less abrupt and milder in course, in comparison to gonococcal urethritis. A low-grade urethritis, with scanty to moderate, mucoid urethral discharge, unlike the profuse purulent gonococcal discharge. Subclinical infection is also common. Complaints include dysuria, hematuria, or pyuria.
- *Littritis*: It presents as urethral inflammation with no specific symptoms. Threads or grains can be found in the urine.
- *Epididymitis*: It presents with unilateral scrotal pain, tenderness, swelling, and fever.
- *Prostatovesiculitis*: It is characterized by diffuse pain in the perineal and suprapubic region, fever, malaise, and dysuria. Painful urination with muscle spasm of the urethra resulting in urinary retention, tenesmus, and difficult defecation can occur.
- *Proctitis*: It presents with symptoms such as rectal pain, bleeding, mucous discharge, and diarrhea.
- *Reiter's syndrome* [diagnostic triad of urethritis, arthritis, and conjunctivitis with typical mucocutaneous findings (diagnostic tetrad)] or sexually acquired reactive arthritis (SARA) has been associated with Chlamydial genitourinary infection (present or past).

Infection in women:
- *Cervicitis*: It usually goes unnoticed or may present with mucopurulent discharge and hypertrophic friable cervix.
- *Urethritis*: It is infrequent in women in the absence of cervical involvement.
- *Bartholinitis* is purulent exudative infection of Bartholin's ducts.

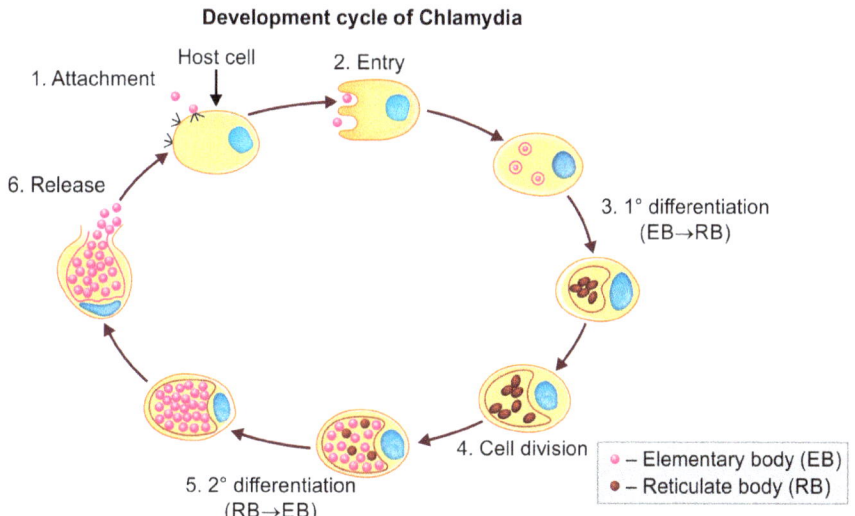

FIG. 5: Life cycle of chlamydia.

- *Endometritis* is characterized by abnormal vaginal bleeding, menorrhagia, and metrorrhagia.
- *Salpingitis/pelvic inflammatory disease* is associated with absent or mild signs and symptoms (silent salpingitis) but can cause long-term sequela of tubal scarring resulting in ectopic pregnancy or infertility.
- *Perihepatitis (Fitz-Hugh-Curtis syndrome)* is more commonly caused by *C. trachomatis*. It simulates acute cholecystitis with fever, nausea, vomiting, and right upper quadrant pain.

Other infections (both men and women):
- Conjunctivitis commonly seen in neonates and children
- Pharyngeal involvement in those involved in oral sex
- Systemic involvement gives rise to endocarditis, pneumonitis, meningoencephalitis, and peritonitis.

Diagnosis

- *Direct microscopy*: Presence of mucopurulent discharge with Gram staining showing more than 5 WBC/HPF (penile) or more than 30 WBC/HPF (endocervical specimens) can help presumptive diagnosis. Persistent pyuria in first voided urine or positive leukocyte esterase test is helpful for a presumptive diagnosis.
- *Cytology* detects intracytoplasmic inclusions in exfoliated epithelial cells by Giemsa stain, immunofluorescence, immunoperoxidase, or iodine staining methods.
- *Cell culture* performed in embryonated chicken eggs, McCoy cell line, Monkey kidney, HeLa, and HEp-2 cell lines has been used for isolation.
- *Nonculture tests* include antigen detection tests, nucleic acid detection tests (amplification type or hybridization type), urethral lymphocyte isolation, or nonspecific tests such as leukocyte esterase test (considered the best screening test for adolescent males).

Based on diagnostic tests, case classification for chlamydial infections proposes a confirmed case being the one that is laboratory confirmed by:
- Isolation of *C. trachomatis* by culture
- Demonstration of *C. trachomatis* in a clinical specimen by detection of antigen or nucleic acid

Treatment Recommendations

Coinfection with *C. trachomatis* frequently occurs in patients with gonococcal infection; therefore, presumptive treatment of such patients for chlamydia is appropriate. Centers for Disease Control and Prevention (CDC) 2021 recommendations for the treatment of Chlamydia are as follows:
- *Uncomplicated C. trachomatis infections (urethral, endocervical, and rectal)*:
  - Recommended regimen doxycycline 100 mg orally twice a day for 7 days.
  - Alternative regimens are azithromycin 1 g orally, single dose or levofloxacin 500 mg orally daily for 7 days.
- *C. trachomatis infection in pregnancy*:
  - Recommended regimen is azithromycin 1 g orally in a single dose.
  - Alternative regimen is amoxicillin 500 mg orally three times a day for 7 days.
- *Chlamydia infection in neonates*:
  - Erythromycin base or ethyl succinate 50 mg/kg/day, orally, divided into 4 doses daily, for 14 days
  - Due to the association between oral azithromycin and erythromycin with infantile hypertrophic pyloric stenosis (IHPS) in infants <6 weeks, infants treated with either of these antibiotics should be followed up for IHPS signs and symptoms.
- *Chlamydia infection in infants*:
  - Erythromycin base or ethyl succinate 50 mg/kg/day, orally, divided into 4 doses daily, for 14 days
  - *Alternative regimen*: Azithromycin suspension 20 g/kg/day orally, single dose daily, for 3 days
- *Children who weigh less than 45 kg*:
  - Recommended regimen is erythromycin base or ethylsuccinate 50 mg/kg/day orally divided into 4 doses daily for 14 days.
  - Data is limited regarding azithromycin.
- *Children who weigh >45 kg but aged <8 years*:
  - Recommended regimen of azithromycin 1 g orally in a single dose
  - *Alternative*: Doxycycline 100 mg orally twice a day for 7 days

Follow-up

- Test of cure (at 3–4 weeks after completing therapy) is recommended for pregnant women, with questionable therapeutic compliance, persistent symptoms, or reinfection.
- Retesting is recommended 3 months after treatment, or whenever on the next visit in 12 months posttreatment, regardless of the sex partner management.

Management of sex partner:
- All sex partners during the 60 days preceding the onset of the symptoms or chlamydia diagnosis should be evaluated, tested, and treated.
- Abstinence until 7 days after a single dose regimen or completion of a multiple dose regimen

Chancroid

It is an acute, autoinoculable GUD caused by the bacterium *Haemophilus ducreyi*. It is a major cause of GUDs worldwide, with a high prevalence in developing countries of Africa, Asia, and Caribbean islands (23–56% of GUDs).

Clinical Features

- The incubation period (1–10 days) is followed by the appearance of a small erythematous papule that progresses to a pustule and ulcer.
- Subsequently, multiple, painful nonindurated ulcers varying in size from 3 mm to 2 cm with ragged undermined edges appear **(Fig. 6)**. The floor is covered with yellow necrotic exudate and vascular granulation tissue which bleeds on gentle manipulation.
- These may present anywhere on anogenital skin, rarely extragenital sites including breast, lips, tongue, and oropharynx.
- Classic chancroid triad of "undermined ulcer edge, purulent dirty gray base, and moderate-to-severe pain" is found in most ulcers.
- Clinical variants include follicular, dwarf, transient, papular, giant, or phagedenic chancroid **(Fig. 7)**
- Tender, unilateral, inguinal lymphadenitis develops in 30–60% of patients **(Fig. 8)**.
- In upto 25% cases, suppuration and formation of a unilocular abscess in the regional lymph node, occurs. It is called a bubo **(Fig. 9)**.
- Other complications include phimosis, paraphimosis, urethral fistula, and phagedenic ulcers. Untreated ulcers take several weeks or months to resolve.

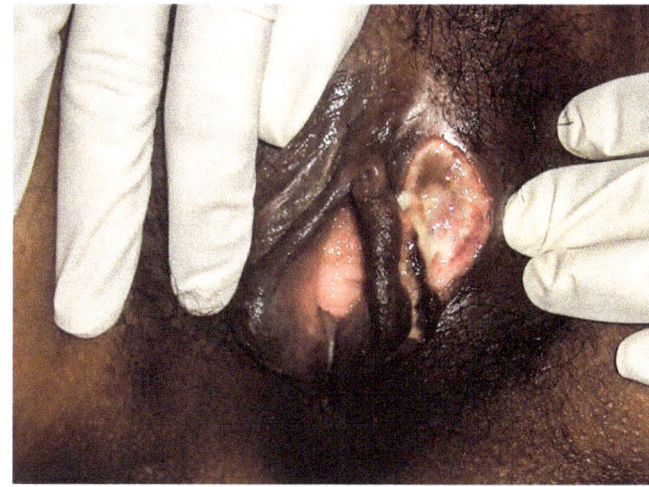

FIG. 7: Phagedenic chancroid.

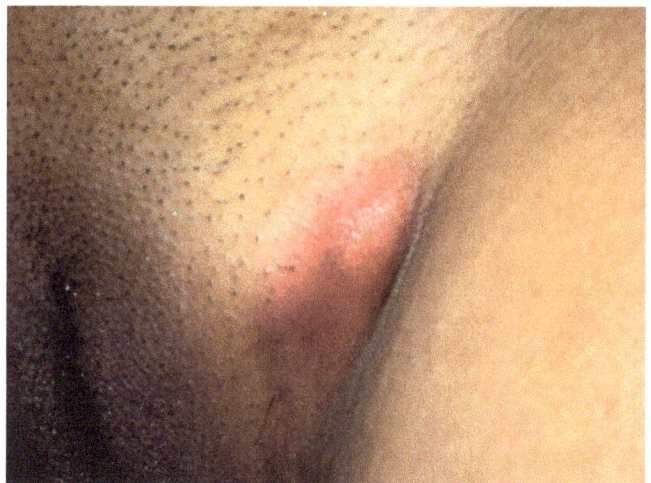

FIG. 8: Unilateral lymphadenitis.

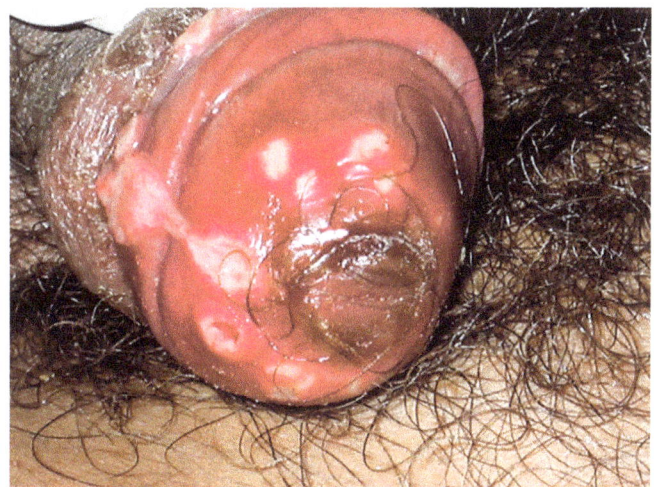

FIG. 6: Multiple, painful, and nonindurated ulcers.

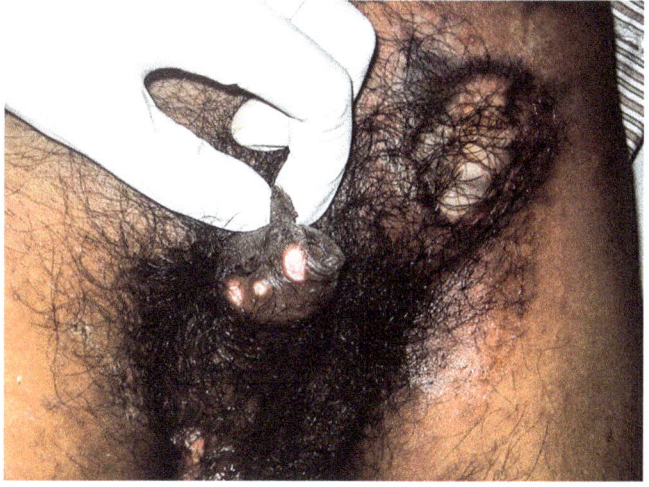

FIG. 9: Chancroid with inguinal bubo.

Diagnosis

- Smears of scrapings from the ulcer base, or pus aspirate from bubo, stained with Gram stain, show a "school of fish" appearance (gram-negative coccobacilli arranged in short parallel chains). Direct microscopy has low sensitivity (10–63%) and specificity.
- The gold standard for diagnosis is culture on selective media such as enriched gonococcal agar base or enriched Mueller–Hinton agar.
- Monoclonal antibody-based direct and indirect immunofluorescence assays have high sensitivity.
- DNA amplification techniques have a high sensitivity of 83–96%.
- Multiplex PCR for *H. ducreyi*, *Treponema pallidum*, and herpes simplex virus is available.

Treatment Recommendations

Single-dose therapies are preferred to improve compliance. CDC 2021 recommendations for the management of chancroid include:

- Recommended regimen is azithromycin 1 g orally, single dose or ceftriaxone 250 mg IM, single dose or ciprofloxacin 500 mg orally twice a day for 3 days (contraindicated for pregnant and lactating women), or erythromycin base 500 mg orally three times a day for 7 days.
- The fluctuant bubo should be aspirated from the nondependent part.
- Patients should be examined 3–7 days after the treatment. Complete healing of an ulcer takes approximately 2 weeks, while lymphadenopathy may take another week.

Lymphogranuloma Venereum

It is a chronic systemic STI primarily infecting lymphatics. It is caused by *C. trachomatis* biovars L1–L3. LGV proctitis has emerged among HIV seropositive patients predominantly in the Western world, making it one of the major re-emerging infections.

Clinical Features

- It is more common in males with a peak incidence in 15–40 years individuals.
- Males commonly present with acute form, while females present with late complications.
- Classical LGV presents in three clinical stages:
    i. The first stage is characterized by a small, often unnoticed transient ulcer over the genitalia at the site of inoculation. With rectal transmission, acute proctitis may be the initial manifestation presenting with a mucoid, purulent or bloody anal discharge with excruciating pain, tenesmus, and constipation.
    ii. The second stage, the inguinal stage, develops 2–6 weeks later when initial ulceration has resolved. It presents with firm, enlarged, painful, and tender regional lymph nodes (buboes) associated with fever and malaise. Inguinal and femoral lymph nodes are most commonly involved with painful, elongated, unilateral, sausage-shaped swellings above and below the Poupart's ligament (the "groove sign"). Involved lymph nodes may suppurate and rupture in one-third of cases and discharge purulent material from multiple fistulous orifices. Most buboes ultimately heal without complications; some may progress to chronic sinus formation.
    iii. Third stage (genitoanorectal syndrome) in MSM and females engaging in anal intercourse, leads to distortion of anal and rectal anatomy. This can lead to sequelae such as stricture formation, fistulae, and abscesses, associated with rectovaginal, rectovesical, and fistula in ano.
- Chronic inguinal lymphadenitis leads to genital elephantiasis, leading to woody hard genital tissue with a verrucous surface, due to lymphangiectatic papules. The penis may assume the shape of a "ram horn" or a "saxophone" while in women, "esthiomene" results **(Fig. 10)**.

Diagnosis

- Direct staining of smears with Giemsa or Fuchsin stain may reveal the intracellular corpuscles or Miyagawa bodies, suggestive of this infection.

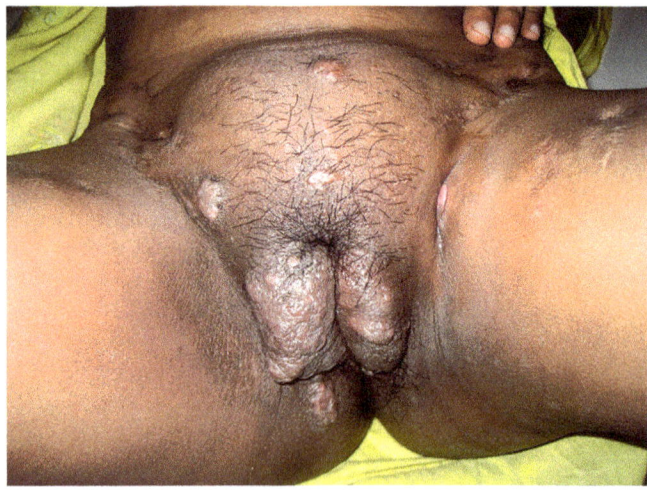

FIG. 10: Esthiomene in a female patient present with enlargement of genitalia. Note the scarring in the bilateral inguinal area.

- Serology using complement fixation test and microimmunofluorescence is useful in detecting immunoglobulin G (IgG) antibodies.
- Culture is the most specific method of diagnosis but is technically demanding, expensive and not readily available. It requires specific cyclohexamide treated McCoy cells or diethylaminoethyl-treated HeLa cells.
- NAAT is available for detecting all serovars of *Chlamydia* including LGV serovars and is the investigation of choice.

Treatment Recommendations

The CDC 2021 recommendations for the treatment of LGV include:
- Recommended regimen is doxycycline 100 mg orally twice a day for 21 days.
- Alternative regimen is azithromycin 1 g orally daily for 21 days or erythromycin base 500 mg orally four times a day for 21 days.
- Azithromycin regimen, if used, necessitates a test-of-cure with *C. trachomatis* NAAT, 4 weeks after completion of therapy.
- Fluctuant lymph nodes should be aspirated through healthy skin and not incised and drained.
- Patients without residual sequela usually will not require follow-up. In the case of sinus formation, strictures, or fistulae, surgical correction is indicated, and the patient should be followed up till these are asymptomatic.

Syphilis

It is an STI that causes a chronic, systemic infection capable of involving every organ in the body. The disease has been prevalent for centuries and still continues to be a challenge in STI control. The distribution of syphilis is worldwide, and resurgence has been documented with the HIV epidemic. There are two broad stages of syphilis—early and late (cut off being taken as 2 years by CDC and 1 year by WHO):
1. Early-stage syphilis manifests as:
   a. Primary syphilis presenting with chancre and lymphadenopathy
   b. Secondary syphilis with pleomorphic cutaneous and systemic presentations
   c. Latent syphilis as an extended asymptomatic phase with serological positivity
2. Late-stage syphilis manifests as:
   a. Late latent syphilis which may persist and progress without any clinical manifestations.
   b. Tertiary syphilis—clinically manifested as tertiary gummatous syphilis, neurosyphilis, or cardiovascular syphilis.

Clinical Features

Syphilis is also known as the "great mimic" as it presents with a variety of clinical features across the spectrum of the disease.

Primary Syphilis

- After a highly variable incubation period (9–90 days), a primary chancre appears at the site of inoculation as a single, painless, button-like indurated, round to oval, clearly defined ulcer **(Fig. 11)**.
- The sites of predilection include prepuce, coronary sulcus, frenulum, or glans in males and labia in females **(Fig. 12)**.
- Special attention should be given to anal chancres, and extragenital sites such as lips, tongue, nipples, or hands. Kissing ulcers occur in the urethral meatus and coronal sulcus **(Fig. 13)**.
- The ulcer is accompanied by firm, nontender, regional lymphadenopathy.
- Spontaneous resolution of the chancre and lymphadenopathy usually occurs within 4–6 weeks leaving a depressed scar.

Secondary Syphilis

- After 6 weeks to 6 months, 40% of untreated infected individuals go on to develop secondary syphilis signified by flu-like prodrome with fever, malaise,

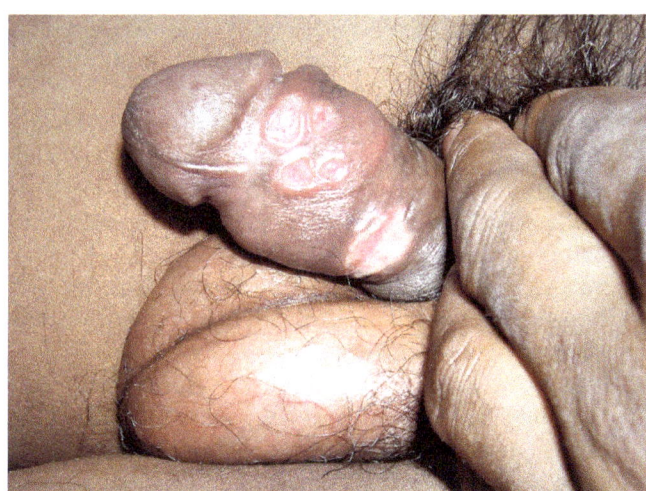

FIG. 11: Primary chancres on the penile shaft.

CHAPTER 16: Sexually Transmitted Infections

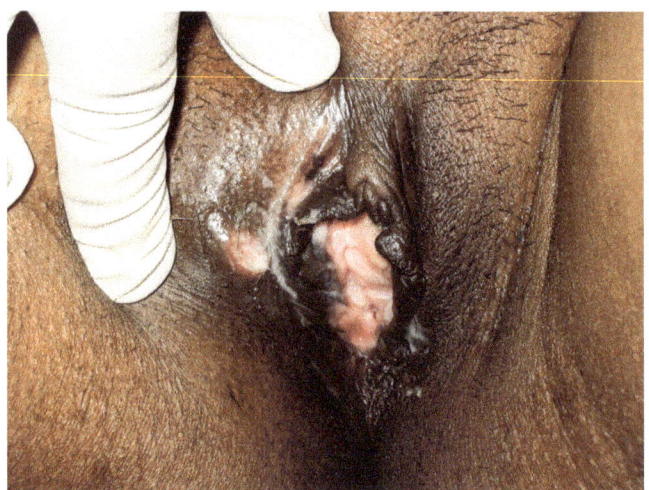

FIG. 12: Primary chancre in a female patient.

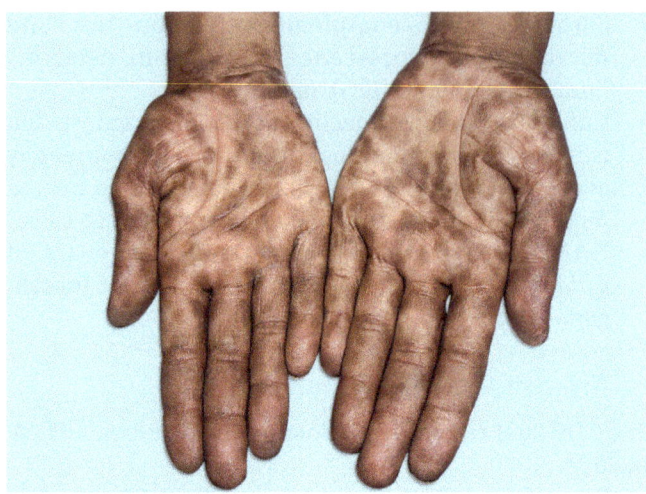

FIG. 14: Lesions of secondary syphilis involving palms.

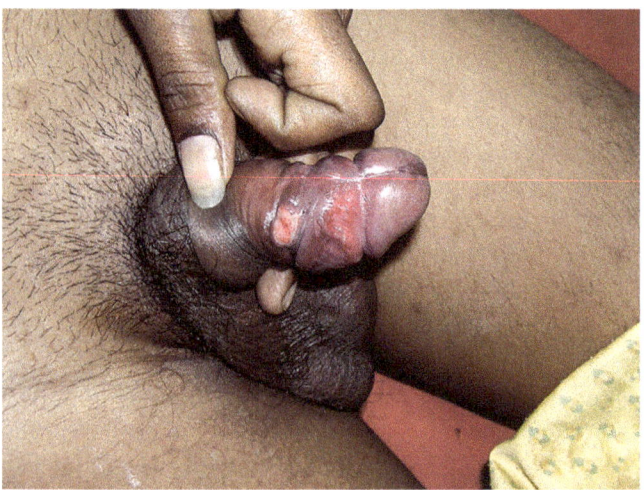

FIG. 13: "Kissing" chancre.

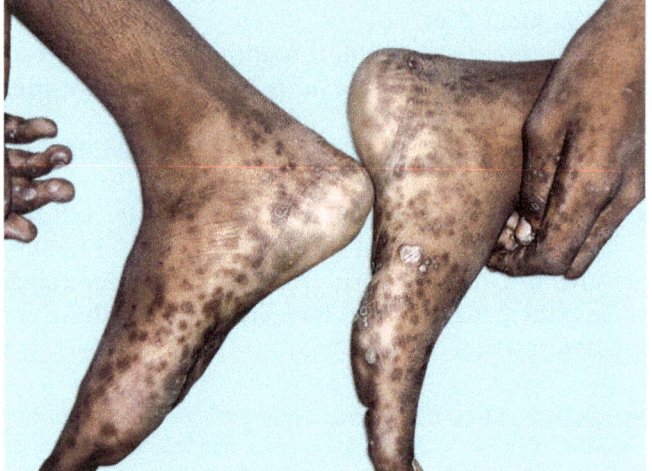

FIG. 15: Syphilides over bilateral soles.

- stiffness, myalgia, arthralgia, and generalized, nontender lymphadenopathy.
- Initial eruption is a faint pink, macular rash (lasting for up to 3 weeks) followed by a copper-colored, maculopapular eruption in about 50% of patients involving the trunk, flexors of upper extremities, and palms and soles **(Figs. 14 and 15)**.
- Subsequent lesions can include papulosquamous exanthema mimicking psoriasis, lichen planus, or the "fir-tree pattern" of pityriasis rosea.
- The corresponding lesions in the warm and moist areas are large, moist, and referred to as condyloma lata **(Figs. 16 to 18)** and are highly infectious.
- Papules along the hairline in a crown-like pattern (corona veneris), or scalp lesions associated with moth-eaten alopecia may occur.

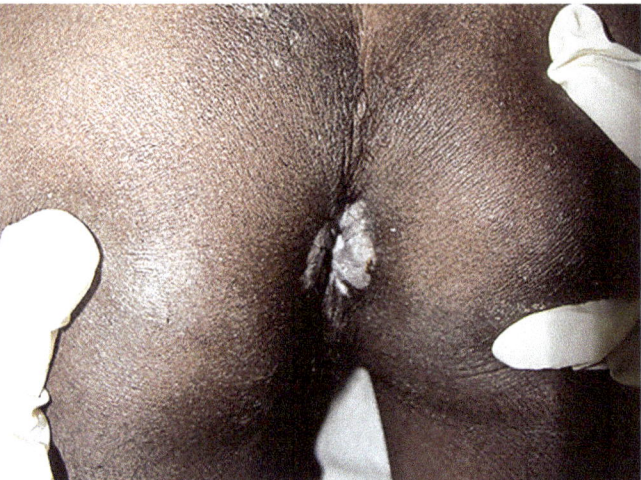

FIG. 16: Condyloma lata in the perianal area.

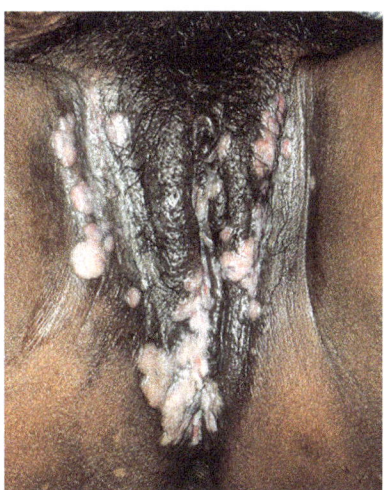

FIG. 17: Condyloma lata involving external genitalia in a female patient.

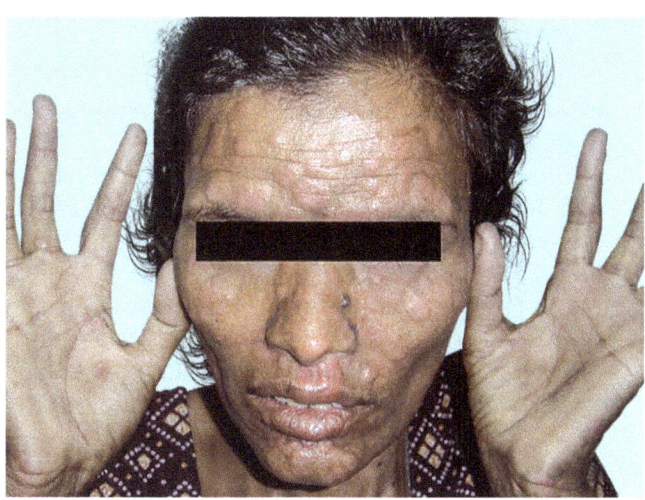

FIG. 19: Nodular syphilid.

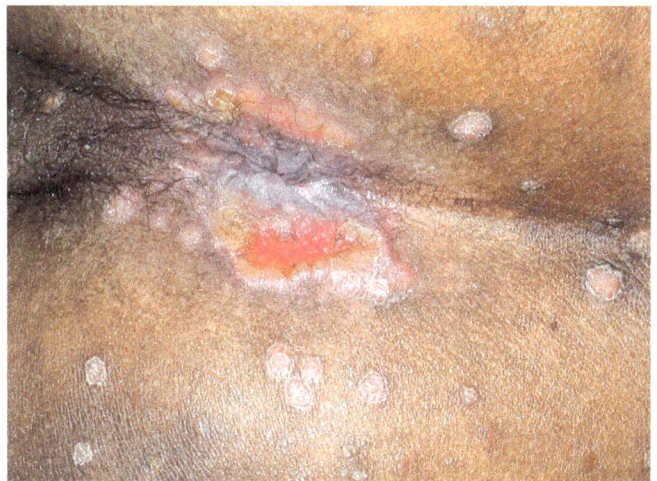

FIG. 18: Moist eroded plaque with peripheral drier lesions in a human immunodeficiency virus (HIV)-positive patient.

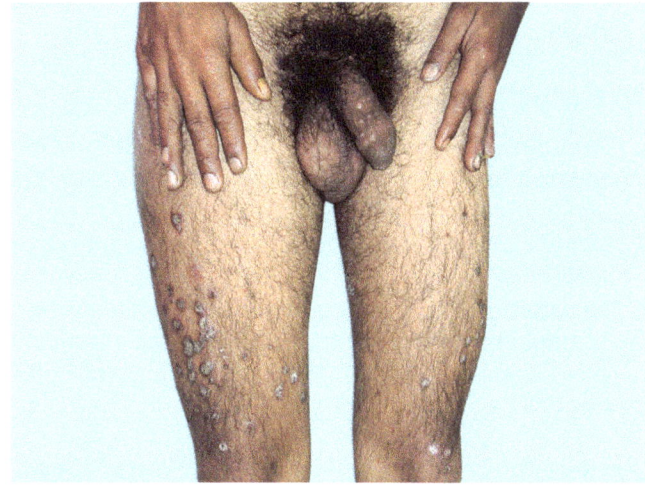

FIG. 20: Psoriasiform syphilid.

- Pressure with the blunt side of the pin over a papule elicits deep dermal tenderness (Buschke Ollendorff sign)
- The rash can also present as nodular **(Fig. 19)**, pustular, follicular, lichenoid, psoriasiform **(Fig. 20)**, corymbiform, or annular lesions.
- Mucous patches are intraoral plaques (snail-track ulcers) with slightly raised grayish-white margins and frequent ulcerations **(Fig. 21)**.
- Systemic features include mild hepatitis, neurologic signs (headache, meningismus, meningitis, cranial nerve disorders, cerebrovascular accident), periostitis, iritis, uveitis, arthritis, parotitis, and glomerulonephritis.
- Without treatment, the secondary stage resolves in 3–6 weeks, becoming asymptomatic (latent) syphilis with no clinical manifestations, and a positive serology.

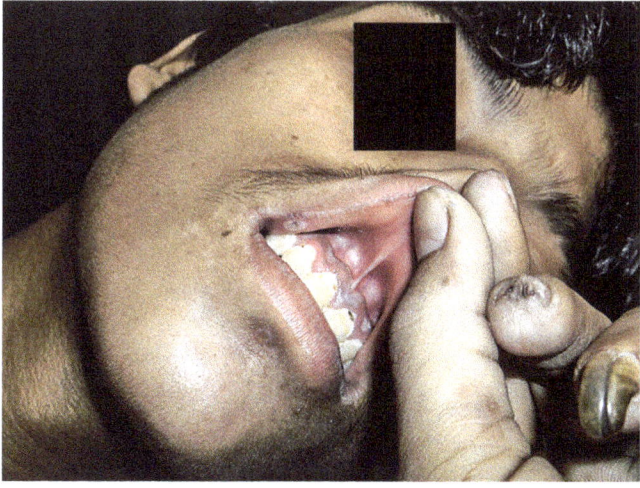

FIG. 21: Mucous patches in a case of secondary syphilis.

Late Syphilis

- Progression to tertiary syphilis (gummatous, cardiovascular, or neurosyphilis) is seen in one-third of untreated late latent syphilis.
- *Neurosyphilis*: Meningovascular involvement (stroke and nerve palsies) or parenchymal involvement (general paresis of insane and tabes dorsalis) may occur.
- Cardiovascular syphilis affects the proximal aorta with features of aortic incompetence, coronary ostial stenosis (angina), and aortic medial necrosis (leading to aneurysms).

Congenital Syphilis

- This represents a failure of appropriate case detection and treatment in the antepartum period. Vertical transmission can occur ante-, intra-, or post-partum.
- It can be divided into early, late syphilis, or syphilis stigmata **(Table 2)**.

Early Congenital Syphilis

- Arbitrarily, the first 2 years with infectious lesions are referred to as early congenital syphilis. It resembles acquired secondary syphilis.
- Infants are irritable and have low birth weight with a feeble cry.
- Generalized lymphadenopathy, hepatosplenomegaly, lacrimation, rhinitis (snuffles), and mucosal ulceration may be present **(Fig. 22)**. The skin is dry and wrinkled.
- Common skin lesions include macular, papular, coppery red, and scaly rash. These are predominantly present involving palms, soles, and diaper areas **(Figs. 23 to 25)**.
- Bullous lesions (pemphigus syphiliticus) **(Fig. 26)**, syphilitic alopecia, condyloma lata, purpura, and paronychia may be present.
- Radiating fissures at an angle of mouth, nares, and anus may heal leaving linear scars (rhagades).
- Involvement of long bones (osteochondritis) or syphilitic epiphysitis causes local pain and tenderness with the limb being held immobile (pseudoparalysis of Parrot).
- Wimberger's sign is radiological loss of density on the medial side of the upper end of the tibia.

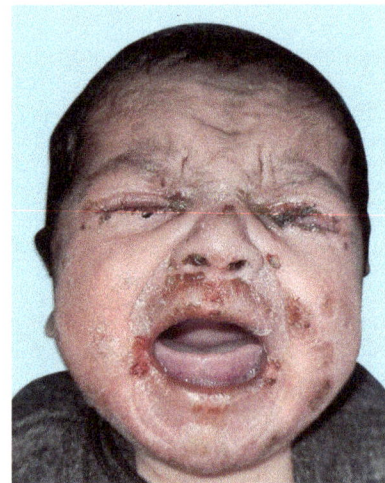

FIG 22: Neonate with early congenital syphilis.

TABLE 2: Features of congenital syphilis.

Early congenital syphilis	Late congenital syphilis	Stigmata of congenital syphilis
• Snuffles	• Gumma	• Saddle nose
• Rhagades	• Hutchinson's triad	• Frontal bossing of Parrot
• Pemphigus syphiliticus	• Interstitial keratitis	• Short maxillae
• Syphilitic alopecia	• Hutchinson's teeth	• Bulldog jaws
• Condyloma lata	• 8th nerve deafness	• High-arched palate
• Pseudoparalysis of Parrot	• Salmon patch	• Hutchinson's teeth
• Wimberger's sign	• Mulberry/Moon molars	• Moon molars
• Onion peel periosteum	• Parrot's nodes	• Saber tibia
	• Clutton joints	• Higoumenaki's sign
	• Juvenile paresis	• Scaphoid scapula
		• Clutton's joint
		• Corneal opacities
		• Optic atrophy
		• Deafness
		• Hydrocephalus

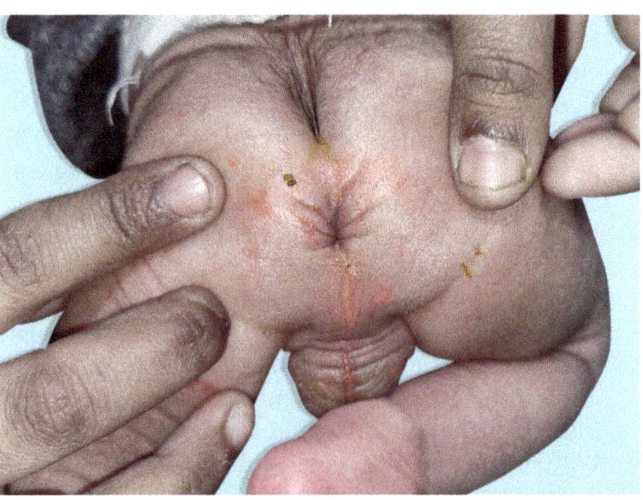

FIG. 23: Lesions of early congenital syphilis.

- Nervous system involvement [abnormal cerebrospinal fluid (CSF)] is seen in 40–60% of infected infants.
- Leptomeningitis or encephalitis presents with seizures, bulging fontanelles, neck rigidity, and hydrocephalus.
- Choroiditis, glaucoma, and uveitis can rarely be seen.

Late Congenital Syphilis

- These are lesions presenting after 2 years of age and are noninfectious.
- Subcutaneous/submucous gummata of soft tissue appear from 5 years of age, resulting in ulceration of the soft palate and nasopharynx.
- Hutchinson's triad is pathognomonic and comprises interstitial keratitis, Hutchinson's teeth **(Fig. 27)**, and eighth nerve deafness.
- Interstitial keratitis is the most common presentation, associated with uveitis, photophobia, blurred vision, and circumcorneal vascularization ending in a corneal ground glass appearance and blindness.
- Vertigo, nausea, and tinnitus may result due to osteochondritis of otic capsule at puberty. It can lead to bilateral high tone neural deafness.
- Bone involvement in the form of sclerosis and new bone formation can result in saber tibia and Higoumenakis' sign **(Fig. 28)**.
- Osteoperiostitis of skull bones leads to rounded bony swelling, called Parrot's nodes.
- Knee joints may show symptomless effusion (Clutton's joints).
- Neurosyphilis may cause juvenile paresis or juvenile tabes dorsalis.
- Cardiovascular syphilis is very rare.

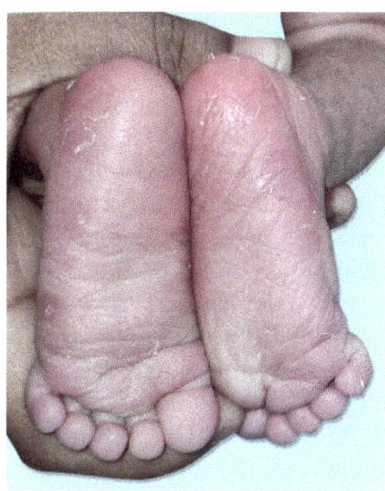

FIG 24: Involvement of soles with desquamation.

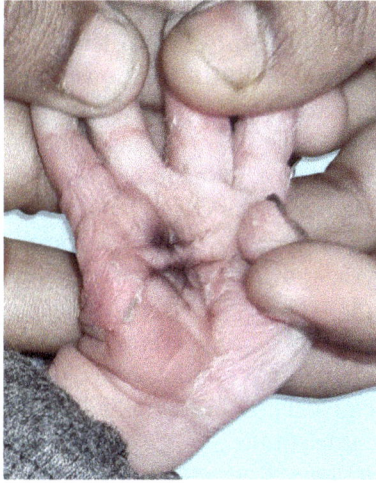

FIG 25: Palmar involvement in congenital syphilis.

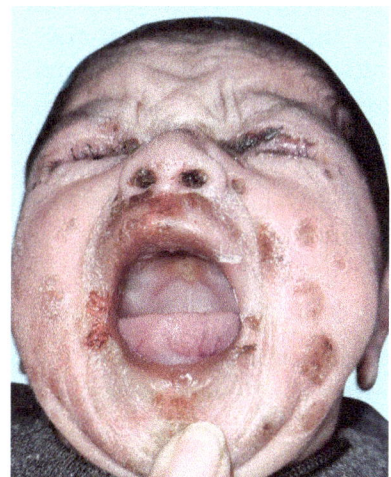

FIG 26: Multiple bullous lesions, with rupture and secondary erosions in congenital syphilis.

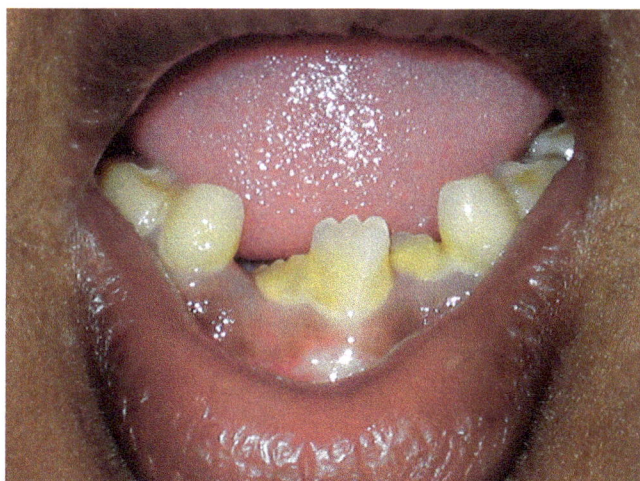

FIG. 27: Hutchinson's teeth.

Stigmata of Congenital Syphilis

Stigmata are scars from early or late congenital syphilis and represent permanent evidence of the infection.

Syphilis and Human Immunodeficiency Virus

- Syphilitic ulcers increase transmission of HIV.
- In the presence of HIV, syphilis may present with multiple and atypical chancres, early progression to neurosyphilis, pustular or malignant syphilis **(Figs. 29A and B)**, multiorgan involvement in the secondary stage, and misleading serological tests (including false negative results).
- Also, a higher rate of failure to clear antitreponemal antibodies after treatment has been observed in HIV-positive individuals.

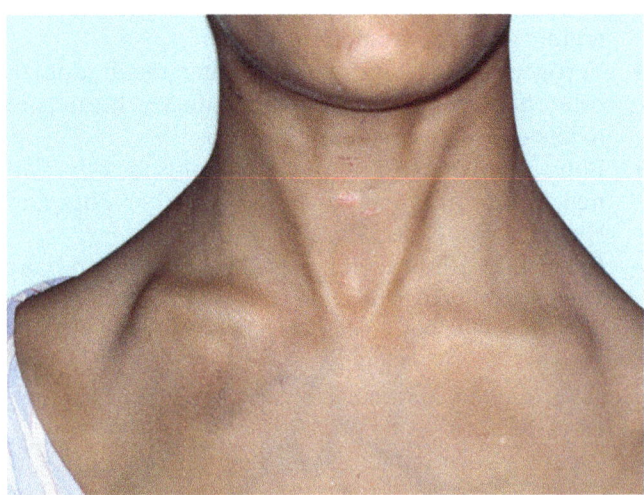

FIG. 28: Higoumenaki's sign.

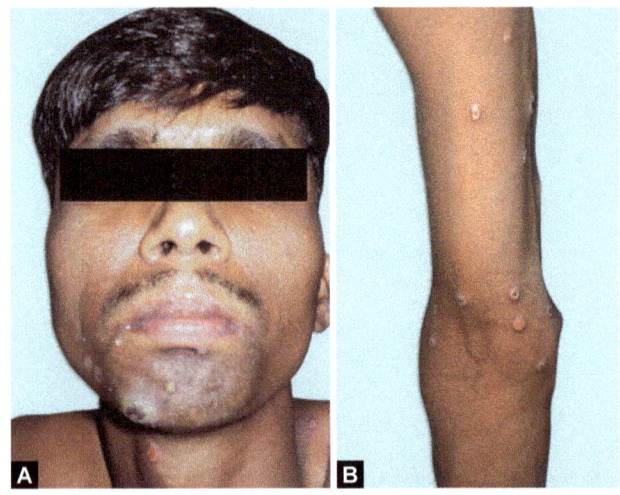

FIGS. 29A AND B: Extensive syphilis in a human immunodeficiency virus (HIV)-positive man.

Diagnosis

Treponema pallidum is not easy to cultivate or stain. The following tests have been developed for the diagnosis of various stages of syphilis:

- *Direct identification of T. pallidum*:
  - Dark ground microscopy allows immediate diagnosis of infectious lesions of early syphilis. Disadvantages include the need for special apparatus, technical expertise, and the lack of specificity for oral and rectal samples.
  - Direct fluorescent antibody testing (DFAT) has a sensitivity of 73–100% and a specificity of 87–100%.
  - NAAT: PCR has a high sensitivity (94.7%) and specificity (98.6%) and is considered the gold standard for diagnosis.
- *Serology forms the mainstay of diagnosis. It can be classified as*:
  - Nontreponemal tests include the venereal disease research laboratory (VDRL) test and the rapid plasma reagin (RPR). Caution is required in the interpretation of prozone phenomenon and biological false positive reactions. All serological tests are positive in secondary syphilis.
  - Treponemal tests include *T. pallidum* hemagglutination (TPHA), *T. pallidum* particle agglutination (TP-PA), and fluorescent treponemal antibody-absorption (FTA-ABS) test. The sensitivity of these tests in tertiary syphilis varies from 97 to 100%.
  - Treponemal IgM antibody detection is of value in early cases of primary syphilis, congenital syphilis, and neurosyphilis.
- *Histopathology*: Primary lesions have erosion or ulceration with a dense inflammatory infiltrate. Secondary syphilis shows a wide variety of histological changes including involvement of blood vessels, seen as marked endothelial swelling and proliferation. Treponemes may be demonstrated perivascularly or at the dermal-epidermal junction zone, with the help of special stains. The inflammatory infiltrate presents perivascularly in a coat-sleeve-like pattern. Presence of plasma cells and lymphocytes is characteristic **(Figs. 30A and B)**.

Treatment Recommendations

The CDC 2021 recommendations for the treatment of various stages and manifestations of syphilis include:

Primary and secondary syphilis:
- Recommended regimen for adults is benzathine penicillin G 2.4 million units IM in a single dose after the test dose.

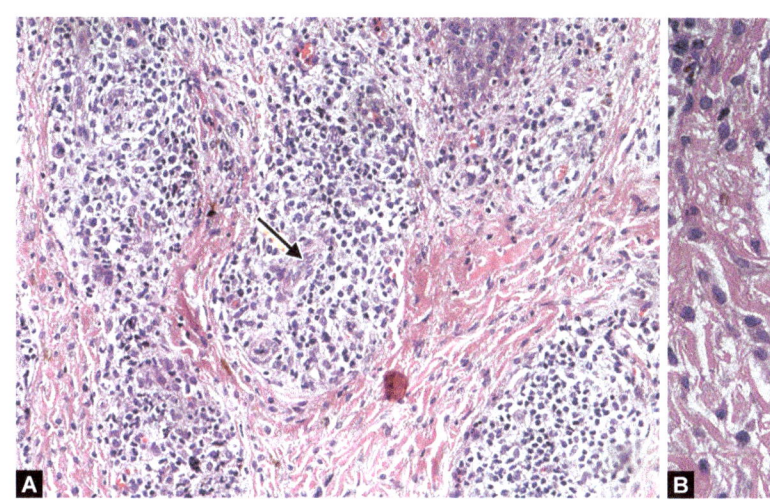 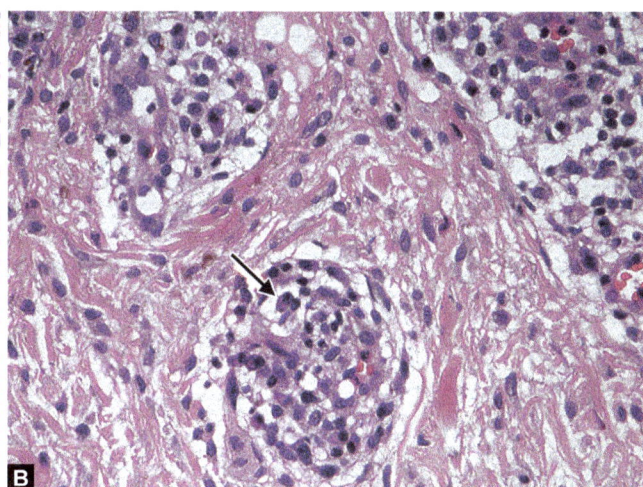

FIGS. 30A AND B: Histopathological features of secondary syphilis [hematoxylin and eosin (H&E) at 100× (A) and 400× (B)].

- Recommended regimen for infants and children is benzathine penicillin G 50,000 units/kg up to a maximum of 2.4 million units IM in a single dose after the test dose.
- Alternative regimen for penicillin-allergic nonpregnant patients is doxycycline, 100 mg orally, twice daily for 14 days or tetracycline, 500 mg orally, 4 times daily for 14 days.
- Alternative regimen for penicillin-allergic pregnant patients is desensitization and treatment with penicillin G.
- Persons with a penicillin allergy whose compliance with therapy or follow-up cannot be ensured should be desensitized and treated with benzathine penicillin G.

Early latent syphilis:
- Benzathine penicillin G 2.4 million units IM in a single dose.

Late latent syphilis or latent syphilis of unknown duration:
- Benzathine penicillin G 7.2 million units total, administered as 3 doses of 2.4 million units IM each at 1-week intervals

Tertiary syphilis:
- All persons who have tertiary syphilis should receive a CSF examination before therapy is initiated and have an HIV test.
- *With normal CSF examination*: Benzathine penicillin G 7.2 million units total, administered as 3 doses of 2.4 million units IM each at 1-week intervals
- *Persons with CSF abnormalities*: Treated with a neurosyphilis regimen
- Certain providers treat all persons who have cardiovascular syphilis with a neurosyphilis regimen.

Neurosyphilis, ocular syphilis, and otosyphilis in adults:
- Recommended regimen is aqueous crystalline penicillin G 18–24 million units per day, administered as 3–4 million units IV every 4 hours or continuous infusion, for 10–14 days.
- If compliance can be ensured, then the alternative regimen is procaine penicillin 2.4 million units IM once daily plus probenecid 500 mg orally four times a day, both for 10–14 days.

Syphilis in pregnancy:
- Should be treated with the recommended penicillin regimen for their stage of infection.
- Additional therapy may be beneficial for pregnant women to prevent congenital syphilis. Hence, a second dose of benzathine penicillin G 2.4 million units IM can be administered 1 week after the initial dose for early syphilis.
- Syphilis diagnosis during the second half of pregnancy necessitates sonographic fetal evaluation for congenital syphilis. Sonographic signs of fetal or placental syphilis (e.g., hepatomegaly, ascites, hydrops, fetal anemia, or a thickened placenta) indicate a greater risk for fetal treatment failure. A second dose of benzathine penicillin G 2.4 million units IM after the initial dose might be beneficial for fetal treatment in these situations.
- Women treated for syphilis during the second half of pregnancy are at risk for premature labor or fetal distress (Jarisch–Herxheimer reaction) hence should be treated under fetal monitoring and obstetric care. Stillbirth is a rare complication; however, it should not delay necessary treatment.
- Missed doses (>9 days between doses) are not acceptable for pregnant women receiving therapy

for late latent syphilis. Such a scenario necessitates a repeat of the full course of therapy.
- All women who have syphilis should be offered testing for HIV at the time of diagnosis.

Congenital syphilis:
- For treatment purposes, congenital syphilis is classified as:
  o **Confirmed proven or highly probable congenital syphilis**: This includes any neonate with either of the following:
    – An abnormal physical examination that is consistent with congenital syphilis.
    – Serum quantitative nontreponemal serologic titer is fourfold or higher than the mother's titer at delivery.
    – One of the following findings (a positive dark-field test or PCR of placenta, cord, lesions, or body fluids OR a positive silver stain of the placenta or cord).
- The recommended evaluation in such a neonate includes:
  o CSF analysis for VDRL, cell count, and protein
  o Complete blood count (CBC), differential blood count and platelet count
  o Long-bone radiographs
  o Other tests as clinically indicated (e.g., chest radiograph, liver function tests, neuroimaging, ophthalmologic examination, and auditory brain stem response)
- The recommended treatment for such a neonate is:
  o Aqueous crystalline penicillin G 100,000–150,000 units/kg/day administered as 50,000 units/kg/dose IV every 12 hours for the first 7 days and every 8 hours for the next 3 days.
  o Procaine penicillin G 50,000 units/kg/dose IM in a single daily dose for 10 days.
  o **Possible congenital syphilis**: This includes any neonate with:
    – Normal physical examination
    – Serum quantitative nontreponemal serologic titer equal to or less than fourfold of the maternal titer at delivery
    – And one of the following (mother not treated, inadequately treated, or has no documentation of having received treatment; mother treated with erythromycin or a regimen other than those recommended in these guidelines; mother received the recommended regimen, but treatment was initiated <30 days before delivery.

- The recommended evaluation in such a neonate includes the following:
  o *CSF analysis for VDRL, cell count, and protein*: A lumbar puncture might document CSF abnormalities that would prompt close follow-up.
  o CBC, differential, and platelet count can further support a diagnosis of congenital syphilis.
  o Long-bone radiographs can further support a diagnosis of congenital syphilis.
- The recommended treatment for such a neonate is:
  o Aqueous crystalline penicillin G 100,000–150,000 units/kg/day administered as 50,000 units/kg/dose IV every 12 hours for the first 7 days and every 8 hours for the next 3 days
  o Or procaine penicillin G 50,000 units/kg/dose IM in a single daily dose for 10 days
  o Or benzathine penicillin G 50,000 units/kg/dose IM in a single dose

Follow-up

- Early syphilis should be followed up to ensure healing of ulcer or rash.
- A fourfold fall of VDRL titer at or before 6 months is considered an adequate treatment response.
- Serological testing is repeated at 3, 6, and 12 months for primary syphilis and up to 24 months for secondary syphilis.
- In HIV coinfected, the decline in titers may be less predictable.

Partner treatment: Presumptive treatment with single dose benzathine penicillin 2.4 million units IM should be given to all sex partners exposed in the last 90 days.

Granuloma Inguinale (Donovanosis)

- It is a genital ulcerative disease characterized by chronic, progressively destructive granulomas and ulcerative lesions of the genitals.
- The causative organism is the intracellular gram-negative bacterium *Klebsiella granulomatis*, formerly known as *Calymmatobacterium granulomatis*.

Clinical Features

- Initial lesions are painless, slowly progressive, papules, or nodules which may subsequently ulcerate, involving the genitals and perineum. They are highly vascular, beefy-red, bleeding easily on contact **(Fig. 31)**.

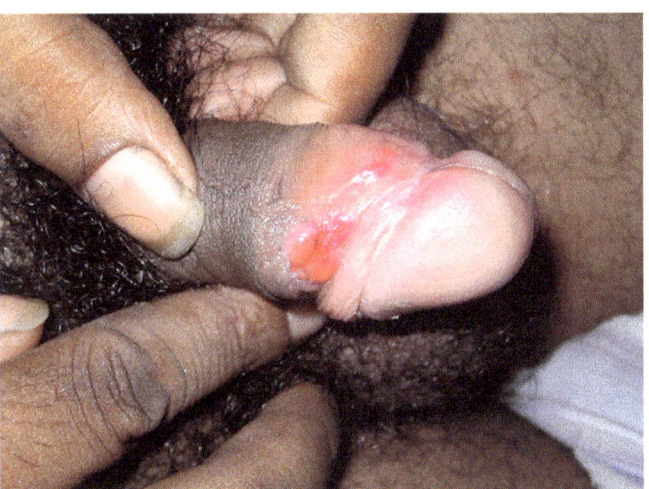

FIG. 31: Beefy red ulcers of donovanosis.

- The ulcers, when formed, are clean based, irregularly bordered without associated lymphadenopathy.
- Untreated ulcers progressively erode underlying structures, resulting in extensive mutilation which is the key hallmark of this disease.
- There may also be verrucous lesions, necrotic or phagedenic ulcers, and sclerotic lesions.
- A characteristic feature is the absence of lymph node involvement.
- An occasional deep granuloma in the inguinal area is known as a pseudobubo.
- In long-standing cases, dissemination to the extra-genital area such as pelvis, intra-abdominal, or metastatic hematogenous spread may occur.

Diagnosis

- *Direct microscopy* of crush smears obtained from the fleshy exuberant ulcers, stained with Giemsa or Leishman's stain, shows "Donovan bodies" seen as large blue-purple coccobacilli with a "safety pin" configuration.
- *Histopathology* from the ulcer edge shows pseudo-epitheliomatous hyperplasia, multiple neutrophilic microabscesses, and multiple mononuclear cells with intracellular Donovan bodies.
- *Culture* is difficult with duck embryo yolk sac being used as a culture medium.
- *Serological diagnosis* with PCR assay and complement fixation test has been suggested.

Treatment Recommendations

Generally, a prolonged therapy is required, with a risk of relapse even 6–18 months after apparently effective therapy. The CDC 2021 recommendations are as follows:
- *Recommended regimen*: Azithromycin 1 g orally once/week or 500 mg daily, for >3 weeks until all lesions have completely healed.
- *Alternative regimens*:
  o Doxycycline 100 mg orally twice a day
  o Erythromycin base 500 mg orally four times a day
  o Trimethoprim-sulphamethoxazole DS (160 mg/800 mg) orally two times a day
- For at least 3 weeks and until all lesions have completely healed

Pregnancy:
- Patients should be treated with an erythromycin regimen.
- Additional use of parenteral aminoglycoside may be considered.
- Azithromycin is another useful option.

Human immunodeficiency virus:
- Patients should receive the same regimens as those for HIV negative.
- Addition of a parenteral aminoglycoside (e.g., gentamicin) is recommended by CDC.

Follow-up

- Patients should be followed clinically until signs and symptoms have resolved.
- Additional aminoglycoside (especially gentamicin 1 mg/kg IV every 8 hours) is recommended if there is no improvement in the first few days.

Management of sex partners: Persons with a history of sexual contact within the last 60 days should be examined and offered therapy.

Complications

- Carcinoma is the most serious complication but is relatively rare. The histological distinction between squamous cell carcinoma and donovanosis may be difficult.
- Surgery may be required for advanced intractable lesions, causing tissue destruction.

CHAPTER 17: Human Immunodeficiency Virus and Related Infections

Introduction

Human Immunodeficiency Virus (HIV) is the causative agent of the Acquired Immunodeficiency Syndrome (AIDS). The disease was first recognized in 1981 among young homosexual men. Since then, it went on to attain pandemic proportions. Mucocutaneous manifestations are among the first recognized clinical manifestations of HIV/AIDS. HIV belongs to the family of retroviruses, subfamily lentiviruses **(Fig. 1)**. HIV virion is a 120 nm icosahedron, enveloped ribonucleic acid (RNA) virus.

Clinical Features

Human Immunodeficiency Virus produces a spectrum of diseases progressing from clinically latent/asymptomatic state to AIDS as a late manifestation **(Table 1)**.

The staging for HIV infection has also been simplified into three stages:
1. *Acute HIV infection*: This is the same as the stage of primary HIV infection, developing 2–4 weeks after exposure and characterized by flu-like symptoms.
2. *Chronic HIV infection*: This comprises asymptomatic HIV infection and clinical latency period. These patients may not have any HIV-related symptoms, and viral multiplication is at very low levels. People on antiretroviral therapy (ART) may remain in this stage

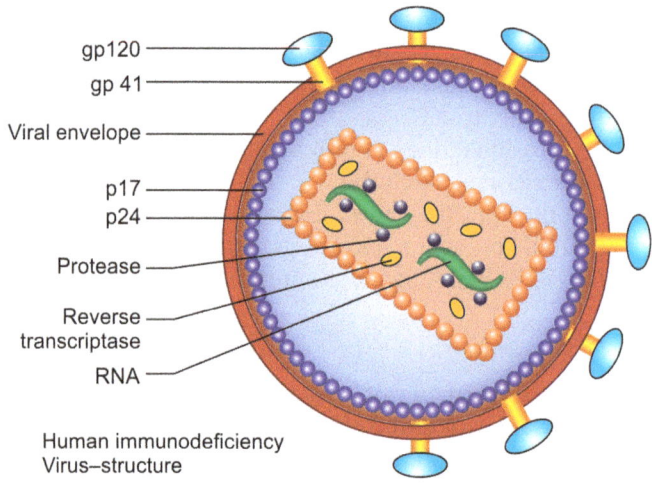

FIG. 1: Structure of human immunodeficiency virus.

TABLE 1: Various clinical stages through which HIV infection passes before reaching full-blown AIDS.	
Stage of HIV infection	**Clinical features**
Primary HIV infection	Asymptomatic, acute retroviral syndrome
Clinical stage 1	Asymptomatic, persistent generalized lymphadenopathy (PGL)
Clinical stage 2	Moderate unexplained weight loss (<10%), recurrent respiratory tract infections, herpes zoster, angular cheilitis, recurrent oral ulcers, papular pruritic eruption, and seborrheic dermatitis
Clinical stage 3	Severe weight loss (>10%), unexplained chronic diarrhea (>1 month), unexplained persistent fever (>1 month), oral candidiasis, unexplained anemia (<8 g/dL), neutropenia (<500/mm^3), thrombocytopenia (<50,000/mm^3) for more than 1 month
Clinical stage 4	HIV wasting syndrome, pneumocystis pneumonia, chronic herpes simplex, esophageal candidiasis, extrapulmonary tuberculosis, Kaposi's sarcoma, extrapulmonary cryptococcosis, disseminated nontuberculous mycobacteria, candida of trachea, bronchi or lungs, cryptosporidiosis, visceral herpes simplex infection, cytomegalovirus infection, and disseminated mycosis

for decades, while those not on therapy advance to the next stage over 10 years or longer. Viral loads may remain undetectable, especially in those compliant with therapy.

3. *AIDS*: This is the final, most severe stage of HIV infection characterized by opportunistic infections, and CD4 counts of less than 200 cells/mm^3. They have high viral loads and a high risk of transmission. Survival is typically 3 years.

The goal of evaluation of a patient with HIV is to confirm the presence of HIV infection, obtain appropriate baseline historical and laboratory data, ensure patient understanding about HIV infection and its transmission, and initiate care as recommended by established guidelines. This includes a complete medical history, physical examination, and laboratory evaluation along with counseling.

Diagnosis

Various investigations required in a patient are as follows:
- HIV antibody testing includes screening tests [such as rapid tests and enzyme-linked immunosorbent assays (ELISA)] and confirmatory/supplemental tests [such as 3rd/4th generation ELISA, Western blot assay, and the nucleic acid amplification test (NAAT)]. For symptomatic persons, the sample should be reactive with two different kits, to finalize the diagnosis.
- CD4 T-cell count is one of the key factors in deciding whether to initiate ART and prophylaxis for opportunistic infections. It is the strongest predictor of subsequent disease progression and survival.
- Plasma HIV RNA involves viral load testing as a surrogate marker for treatment response and predictor of clinical progression.
- Complete blood count, chemistry profile, transaminase levels, blood urea nitrogen (BUN), creatinine, urinalysis, and serologies for hepatitis A, B, and C viruses are important to stage the disease and decide therapy.
- Fasting blood glucose and serum lipids
- If possible, genotypic resistance testing at entry into care, regardless of whether ART will be initiated immediately
- Other tests, including screening for sexually transmitted infections (STIs) and tests for determining the risk of opportunistic infections and the need for prophylaxis

Treatment

The goals of ART are to reduce HIV-associated morbidity, prolong the duration and quality of survival, restore and preserve immunologic function maximally, durably suppress plasma HIV viral load, and prevent HIV transmission. **Table 2** enumerates the drugs that can be given as a part of Highly Active Antiretroviral Therapy (HAART). Regimens should be tailored for individual patients.

The recommended starting regimens for the majority of patients with HIV-1 (treatment naïve patients) are:
- Bictegravir, tenofovir alafenamide (TAF), and emtricitabine
- Dolutegravir, emtricitabine or lamivudine, and TAF (or TDF)

TABLE 2: Various classes of antiretroviral drugs.

Nucleoside reverse transcriptase inhibitors	Nonnucleoside reverse transcriptase inhibitors	Protease inhibitors
- Abacavir	- Efavirenz	- Atazanavir
- Emtricitabine	- Etravirine	- Darunavir
- Lamivudine	- Nevirapine	- Fosamprenavir
- Tenofovir disoproxil fumarate (TDF)	- Rilpivirine	- Ritonavir
- Tenofovir alafenamide (TAF)	- Delavirdine	- Saquinavir
- Zidovudine	*Integrase inhibitors*	- Tipranavir
- Stavudine	- Dolutegravir	- Nelfinavir
- Didanosine	- Raltegravir	- Amprenavir
- Zalcitabine	- Elvitegravir	- Indinavir
Postattachment inhibitors	- Bictegravir	- Lopinavir
- Ibalizumab	*CCR5 antagonist*	*Pharmacokinetic enhancers*
Fusion inhibitors	- Maraviroc	- Cobicistat
- Enfuvirtide		

Immune Reconstitution Inflammatory Syndrome (IRIS): This may occur as an unmasking of a previously untreated opportunistic infection (OI), the paradoxical reaction in a patient receiving appropriate antimicrobial therapy, or as an autoimmune condition.

Criteria for diagnosis of IRIS are:
- A patient must be HIV positive and receiving HAART.
- Have a decreasing HIV viral load with or without an increase in CD4 cell count from baseline.
- Have clinical symptoms consistent with an inflammatory process where the clinical course is not consistent with the expected course of a previously diagnosed OI, expected course of newly diagnosed OI, or drug toxicity.

Dermatologic Infections Associated with HIV/AIDS

In the context of HIV, cutaneous infections can present with atypical manifestations such as unusual anatomical sites, increased severity, unusual clinical appearance, and treatment failure. These infections can be of the following types.

Bacterial Infections

Bacterial infections in the setting of HIV include those caused by both common and uncommon organisms.

Staphylococcal, Streptococcal Skin and Soft Tissue Infections

Clinical Features

- Skin and soft tissue infections (SSTIs) develop in 20% of HIV patients, which is higher compared to the general population. The rates can be higher due to higher rates of recurrent or chronic nasal carriage including methicillin-resistant *Staphylococcus aureus* (MRSA).
- These include the usual manifestations, which are seen in immunocompetent patients like ecthyma **(Fig. 2)**, folliculitis **(Fig. 3)**, and also uncommon disease manifestations seen in the setting of immunosuppression such as plaque folliculitis, pyomyositis, and botryomycosis.
- Botryomycosis manifests as a chronic, granulomatous, suppurative infection following skin trauma. It presents as subcutaneous nodules to plaques with ulcers,

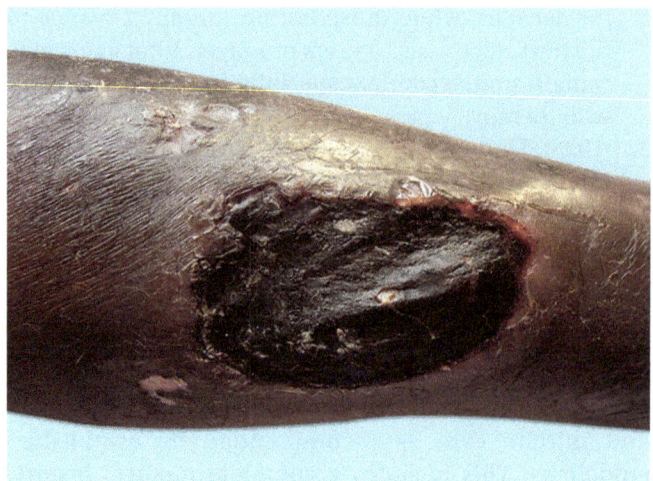

FIG. 2: Ecthyma presenting as a necrotic ulcer with central black eschar and surrounding erythema over the lower leg in a HIV patient.

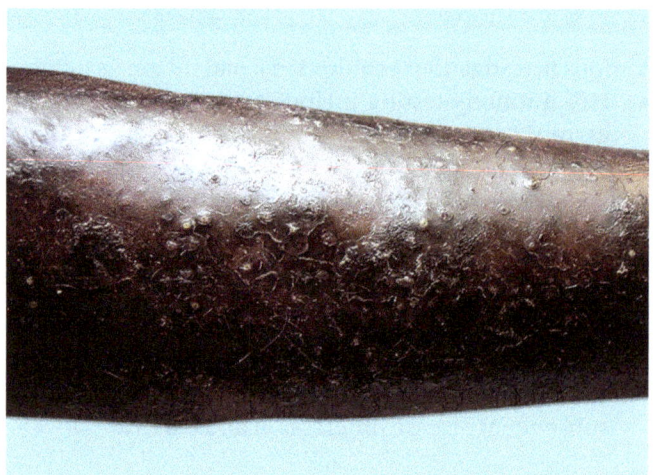

FIG. 3: Folliculitis, multiple small follicular pustules with exfoliating scales over the lower limb in an HIV patient.

purulent secretions, fistulae, and "sulfur-like" grains, presenting over the scalp, axillae, and groins. It is caused by *Staphylococcus aureus* and *Staphylococcus epidermidis* (most commonly), *Pseudomonas aeruginosa, Escherichia coli, Proteus, Bacteroides*, and some other bacteria.

Diagnosis

Diagnosis of SSTI can be established by Gram stain and bacterial culture from the lesions. In botryomycosis, histopathologic examination of skin biopsy helps confirm the diagnosis.

Treatment

Treatment in the setting of HIV is not different from that for the immunocompetent host. Penicillins and cephalosporins are the first-line agents. In MRSA infections, or patients with penicillin allergy, clindamycin and trimethoprim/sulfamethoxazole may be used. For severe infections, intravenous vancomycin is the drug of choice. For recurrent infections, rifampicin 600 mg once daily for 10–14 days may be tried.

Bacillary Angiomatosis

Clinical Features

- It is caused by *Bartonella henselae* and has a moderately strong association with HIV infection. It is seen at CD4 cell counts <100 cells/mL.
- It presents as solitary to multiple, small, purple-red papules, nodules, and subcutaneous cystic nodules, which enlarge to form exophytic, friable nodules, with a collarette scale.
- Rarely, disseminated lesions may occur.

Diagnosis

Diagnosis requires histopathologic examination. Warthin–Starry stain reveals typical clumps of tangled bacteria.

Treatment

Treatment involves administration of erythromycin (2 g/day) or doxycycline (100 mg twice daily) for 2–3 months.

Cutaneous Tuberculosis

Clinical Features

- The HIV pandemic has contributed greatly to the worldwide increase in rates of tuberculosis, especially pulmonary tuberculosis.
- Most common variants of cutaneous tuberculosis are scrofuloderma (**Fig. 4**), lupus vulgaris, tuberculosis verrucosa cutis, lichen scrofulosorum, papulonecrotic tuberculids, erythema nodosum, and erythema induratum of Bazin.
- The most characteristic cutaneous tuberculosis associated with HIV is miliary tuberculosis, usually seen with CD4 <100 cells/mm^3.
- In a patient with cutaneous tuberculosis, one should suspect the coexistence of HIV, in cases with widespread lesions, involvement of more than one site, involvement of more than one underlying structure, miliary tuberculosis, or metastatic tubercular abscess.

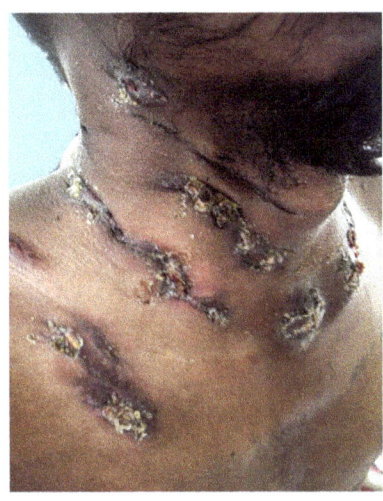

FIG. 4: Scrofuloderma presenting as multiple discharging sinuses over the neck and chest, surmounted by crust, ulceration, and peripheral erythema.

Diagnosis

Diagnosis requires Mantoux testing (may be false negative), chest X-ray, skin biopsy and histopathology, sputum smear examination, culture (Gold standard), and CB-NAAT.

Treatment

Treatment is similar to those patients who are HIV negative, involving the administration of 4 drugs (isoniazid, rifampicin, pyrazinamide, and ethambutol) for 2 months and continuing 3 drugs (isoniazid, rifampicin, and ethambutol) for another 4 months. In general, there is a good response to anti-tubercular treatment in most cases.

Leprosy

Clinical Features

Leprosy per se has not shown any significant association with HIV infection. However, immune-mediated reaction occurs at a higher frequency in coinfected patients. Leprosy can present as an IRIS among patients started on ART (**Fig. 5**). HIV infection is a risk factor for developing erythema nodosum leprosum (ENL), recurrent reversal reactions, neuritis, and mortality.

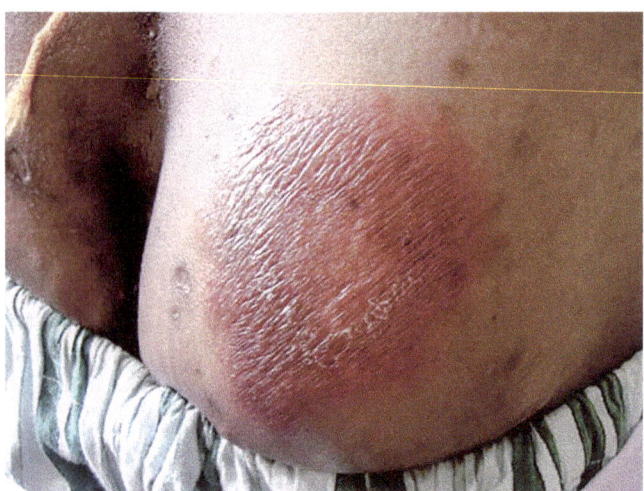

FIG. 5: Leprosy as immune reconstitution syndrome, note the erythematous annular plaque of borderline leprosy with overlying erythema, scaling, and edema.

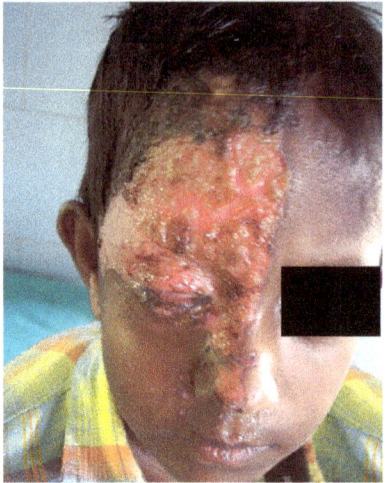

FIG. 6: Herpes zoster ophthalmicus; necrotic ulcerated crusted plaque involving the right half of forehead, eye, and dorsum of the nose, with few discrete small vesicles and papules. Note the complete destruction of the right eyelid and sharp midline demarcation.

Treatment

All dual infection cases require regular treatment with multidrug therapy. However, a longer duration of surveillance is needed for detection of early relapse.

Viral Infections

This section describes the unique or common manifestations of viral infections in HIV patients.

Varicella Zoster Virus

Clinical Features

- Varicella zoster virus (VZV) and herpes zoster infection may present with atypical features in HIV-infected patients. The disease may be very severe, or even fatal, and have internal organ involvement causing pneumonitis, pancreatitis, encephalitis, and disseminated varicella.
- Zoster in an HIV-infected person may present with unusual lesions such as follicular zoster, verrucous zoster, and erythematous, crusted, or punched-out ulcerations **(Figs. 6 and 7)**.
- Disseminated zoster refers to lesions extending over three contiguous dermatomes or more than 20 lesions outside the initial dermatomes.
- Zoster can be a complication of immune reconstitution in both children and adults.

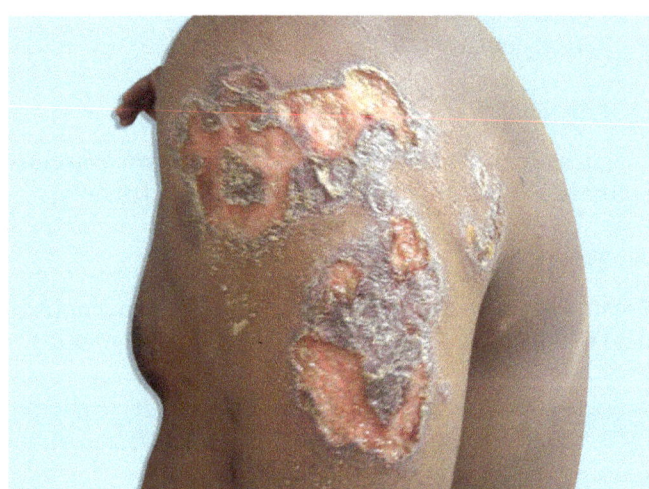

FIG. 7: Dermatomal involvement of right arm and shoulder, in the form of erythematous crusted plaques with central necrotic polycyclic ulceration.

- Postherpetic neuralgia complicates zoster in a significantly higher proportion of HIV patients.

Diagnosis

Diagnosis can be done bedside with the help of a Tzanck smear showing multinucleated giant cells. Direct fluorescent antibody (DFA), cell culture, or PCR may be needed in cases with atypical presentations.

Treatment

Treatment of choice is acyclovir and its congeners, such as famciclovir or valacyclovir, given orally in uncomplicated cases. Intravenous therapy is reserved for disseminated zoster or zoster ophthalmicus. In patients with acyclovir resistance, foscarnet may be used. HIV-infected patients exposed to VZV for the first time may receive VZV immunoglobulin within 96 hours of exposure.

Molluscum Contagiosum

Clinical Features

- Molluscum contagiosum, especially facial lesions in an adult, is considered a cutaneous marker for advanced HIV infection (CD4 count < 50 cells/cm^3).
- Lesions begin as discrete, grouped, or disseminated, pearly to flesh-colored, dome-shaped papules of 3–10 mm in diameter, often with central umbilication **(Fig. 8)**.
- Giant molluscum more than 1 cm in size may occur in the setting of HIV.
- Molluscum-like lesions may be seen in deep fungal infections among HIV patients.

Diagnosis

Diagnosis is clinical or by extirpation. Histopathologic examination can be used to confirm diagnosis.

Treatment

A limited number of lesions of molluscum respond well to destructive modalities such as cryotherapy with liquid nitrogen, curettage, or electrodesiccation. However, treatment of extensive lesions is difficult.

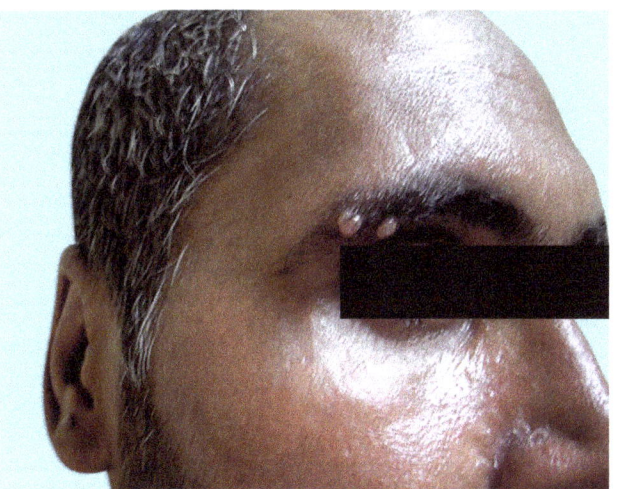

FIG. 8: Molluscum contagiosum, fleshy hypopigmented umbilicated papules right eyebrow.

Kaposi's Sarcoma

Clinical Features

It is the most common HIV-related malignancy, which, if left untreated has a median survival of 18 months. It occurs due to poor control of the *Human Herpes Virus 8 (HHV-8)* infection.

- It starts as asymptomatic erythematous macules or papules over the trunk, leg, arm, and face which enlarges gradually to become violaceous nodules and plaques, with a yellow-green bruise-like halo.
- The lesions may be solitary or in a follicular or pityriasis rosea-like pattern.
- Oral (macular stain over hard palate), gastrointestinal, and lymph node involvement is common.

Diagnosis

Diagnosis is confirmed by histopathology.

Treatment

- Local therapy is reserved for patients with minimal cutaneous disease or as palliative therapy. This includes cryotherapy and excisional surgery; alitretinoin gel 0.1%, intralesional vincristine, vinblastine, bleomycin/interferon.
- Radiotherapy is an effective palliative treatment.
- ART plus chemotherapy may be beneficial in reducing disease progression. There is no difference between different chemotherapy regimens using liposomal doxorubicin, liposomal daunorubicin, and paclitaxel.

Fungal Infections

This section describes unique manifestations of fungal infections in HIV patients. Diagnosis and treatment are covered in relevant chapters on fungal infections.

Cryptococcosis

It is one of the most common invasive fungal infections in HIV-infected patients with a CD4 cell count of <100 cells/mL. Disseminated cutaneous cryptococcosis is an AIDS-defining illness.

Clinical Features

Clinically, varied cutaneous lesions may be seen including molluscum-like umbilicated papules and nodules; cellulitis-like features; erythematous papules, nodules, pustules, and ulcers; herpetiform vesicles; and subcutaneous swelling.

Histoplasmosis

It is a frequent OI in HIV-infected patients in endemic areas. Cutaneous lesions that manifest at CD4 counts of <150 cells/mL are protean.

Clinical Features

- Cutaneous lesions include nodules, plaques, vesicles, hemorrhagic macules, papules, and pustules, with or without ulceration.
- Erythematous scaly plaques, pyoderma gangrenosum-like lesions, erythroderma, cellulitis, petechiae, purpura, ecchymoses, and necrotizing vasculitis also have been described.

Talaromyces marneffei

It is the third most common opportunistic infection, after tuberculosis and cryptococcosis.

Clinical Features

- Specific cutaneous lesions appear in three-fourths of patients, characteristically seen as umbilicated papules with a necrotic center over the face and neck, upper extremities, and trunk.
- Other presentations include ecthyma-like lesions, folliculitis, subcutaneous nodules, and morbilliform eruptions.

Candidiasis

Most commonly, infections are caused by *Candida albicans*. However, *Candida glabrata*, *Candida tropicalis*, *Candida parapsilosis*, *Candida krusei*, and *Candida dubliniensis* are emerging pathogens.

Clinical Features

- Common manifestations are pseudomembranous oral candidiasis (thrush), erythematous or atrophic candidiasis, angular cheilitis, and vulvovaginal candidiasis.
- Oropharyngeal involvement is an important reservoir for disseminated infection in the setting of further immune suppression (**Fig. 9**).
- Disseminated cutaneous disease may present as asymptomatic pustules on an erythematous base, nodules with central necrosis, chronic paronychia, onychodystrophy, distal urethritis, persistent intertriginous, and complicated vulvovaginal infection.

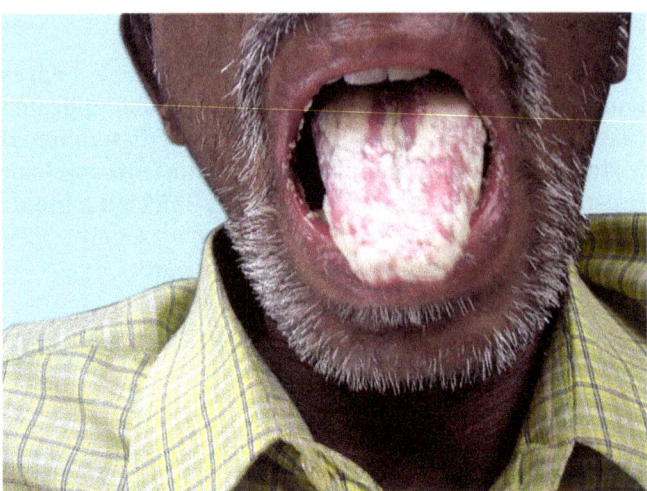

FIG. 9: Oral thrush; note the coating of the tongue with the whitish pseudomembrane.

Dermatophytosis

Dermatophytosis, most commonly caused by *Trichophyton rubrum*, is more common in the HIV-positive population.

Clinical Features

- These superficial infections may be widespread (**Fig. 10**).
- Uncommonly, they may present as deep dermal dermatophytosis with multiple fluctuant erythematous ulcerative nodules or as follicular, violaceous nodules and papules (Majocchi's granuloma).
- Onychomycosis is common with proximal subungual (**Fig. 11**) and superficial white onychomycosis being the characteristic morphology seen in AIDS patients.

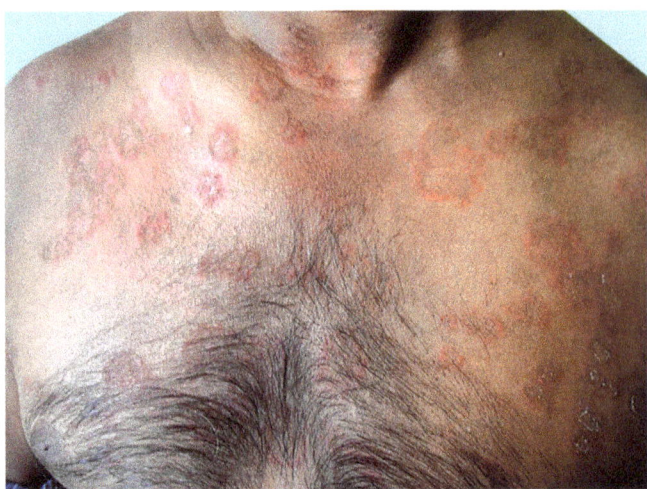

FIG. 10: Tinea corporis; widespread erythematous annular plaques over the chest, with peripheral activity and central clearing.

CHAPTER 17: Human Immunodeficiency Virus and Related Infections

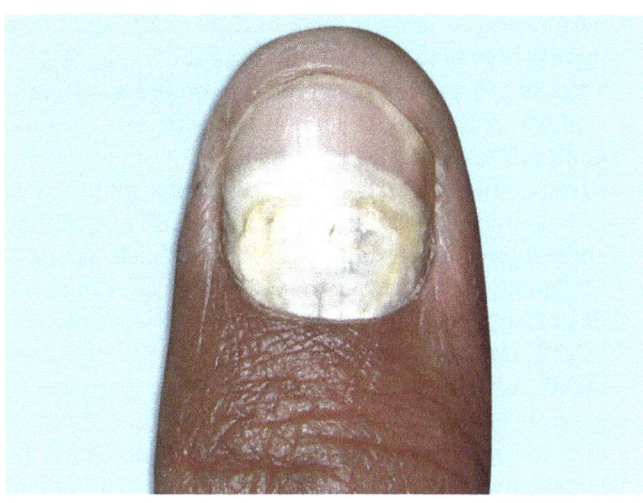

FIG. 11: Proximal subungual onychomycosis; involvement of thumbnail in the form of whitish discoloration in the proximal portion of the nail plate.

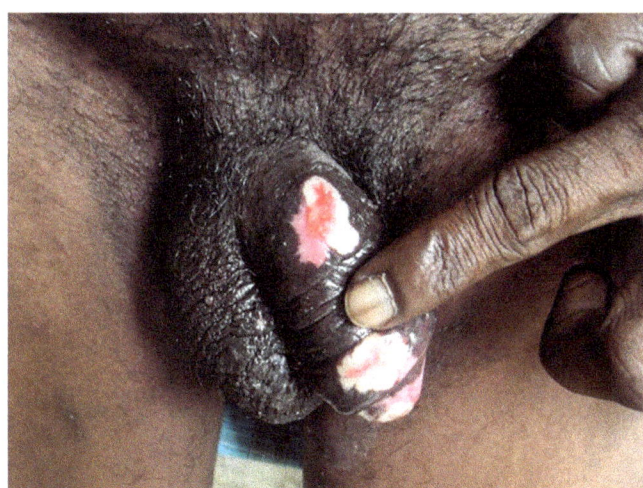

FIG. 12: Herpes genitalis seen as polycyclic erosions of size 3–4 cm, with a necrotic base over the shaft of the penis and the glans penis.

HIV and Sexually Transmitted Diseases

Sexually transmitted disease (STD) increase the risk of HIV transmission by 3- to 5-fold by:
- Reducing physical and mechanical barriers to the virus
- Increasing the number of receptor cells or density of HIV receptors by causing persistent inflammation in the genital region
- Producing a vaginal environment that is more conducive to transmission

HIV in turn facilitates the transmission of STDs and makes them atypical and poorly responsive to treatment. Unique features of STDs in HIV patients are described here. Please refer to the chapter on Sexually Transmitted infections for management considerations in HIV patients.

Genital Herpes

HIV infected patients may experience an increase in the number and size of lesions, in patients with either primary or reactivated herpes simplex virus (HSV) infections. HSV shedding increases in HIV-infected patients making them more contagious.

Clinical Features
- Vesicles and ulcers are more painful and heal slower (Figs. 12 to 14).

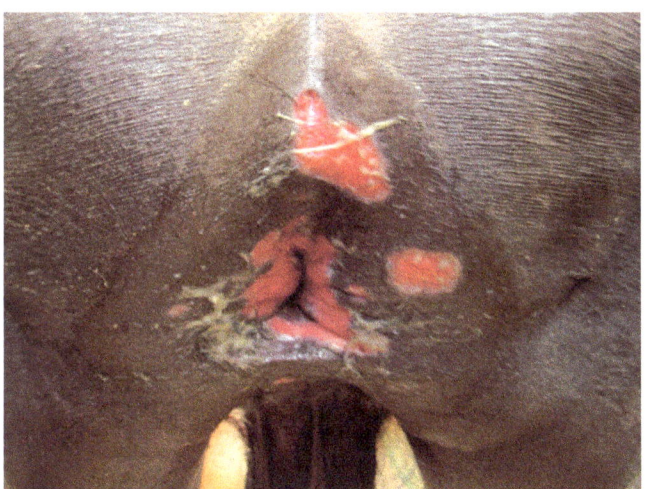

FIG. 13: Herpes genitalis with multiple polycyclic erosions of size 3–4 cm, with erythematous base, over the perianal area.

- As immunosuppression worsens, recurrent outbreaks increase in frequency and severity.
- Chronic herpetic ulcers of more than 1-month duration are an AIDS-defining illness in the HIV-infected persons.
- Ulcers may also become impetiginized.
- HSV may also cause esophagitis, hepatitis, pneumonitis, or life-threatening disseminated infections in AIDS patients.
- Patients may also develop recurrent herpes labialis (Fig. 15).

CHAPTER 17: Human Immunodeficiency Virus and Related Infections

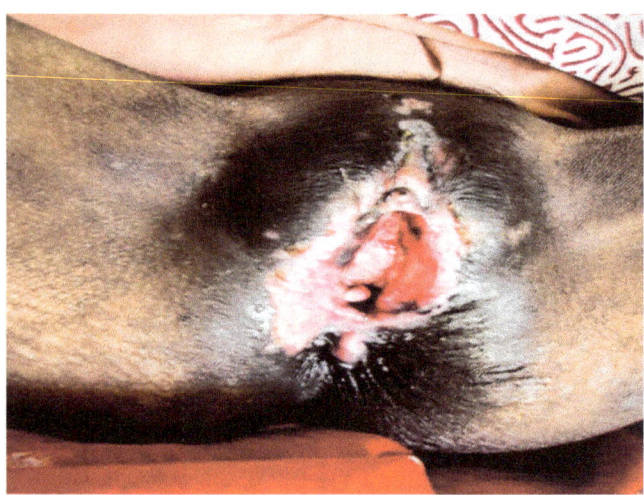

FIG. 14: Herpes genitalis showing a single large erosion, with an erythematous base, over labia majora and minora, extending up to the clitoris. Note multiple small hypopigmented scars in the perineum area.

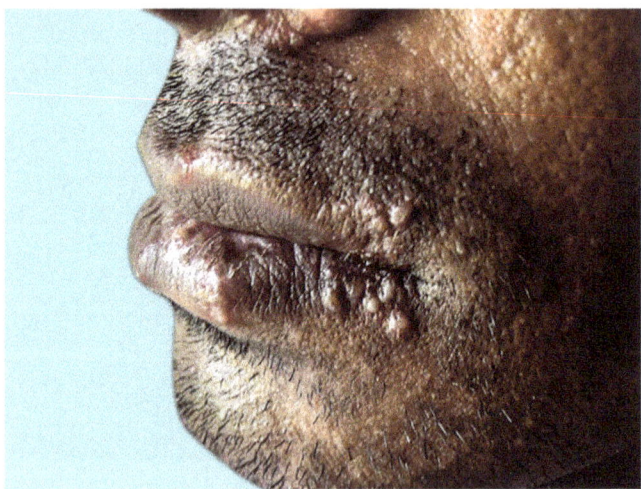

FIG. 15: Herpes labialis with multiple small vesicular lesions with surrounding erythema over both lips and nose.

Syphilis

Syphilis in HIV patients may progress more rapidly, may have an atypical clinical presentation, may have a refractory course after appropriate penicillin therapy, and may lead to unusual serologic test results.

Clinical Features

- Primary syphilis may present with multiple or more extensive chancres, which may be more extensive. Aggressive chancres may be associated with perforation of labia majora and prepuce. They take increased time to heal after treatment.
- Secondary syphilis is more likely to progress to neurosyphilis in the first 2 years after diagnosis, despite appropriate therapy.
- Unusual manifestations of neurosyphilis, gummatous lesions, rapidly developing ocular syphilis, syphilitic aortitis, encephalitis, and arteritis have been reported.
- Malignant syphilis (lues maligna) is a rare extensive, ulcerating secondary syphilis where initial papulopustular lesions rapidly enlarge into sharply bordered ulcers, which crust and are likened to chancres of primary syphilis. Fever, malaise, ocular disease, and strongly positive serology are present. Jarisch–Herxheimer reaction and a clear response to treatment are presently seen.
- Prozone phenomenon (a weakly reactive or falsely negative) reaction might occur more frequently in HIV-infected persons. Seronegative syphilis can be seen due to the prozone phenomenon.
- CSF should be evaluated among HIV-infected adolescents with acquired syphilis of unknown or less than 1 year's duration or if they have neurologic or ocular symptoms or signs. Many clinicians recommend a CSF examination for all HIV-infected patients.

Chancroid

Clinical Features

- In HIV patients, the number of chancroid ulcers may be more, and the duration of the ulcer longer.
- Uncommonly, it may present as a chronic penile ulcer with leg and digital ulcers.

Granuloma Inguinale

Clinical Features

HIV-positive patients have ulcers that persist for a longer duration and may require more intensive antibiotic therapy.

Lymphogranuloma Venereum

Clinical Features

In the MSM population, with HIV positivity, presentation with genital lesions or bloody proctitis may be seen. These cases are mostly caused by L2 strain.

Human Papillomavirus Infection

In HIV patients, biopsy of atypical verrucae may need to be considered before therapy so that an appropriate diagnosis of dysplastic changes or squamous cell cancer can be made.

Clinical Features

- The lesions may be larger, more prolific in number, more verrucous as have a higher risk of malignant transformation.
- The warts tend to be more extensive, refractory to treatment, and associated with a significant risk of transformation into squamous cell carcinoma (SCC) (**Figs. 16 to 18**).

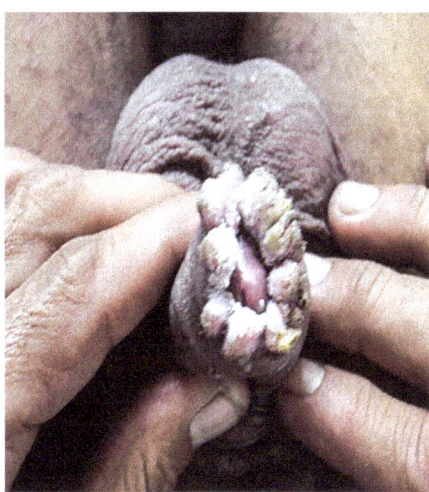

FIG. 16: Genital warts; hyperpigmented verrucous papules, confluent at places, on prepuce, and glans penis.

Treatment

Treatment modalities remain the same in the setting of HIV; however, the success of therapy correlates with the degree of immunosuppression. Dysplastic lesions including cervical and anal squamous intraepithelial lesions (CSIL and ASIL) are associated with HPV types 16, 18, 31, and 45. US Centers for Disease Control and Prevention (CDC) recommends two Pap smears and pelvic examinations during 1st year after diagnosis of HIV and if results are normal, yearly pap smears and pelvic examination.

Other Sexually Transmitted Diseases

- Molluscum in HIV patients appears to be transmitted to both sexual and nonsexual patterns. Lesions occur on the lower abdomen, inner thighs, and genitalia, while those on the face and neck are also common. Lesions can become quite large (up to 2 cm) and numerous (up to the hundreds).
- Bacterial vaginosis appears to be more persistent in HIV-positive women. The treatment regimen in HIV patients recommended is similar to those in HIV-negative women.
- The incidence, persistence, and recurrence of trichomoniasis in HIV-infected women are not correlated with the immune status. The treatment regimen is similar to HIV-negative patients.
- HIV infection can impair the response to hepatitis B vaccination. Hence, HIV patients should be tested for anti-HepB antibodies 1–2 months after 3rd vaccine dose.
- The course of liver disease is more rapid in HIV/hepatitis C virus (HCV) coinfected patients, and the risk for cirrhosis is nearly twice. Treatment of HCV in HIV patients might improve tolerance to ART.

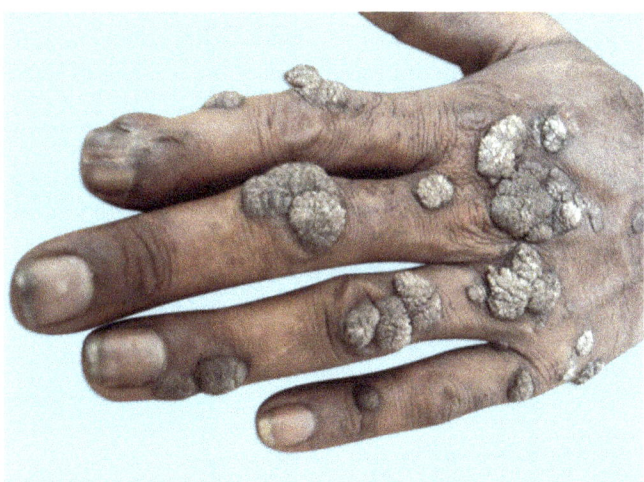

FIG. 17: Verruca vulgaris; multiple hyperpigmented verrucous papules and plaques over dorsum of hand.

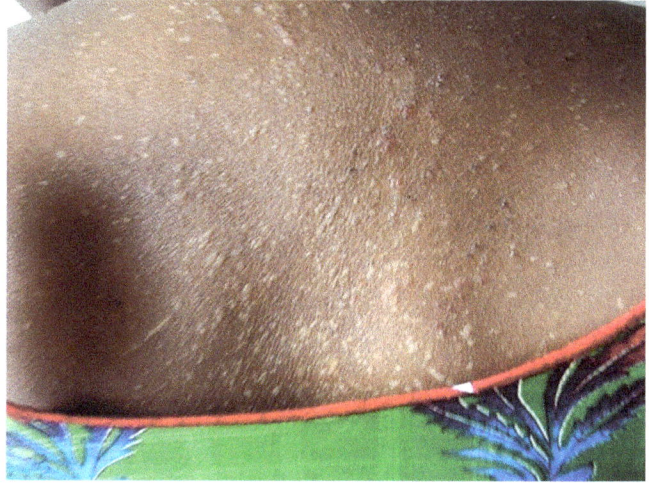

FIG. 18: Plane warts; multiple hypopigmented flat-topped papules over upper back, note evidence of koebnerization.

CHAPTER 18: Cutaneous Manifestations of Coronavirus Disease 2019

Introduction

Coronavirus Disease 2019 (COVID-19) is a highly contagious respiratory tract infection caused by the novel Severe Acute Respiratory Syndrome Coronavirus-2 (SARS-CoV-2). COVID-19 was declared a pandemic by the World Health Organization in March 2020. Since then, it has caused havoc around the globe, before becoming endemic in most areas. Though, it is not a cutaneous infection, an increasing understanding of cutaneous manifestations associated with various types of the disease has emerged, which have a prognostic significance. This chapter summarizes these skin manifestations.

Cutaneous Manifestations of COVID-19

The major skin manifestations related to SARS-CoV-2 infection can be divided across the spectrum as:
- Chilblain-like lesions
- Maculopapular eruption
- Urticarial eruption
- Vesicular eruption
- Livedoid necrosis

Other skin findings reported with COVID-19 are included in **Table 1**.

Familiarity with these changes can aid in early recognition of skin lesions suggestive of COVID-19, particularly in cases with paucisymptomatic infection, as well as in those with progressively worsening disease and potentially bad prognosis.

The estimated incidence of cutaneous manifestations secondary to COVID-19 is 4–20.4%. The dermatologic manifestations may be related to the binding of SARS-CoV-2 to angiotensin-converting enzyme-2 (ACE2) receptors present in cutaneous blood vessels, eccrine gland epithelial cells, and the basal layer of hair follicles. Cutaneous signs may appear a few days before to several days after the diagnosis of COVID-19.

Clinical Features

Clinical presentation of COVID-19 can vary from no symptoms to acute respiratory distress syndrome (ARDS), and multiple organ failure.
- Common symptoms include fever, dry cough, fatigue, sputum production, shortness of breath, loss of sense of smell and taste, and conjunctivitis.

TABLE 1: Cutaneous manifestations of SARS-CoV-2 infection.

Inflammatory reactions	Lesions of vascular origin	Other skin findings
Maculopapular or morbilliform rash	Chilblain-like rashes	Erythema multiforme-like lesions
Urticarial eruption	Petechiae or purpura	Cutaneous manifestations associated with MIS-C or MIS-A
Vesicular rash	Livedo racemosa-like pattern	• Pityriasis rosea • Shingles • Nail changes • Hair changes

(MIS-A: multisystem inflammatory syndrome in adults; MIS-C: multisystem inflammatory syndrome in children; SARS-CoV-2: severe acute respiratory syndrome coronavirus-2)

- Severe disease, is characterized by dyspnea, blood oxygen desaturation, respiratory failure, and venous thromboembolism.

A variety of skin manifestations could be due to:
- The virus infecting through an open skin wound.
- Immune responses.
- Drug-induced changes.

Maculopapular Lesions

- They are the most prevalent cutaneous manifestations seen throughout the pandemic (46–70%).
- They could follow a viral infection, occur as adverse reactions to drugs, or due to the cytokine storm produced by a hyperactive immune system against the virus.
- They are mostly reported in middle-aged patients. Pruritus is present in 56% of patients with maculopapular lesions.
- They are mostly located on the trunk **(Fig. 1)**.
- They could have simultaneous onset with COVID-19 symptoms, or even later onset (average latency 27 days).
- Exanthem lasts for a short period (8–12 days). Possibly associated with greater severity of disease.
- *Histopathology*: Early-onset rash shows epidermal spongiosis, perivascular lymphocytic infiltrate, and eosinophils in the dermis. Late-onset lesions are characterized by mild superficial perivascular lymphocytic infiltrate and histiocytes among collagen fibers, devoid of mucin deposits.

Urticarial Lesions

- One of the most frequent cutaneous manifestations.
- Characterized by an erythematous rash followed by intense pruritus.
- Typically distributed on the trunk or limbs but may be generalized or even localized to the face **(Fig. 2)**.
- Onset is simultaneous with systemic symptoms and it is generally seen in more severe cases.
- *Histopathology*: Perivascular infiltrate of lymphocytes, few eosinophils, and upper dermal edema may be seen.
- Possible pathophysiological mechanisms could include drug-induced allergy, cytokine storm, or direct effect of the virus on the skin.

Chilblain-like Lesions

- These represent late manifestations of COVID-19.
- They are more often reported in children and young adults.
- Pain, pruritus, and burning are the symptoms frequently reported.
- Characteristic lesions are chilblain lesions or pernio, seen as swelling, erythema, and violaceous coloration of extremities such as fingers and toes (COVID toes) **(Fig. 3)**.
- Temporal association with viral infection has been reported.
- These manifestations last longer (1–2 weeks).
- Patients are usually asymptomatic or have mild COVID-19 disease.

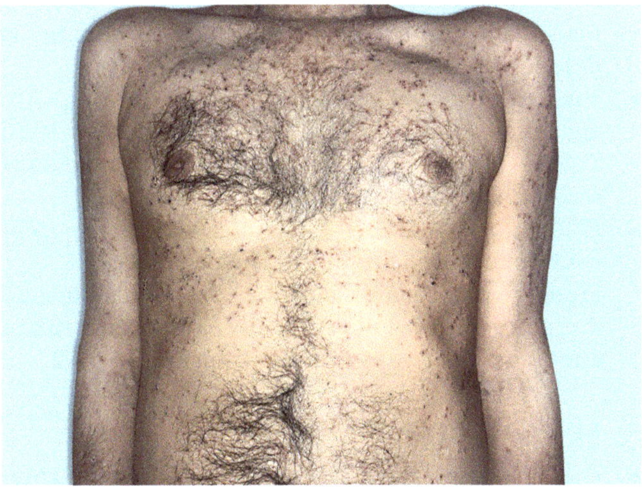

FIG. 1: Extensive maculopapular rash in a patient with coronavirus disease 2019 (COVID-19).

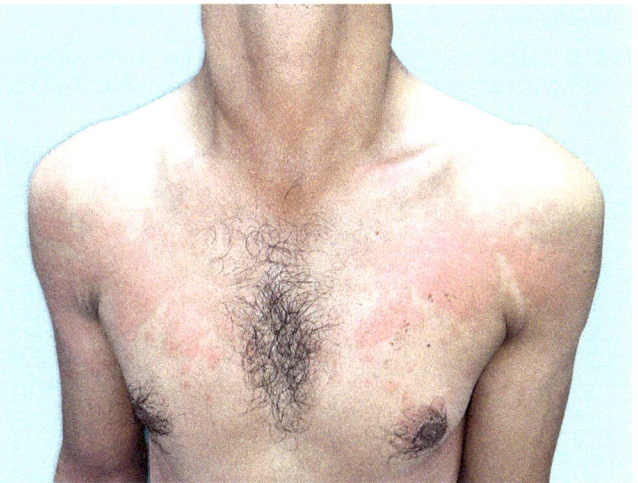

FIG. 2: Urticarial rash in a patient with coronavirus disease 2019 (COVID-19).

- *Histopathology*: Focal vacuolar degeneration of the basal layer, perivascular lymphocytic cuffs in the dermal regions, and microthrombi.
- Pathogenesis could involve host viral response, vasculitis, vessel thrombosis, or neoangiogenesis. They are not considered an accurate indicator for diagnosis of COVID-19.

Vesicular Lesions

- These are less common than the aforementioned manifestations (3.77–15%).
- They are typically seen in middle-aged patients and are described as "specific manifestations" of COVID-19 **(Fig. 4)**.
- Trunk is commonly affected in the localized forms; however, a diffuse pattern with polymorphic lesions, also involving the extremities, is also described.

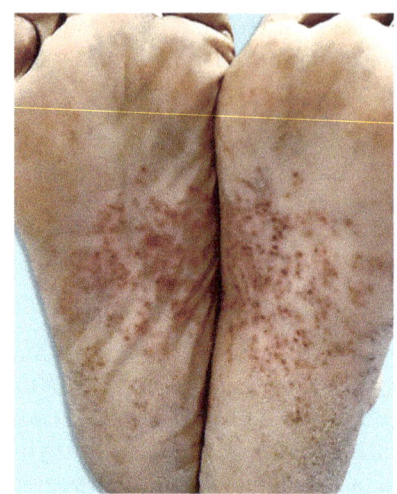

FIG. 5: Plantar involvement in the same patient.

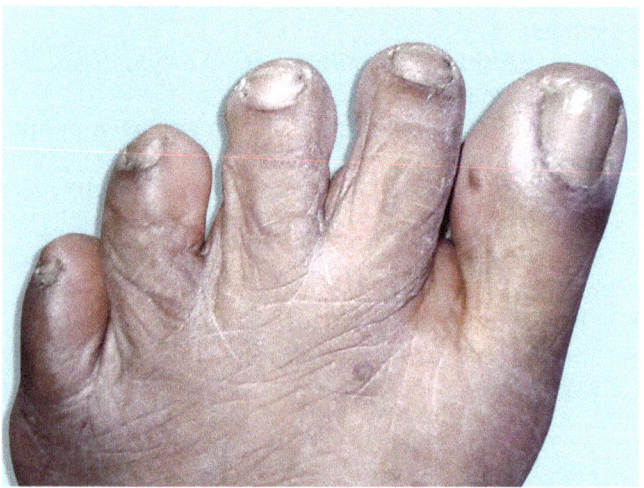

FIG. 3: Sparse, resolving perniotic lesion on the lateral aspect of great toe, in a patient with mild coronavirus disease 2019 (COVID-19).

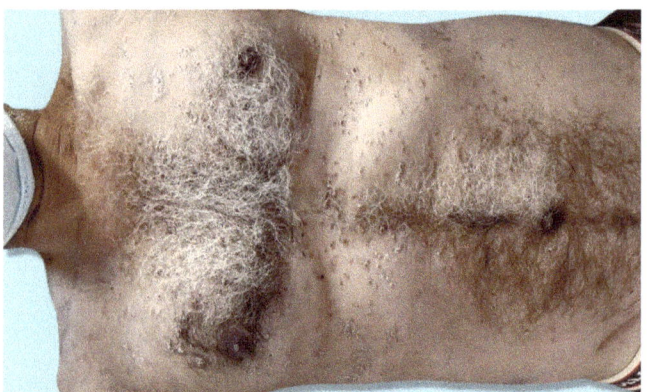

FIG. 4: Vesicular rash in a patient who was later diagnosed with respiratory discomfort and RT-PCR positivity for COVID-19.
(COVID-19: coronavirus disease 2019; RT-PCR: reverse transcriptase–polymerase chain reaction)

- The time of onset from COVID-19 symptoms is 14 days (4–30 days). Duration of rash ranges between 8 and 10 days.
- Vesicular lesions are associated with intermediate severity of disease **(Fig. 5)**.
- *Histopathology* reveals the presence of intraepidermal vesicles with acantholysis, dyskeratosis, and ballooned keratinocytes, with lymphocytic perivascular infiltrate, vascular leak, and edema.
- Pathophysiology involves overactivation of the immune system with "cytokine storm" affecting the skin, or direct cytopathic effect of SARS-CoV-2 on endothelium dermal vessels.

Petechiae/Purpuric Lesions

- Petechiae/purpura are among the less commonly described cutaneous manifestations.
- These are localized on the trunk and extremities.
- The onset is after COVID-19 symptoms.
- They are more frequent in middle-aged patients recovering from severe COVID-19 infections.
- *Histopathology* shows interstitial and perivascular neutrophilia, with prominent leukocytoclasia.
- Proposed pathogenesis involves a pauci-inflammatory thrombogenic vasculopathy, adverse drug effects, or a direct cutaneous manifestation from SARS-CoV-2.

Livedoid Eruption

- These are considered one of the least common cutaneous manifestations associated with COVID-19 (6%).
- They are generally localized on the trunk, flexor surface of forearms, dorsal hand, and dorsal foot.
- They occur at the same time as other COVID-19 symptoms and last for approximately 10 days.

- They are seen in elderly patients with severe infections.
- Pathogenesis could be due to hypercoagulability associated with COVID-19.
- The mortality rate associated with this manifestation is the highest (10%).

Other Skin Manifestations

- Children with COVID-19 have been reported to develop Multisystem inflammatory syndrome with Kawasaki disease-like features (MIS-C). It is characterized by a diffuse polymorphic rash (maculopapular, erythema multiforme-like, or diffuse erythroderma) along with fever, lymphadenopathy, strawberry tongue, and gastrointestinal symptoms.
- COVID-19 has also been associated with telogen effluvium, beginning 50 days after the first symptoms, and affecting 90% of females.
- Alopecia areata with onset 1–2 months following infection has been reported.
- Other rarer manifestations observed include pityriasis rosea, sebopsoriasis, COVID arm, herpes zoster, lichen planus, painful oral ulcers, nail changes including red-half-moon sign **(Fig. 6)**, diffuse pruritic pustular eruption, SDRIFE (symmetrical drug-related intertriginous and flexural exanthema)-like erythematous rash **(Fig. 7)**, pruriginous and painful subcutaneous nodules, eruptive angiomas **(Fig. 8)**, and pseudoherpetic Grover's disease.
- Oral thrush has been reported in patients with severe disease, especially those receiving immunosuppressive therapy, or those with comorbid conditions **(Fig. 9)**. Candidal balanoposthitis was also noted to be a common concern **(Fig. 10)**.

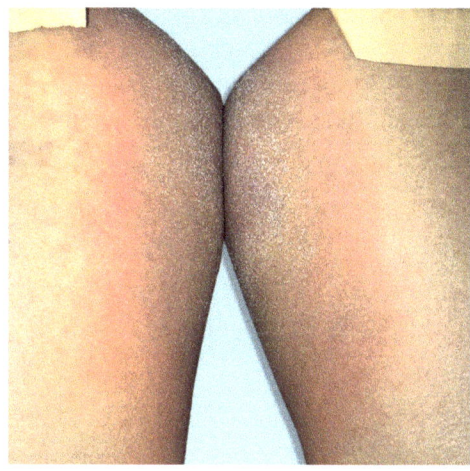

FIG. 7: SDRIFE in a young female with COVID-19.
(COVID-19: coronavirus disease 2019; SDRIFE: symmetrical drug-related intertriginous and flexural exanthema)

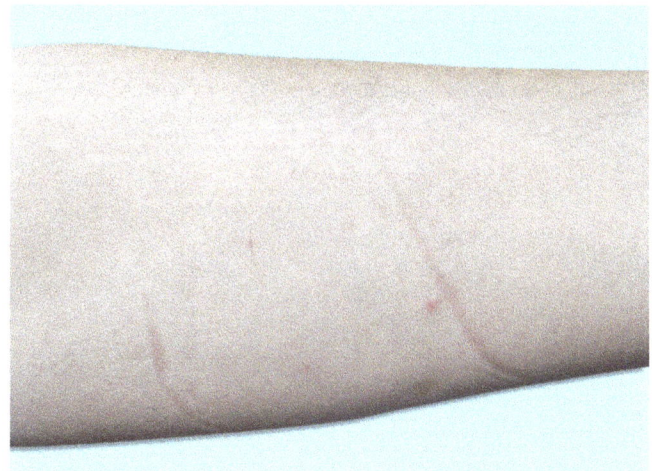

FIG. 8: Eruptive lesions suggestive of angiomas.

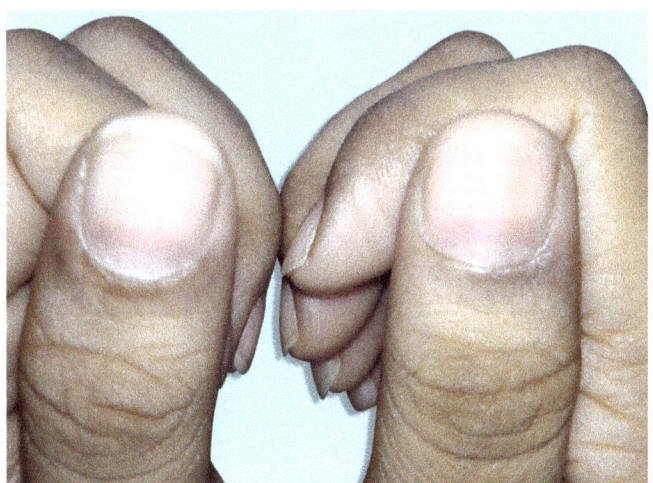

FIG. 6: Red-half-moon lunula in a patient admitted for severe respiratory distress in coronavirus disease 2019 (COVID-19).

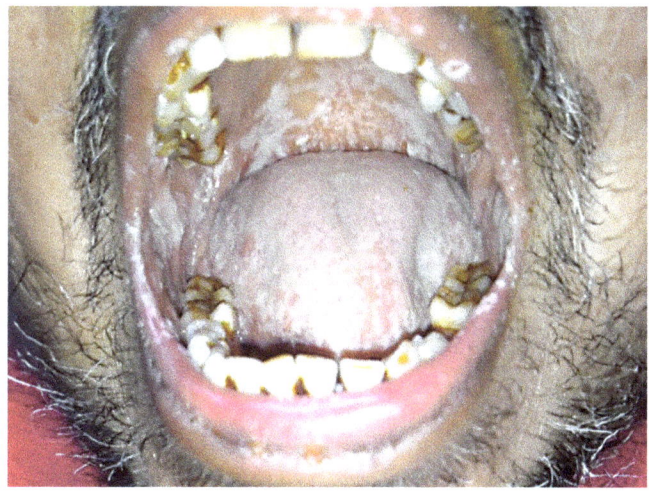

FIG. 9: Severe oral candidiasis in a diabetic male with severe coronavirus disease 2019 (COVID-19).

- Mucormycosis has been reported post-COVID-19 **(Fig. 11)**. It has been implicated on factors related to treatment including the use of steroids and broad-spectrum antibiotics, smoking, and use of oxygen.

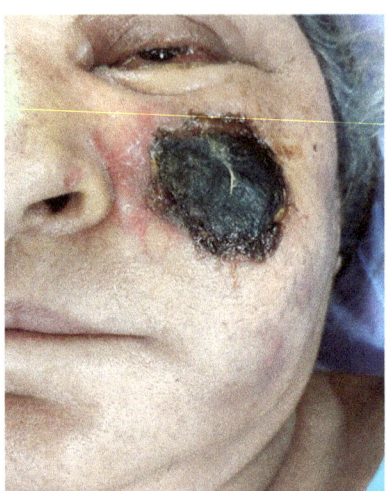

FIG. 11: An obese patient admitted with mucormycosis postrecovery from severe coronavirus disease 2019 (COVID-19). Severe involvement of the nose, maxillary sinus, ocular cavity, and overlying skin can be seen.
Courtesy: Dr Neelima Gupta, Director Professor and Head, Department of Otorhinolaryngology, UCMS and GTB Hospital, Delhi, India.

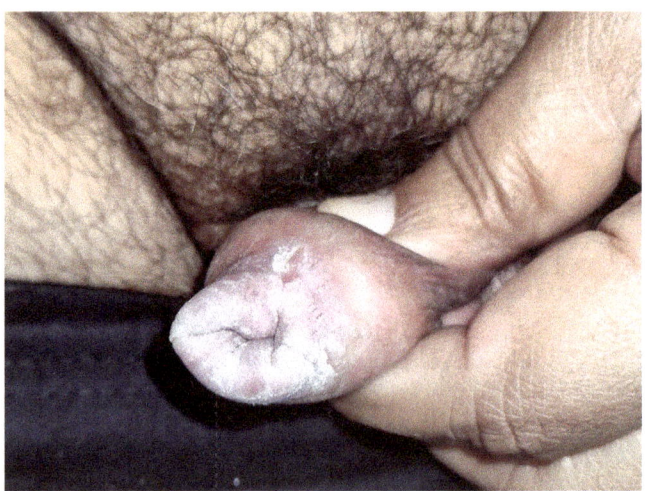

FIG. 10: Candidal balanoposthitis in the same patient.

Index

Page numbers followed by *b* refer to box, *f* refer to figure, and *t* refer to table.

A

Abacavir 183
Abscess 8*f*, 67
    acute neutrophilic 125
    bacterial 126
    cutaneous 8
    metastatic tuberculous 129
    periurethral 166
Absidia 75
Acanthosis 108*f*
Achromicus 115
Acid-fast
    bacilli 114, 120*f*, 124, 135
    Mycobacterium leprae 114
Acne vulgaris 28
Acquired immunodeficiency syndrome 20, 31, 48, 66, 67, 109, 130
Actinomycetoma 62, 63, 63*f*, 64
    features of 63*t*
Actinomycosis 64, 127
Acute neutrophilic abscess 125
    formation 126*f*
Acyclovir 82, 88
Addison's disease 48
Adenosine triphosphate 169
Aedes aegypti 111
African tick bite fever 23
Agammaglobulinemia 85
Albendazole 142, 144, 159
Alcoholism 117
Allergy 85
Allodermanyssus sanguineus 24
Allylamines 46
Alopecia areata 30
Altered sensorium 23
Alternaria 61
Amikacin 15
Amorolfine 46
Amoxicillin 14
Amphotericin B 62, 68
Amprenavir 183
Amyloidosis 117
Anal squamous intraepithelial lesions 191
Ancylostoma duodenale 143
Androgenic alopecia 160
Anesthesia
    conjunctival 118
    corneal 118
Angiomas 195*f*
Angiotensin-converting enzyme-2 192
Angular cheilitis 48, 49*f*
Ankara vaccine 104
Ankles, bilateral 23*f*
Annelida 164
Annular erythema 26
Annular plaques 26
Anthrax 7
Antibiotic
    intravenous 15
    therapy 15
        systemic 14
Antibody testing 68
Antifungal
    agents 46
    effect 46
    systemic 46*t*
    therapy 30
    topical 46*t*
Antigen detection 68
Antileprosy treatment 118
Antimitotic therapy 97
Anti-orthopoxvirus antibodies, serology for 103
Antiretroviral drugs, classes of 183*t*
Antitubercular treatment 125, 127*f*, 133
Antiviral
    agents 109
    drugs, systemic 88
    medications 107
    therapy 81, 84
        systemic 82*t*
Aphthous stomatitis 81
Aphthous ulcers 110
Arthralgia 23
Arthritis 166, 168
    dermatitis syndrome 168
    migratory 111
Arthropod bites 161
Aspergillosis 73
Aspergillus 47
    fumigatus 73
    infection 48
    terreus 73
Aspirin 112
Atazanavir 183
Athlete's foot 32
Atopic dermatitis 1, 13*f*, 30, 78
Atrophy 86*f*
Aurora borealis pattern 43*f*
Autoimplantation therapy 98
Autosomal dominant hypertrophic neuropathy 117
Axillary hair 16*f*
Axillary lymphadenopathy 105
Azelaic acid 160
Azithromycin 170
Azoles 46
    antifungals 16
    medicines 152

B

Babesiosis 163
Bacillary angiomatosis 185
Bacillus Calmette–Guérin vaccination 98, 128*f*, 128
Bacteremia 168
Bacteria 40, 185
Bacterial infection
    Gram-negative 18
    Gram-positive 1, 12
    secondary 13*f*, 83, 156
Bacteroides 184
Baghdad boil 147
Balanitis, candidal 49
Balanoposthitis 49, 166*f*
    candidal 50*f*, 196*f*
Bancroftian filariasis 139
Barefoot walkers, human skin of 144
Bartholin's ducts 165, 169
Bartholinitis 169
Bartonella henselae 185
Basal cell carcinoma 94, 108
Beau's lines post 111*f*
Bedbug
    bites 161, 162*f*
    eradication 162
Bent hair 42*f*
Beta-hemolytic *Streptococcus* 10
Bictegravir 183
Biopsy 58
Bites 161
Bivalent human papillomavirus vaccine 99

Index

Black dot tinea capitis 28, 29f
   linear patch of 29f
Black piedra 54
Blastomyces dermatitidis 68
Blastomycosis 20, 68
   extrapulmonary 68
   primary pulmonary 68
Bleomycin 98
Blepharoconjunctivitis 160
Blister beetle dermatoses 162
Blistering distal dactylitis 12
Blood
   culture 21
   dyscrasias 85
   stained discharge 125f
Bockhart's impetigo 5
Body louse 157, 159
   infestation 159
Boggy swelling 30f
Borderline lepromatous 114, 116
Borderline tuberculoid 114
   Hansen 116f
      dry plaque of 115f
   lazarine leprosy, ulcerated lesion of 118f
Botryomycosis 12, 64, 184
Bowen's disease 92, 94, 95f
   extragenital 94, 95f
Bowenoid papulosis 94, 94f
   pigmented lesions of 94f
Breakfast, lunch, and dinner sign 162, 162f
Brill-Zinsser disease 22
Brincidofovir 104
Broad telangiectatic vessels 45f
Budding yeasts 52f
Buffalopox 100, 104
   papulovesicular lesions of 105f
Bullous impetigo 2, 4
   lesions of 3f
Bullous lesions, multiple 177f
Buruli ulcer 136
Buschke–Löwenstein
   giant condyloma acuminate of 93f
   tumor 93
      long-standing 95f

C

Camelpox 104
   lesions of 104f
   virus 104
Cancer
   cervical 95
   invasive 96f
   penile 95
Candida
   albicans 188
   dubliniensis 48, 188
   glabrata 48, 188

   krusei 48, 188
   parapsilosis 48, 188
   pseudohyphae 52f
   tropicalis 48, 188
Candidemia 74f
Candidiasis 15, 25, 48, 48b, 188
   acute pseudomembranous 48
   cutaneous 52t
   perianal 50, 51f
Cantharidin 97
Cantharis vesicatoria 97
Captain's wheel-like appearance 71f
Carbon dioxide laser 97
Carbuncle 7, 8f
Carcinoma 64
   cervix 96f
   in-situ 94
Cartridge-based nucleic acid amplification testing 124
CD4 T-cell count 183
Cellulitis 10, 11f, 67, 73
   early lesion of 11f
   severe 11
Central necrotic polycyclic ulceration 186f
Central nervous system cryptococcosis 71
Cephalexin 14
Cerebral pheohyphomycosis 62f
Cerebrospinal fluid 19
Cervical lymph nodes 126
Cervicitis 165, 169
Cervix
   anterior lips of 96f
   posterior lips of 96f
   ulcerated 96f
   uncomplicated gonococcal infections of 167
Cestodes 139
Chancre
   primary 173f, 174f
   syphilitic 81
   tuberculous 124
Chancroid 81, 171, 171f, 190
Chemotherapeutic agents, newer 123
Chest, roentgenogram of 133
Chickenpox 82, 102
Chik sign 111, 112f
Chikungunya 111f, 112f
   fever 113
   virus 111
Chlamydia 169
   infection 167, 169, 170
   life cycle of 169f
   trachomatis 165
Chloramphenicol 24
Chloronychia 21
Chromoblastomycosis 56, 58, 59, 60f, 61
Cicatricial hair loss 29f
Ciclopirox 46
Cidofovir 107

Cimex lectularius 161
Cimicosis 161
Ciprofloxacin 21, 137
Cladophialophora 61
Cladosporium 61
   trichoides, culture of 62f
Clarithromycin 136
Clavulanate 14
Clindamycin 14
Clofazimine 123
Clotrimazole 16, 49
Coccidioides
   immitis 69
   thick-walled mature spherules of 69f
Coccidioidomycosis 69, 108
Cold abscess, painless 126f
Colorado tick fever 163
Complement fixation test 68
Compression bandaging 142f
Condyloma lata 174f, 175f
Condylomata acuminata 93
   lesions 93f
Congenital syphilis 176, 176f, 176t, 177f
   stigmata of 176, 178
Congestion, conjunctival 109
Conjunctival effusion 23
Conjunctivitis, gonococcal 166, 168
Contact dermatitis 10, 78
Corneal reflex 118
Coronavirus disease 2019 (COVID-19) 75, 192, 193f, 194, 195, 195f
   clinical presentation of 192
   cutaneous manifestations of 192
   mild 194f
   severe 195f, 196f
Corticosteroid, signs of 40
Corynebacterium 16
   minutissimum 15
Coryneform bacteria 15
Cotrimoxazole 14, 65, 159
Cough 73
Cowper's gland inflammation 166
Cowpox virus 105
Coxsackieviruses 100, 110
Crab louse 159f
Crotamiton 160
Crusted scabies 155, 157
Cryotherapy 97
Cryptococcal spores 72f
Cryptococcosis 71, 108, 187
   disseminated 71
   ocular 71
   pulmonary 71
Cryptococcus gattii 71
Cryptococcus neoformans 71
Cunninghamella 75
Curvularia 61
Cushing's syndrome 48
Cut larva migrans 144f
Cutaneous cryptococcosis 71
   plaques of 71f

Cutaneous leishmaniasis 58, 60, 116, 147, 151
   chronic 149
   diffuse 148, 151
   granulomatous 64
   nodules of 148*f*
   plaques of 147*f*
   volcanic nodule of 148*f*
Cutaneous sporotrichosis 56, 61
   ulcerative variant of 58*f*
Cutaneous tuberculosis 61, 124, 185
   treatment of 133*t*
Cycloheximide 54
Cyclosporine 79*f*
Cysticercosis 144
   subcutaneous 145
Cysticercus cellulosae 145
Cysts 137
Cytomegalovirus 76
Cytotoxic drugs 66

D

Dairy products 135
Dapsone 64, 123
Darier's disease 78
Darling's disease 66
Darunavir 183*t*
Daughter yeast cells 67*f*
Deep folliculitis 6
   lesion of 6*f*
   type of 27
Deep vein thrombosis 10
Delavirdine 183*t*
Delhi boil 147
Demodex 160
   brevis 160
   folliculorum 160
   infestation 160
   mite 160
   rosacea 160
Demodicidosis 160, 160*f*
Dengue 112
   fever 112
   hemorrhagic fever 112, 112*f*
   shock syndrome 112
Deoxycholate amphotericin 59
Deoxyribonucleic acid 73, 89, 100, 132, 162
   double-stranded 100
   non-enveloped 89
   viruses 76
Dermal necrosis 11*f*
Dermatitis
   extensive 163*f*
   perioral 28, 160
   sebaceous 26, 27, 30, 50, 53
Dermato-adeno-lymphangitis, acute 139
Dermatofibroma 118
Dermatophyte
   infections 25, 44*t*
      types of 25
   septate hyphae 45*f*

Dermatophytoma 42, 44*f*
Dermatophytosis 5, 25, 34*f*, 47, 47*f*, 188
   chronic 25
   management of 41
   microbiological resistance of 25
   recurrent 25
Dermatoscopy 41
Dermatoses, severe generalized 7
Dermis 106*f*
Destructive therapy 109
Detritus 67
Dhobi itch 27
Diabetes mellitus 117
Diaper
   candidiasis 52
   dermatitis, candidal 52
Diarrhea 109
Dicloxacillin 14
Didanosine 183
Diethylcarbamazine citrate 141
DiGeorge syndrome 48
Direct fluorescent antibody 186
Direct microscopy 45, 60
Discoid lupus erythematosus 116
Disseminated disease 69
Disseminated intravascular coagulation 84
Dolutegravir 183
Donovanosis 180
   beefy red ulcers of 181*f*
Dorsal radial branch, enlarged 120*f*
Down's syndrome 155
Doxycycline 14, 24, 136, 170, 185
Dysplastic lesions 191

E

Ear pinna 58*f*
Echinocandins 74
Ecthyma 4, 4*f*, 5
   gangrenosum 20, 20*f*
   lesion of 4
   multiple lesions of 5*f*
   typical lesion of 4*f*
Ectropion 118
Eczema 1
   chronic 30
   herpeticum 78, 79*f*, 82, 102
Eczematization 161
Eczematous tinea 34*b*
Edema
   peripheral 104*f*-106*f*
   reactive 103*f*
Edmonston–Zagreb measles virus 108
Efavirenz 183*t*
Ehrlichiosis 163
Electron microscopy 103
Elvitegravir 183*t*
Emtricitabine 183*t*
Endemic mycoses 66
Endemic typhus 22
Endocarditis 168

Endometritis 170
Endonyx 44*f*
   onychomycosis 32*f*, 43
Endophthalmitis 74*f*
Endotoxin layer 18
Enfuvirtide 183*t*
Enterobiasis 142
Enterobius vermicularis 142
   life cycle of 142*f*
Enterovirus 110
Entomophthoromycosis 56
Enzyme-linked immunosorbent assay 64, 68, 80, 108, 140, 167, 183
Eosinophilia, tropical pulmonary 139
Epidemic typhus 22
Epidermal cells 108*f*
Epidermal parasitic skin diseases 154
Epidermis 106*f*
Epidermodysplasia verruciformis 92, 92*f*
Epididymitis 166, 169
Epididymo-orchitis, acute 121, 139
Epithelioid granuloma 129*f*
Epitheliomas 108
Erbium-doped yttrium aluminum garnet 97
Eruptive lesions 195*f*
Erysipelas 10, 10*f*
   hallmark of 10
   recurrent 10
Erythema 11*f*, 44*f*, 104*f*, 162
   annulare centrifugum 116
   induratum of Bazin 130, 132, 185
   infectiosum 113
   migrans 163*f*
   multiforme 110
   nodosum 132, 185
      erythematous tender nodules of 132*f*
   leprosum 121, 122*f*, 185
   peripheral 106*f*
Erythematous 7, 62*f*, 83*f*, 122*f*
   crusted plaques 186*f*
   macules, hyperpigmented 92
   plaque, indurated 131*f*
Erythrasma 15, 15*f*, 16, 27, 50, 53
Erythroderma 7, 67
Erythromycin 14, 16, 168, 170, 185
Escherichia coli 184
Ethambutol 133, 136, 185
Etravirine 183*t*
Eumycetoma 63, 64
   features of 63*t*
Exanthem 100
   subitum 113
Exanthema, flexural 195
Exophiala 61
Extensive perifollicular scaling 42*f*
Extremities, lymphedema of 139
Eye 118
   conjunctival of 105*f*
Eyebrows, loss of 118
Eyelashes, base of 158*f*

F

Facial
　cellulitis, cause of 11
　dermatitis, nonspecific 160, 160f
　nerve palsy 21, 85, 87f, 119, 119f
　pigmentation 111
Facies leprosa 119
Famciclovir 82t, 88
Favus 29
Fever
　hemorrhagic 112
　high 100, 109
　recurrent attacks of 139
　rickettsial 22f
　tickborne relapsing 163
Filariasis 141
　lymphatic 139
Filiform 93
　warts 91, 92f
Fine-needle aspiration cytology 124, 133
Finger-web spaces 154
Fish tank granuloma 135
Fitz–Hugh–Curtis syndrome 170
Flinders island spotted fever 23
Fluconazole 30, 46, 49, 54, 59, 64, 68-70, 152
Fluoroquinolones 24
Fluorouracil 97, 98
Follicular inflammatory lesions 37f
Folliculitis 5, 5f, 6f, 7, 184f
　bacterial 30
　decalvans 30
　herpetic 5
　multiple lesions of 6f
　superficial 5
　types of 5
Folliculocentric papules, multiple 28f
Fonsecaea 61
Foot
　disease 110, 111f
　　lesions of 110f
　dorsal aspect of 33f
　dorsum of 95f
Foreign body
　granuloma 60, 61, 137
　reaction 137
Formaldehyde 98
Formic acid 97
Fosamprenavir 183
Fungal
　culture 45, 47f, 58, 61, 62, 68, 70, 73
　elements 73
　infection 56, 137, 187
　　cutaneous 44
　　deep 66
　　superficial 25
　invasion 46f
Funiculitis 139
Furuncle 7
　classical lesion of 7f

Furunculosis, recurrent 7
Fusarium 47
Fusidic acid 14, 16
Fusion inhibitors 183

G

Gamma benzene hexachloride 159
Gardasil 99
Gastrointestinal system 133
Genital 102
　discharge disease 165
　herpes 76, 81, 189
　　prevention of 81
　　primary 76, 78
　infections 169
　location 156f
　tuberculid 131f
　ulcer disease 165
　warts 191f
　　exuberant 93f
Genitalia 35f
　Bowen's disease of 94
　enlargement of 172f
　external 131f, 175f
Giemsa stain 15
Gingivitis 83f
Gingivostomatitis 77f
Glands, sebaceous 100f
Glans penis 191f
　shaft of 189f
Glomerulonephritis 84
Glucocorticoids 48
Glutaraldehyde, virucidal properties of 98
Goldman-Fox syndrome 21
Gomori methenamine silver stain 69f, 71f
Gonococcal cervicitis, acute 166f
Gonococcal infection, disseminated 166, 168
Gonococci 165
Gonococcus 169
Gonorrhea 165-167
　complications of 166t
Gram stain 6, 15
　smears 5, 7
Granulocyte-macrophage colony-stimulating factor 21
Granuloma
　annulare 116
　faciale 129
　gluteale infantum 52f
　inguinale 180, 190
Granulomatous diseases 137
Granulomatous plaque, large indurated 57f
Great toe, lateral aspect of 194f
Greater auricular nerve, enlarged 117f
Green nail syndrome 20, 21
Griseofulvin 30, 46
Grocott-Gömöri's stains 68

Groins 35f
　faint tender erythema of 9f
Ground itch 144
Guillain-Barré syndrome 85

H

Haemophilus influenzae type B 11
Hailey-Hailey disease 78
Hair
　casts 55
　loss, scaly patches of 28f
　multiple bent 45f
Hand 90f
　bones of 119
　disease 110, 111f
　　lesions of 110f
　dorsae of 18f
　dorsal aspect of 34f
　plaques over dorsum of 191f
Hansen's disease 114, 128
Head louse 157f, 158
Headache, severe 100
Healing 81f
　defect 85
Hebra circle 155f
Hematoxylin 70
Hemoptysis 73
Hemorrhagic blisters 88f
Henderson-Patterson cytoplasmic inclusion bodies 107
Hepatitis
　C virus 191
　subclinical 84
Herpangina 81, 110
Herpes
　anogenital 80
　genitalis 76, 77f, 78f, 82, 189f, 190f
　　recurrent 78f
　gingivostomatitis 76
　gladiatorum 79, 80f
　labialis 76, 77f, 82, 190f
　　recurrent 77f
　simplex
　　disseminated 7, 102
　　infection 4, 76, 80
　　oral lesions of 81f
　　virus 189
　stomatitis 110
　virus 76
　　infection 76, 107
　whitlow 79f
　zoster 85, 85f-88f
　　disseminated 86f
　　necrotic lesions of 88f
　　ophthalmicus 87f, 186f
Herpetic whitlow 79
Heterophile agglutination test 24
Hidradenitis suppurativa 9, 126
Highly active antiretroviral therapy 109
Higoumenaki's sign 178f

Histoid Hansen
　lesions of 118*f*
　succulent cutaneous nodule of 118*f*
Histoid leprosy 117
Histopathology 46, 73
Histoplasma capsulatum 66
Histoplasmosis 66, 108, 188
　cutaneous 67*f*
Honey-colored crusts 2*f*
Hookworm
　disease 143
　life cycle of 143*f*
House dust 135
Human helminthic infections 139
Human immunodeficiency virus 8*f*, 67*f*, 71*f*, 80, 81*f*, 93*f*, 109, 130, 165, 175*f*, 178, 178*f*, 182, 189
　infection 20, 182*t*
　　acute 182
　　chronic 182
　　stage of 182
　pandemic, advent of 100
　structure of 182*f*
Human papillomavirus 89
　infection 191
　structure of 89*f*
　vaccines 98
Humid hot climates 136
Hutchinson's sign 87, 87*f*
Hutchinson's teeth 177*f*
Hybridization techniques 73
Hydrocele 139
Hyperbaric oxygen 137
Hyperpigmentation, diffuse 67
Hyperplasia, sebaceous 108
Hypoalbuminemia 144
Hypoesthesia 118
Hypogammaglobulinemia 85
Hypomelanosis, postinflammatory 115
Hypoparathyroidism 48
Hypopigmentation
　lesional 40
　perilesional 40
Hypopigmented flat, multiple 191*f*
Hypopyon 74*f*
Hypotension 11
Hypothyroidism 48

I

Iatrogenic cushingoid syndrome 41
Ibalizumab 183
Ichthyosis vulgaris 78
Imiquimod 98
　topical 107
Immune reconstitution inflammatory syndrome 184, 186*f*
Immunochromatographic card test 140
Immunofluorescence 109

Immunoglobulin
　A deficiency 85
　G antibodies 70
　M antibodies 70
Immunomodulators, oral 98
Immunosuppression, setting of 66*f*
Immunotherapy 98
Impetigo 1, 4, 30
　contagiosa 2, 3
　contagiosum, localized lesion of 2*f*
　diagnosis of 4
　lesions of 3*f*
　localized nonbullous 2*f*
Indinavir 183*t*
Infections 2*t*, 13*f*, 40*f*, 106, 169
　atypical mycobacterial 127
　bacterial 125, 184
　chronic pulmonary 69
　cutaneous 135
　deep 7
　dermatologic 184
　direct 1
　fungal 56, 137, 187
　genital 169
　meningococcal 18
　nonpurulent 2
　purulent 2
　rickettsial 21, 22, 23*t*
　secondary 1, 13*f*
　severe 73
　treatment of 14
　viral 186
Inflamed epidermoid cyst 9
Inflammatory reactions 192
Ingrown toenail 13*f*
Inguinal bubo 171*f*
Integrase inhibitors 183
Intense erythema 37*f*
Interferon-alpha 98
Intertrigo
　bacterial 50
　candidal 27, 50, 50*f*
　fungal 140*f*
Intracellular diplococci, Gram-negative 167*f*
Intracellular yeasts 67*f*
Intralesional immunotherapy 98
Intravenous vaccinia immunoglobulin 104
Invasion, site of 31
Invasive sinopulmonary aspergillosis 73
Iron
　deficiency anemia 144
　supplementation, oral 144
Irritant dermatitis, signs of 40
Isoniazid 133, 185
Itraconazole 30, 46, 54, 59, 62, 64, 68-70, 152
Ivermectin 144, 159, 160
Ixodes scapularis 163

J

Japanese spotted fever 23
Jaundice 23

K

Kaposi's sarcoma 187
Kaposi's varicelliform eruption 78
Keratoconjunctivitis, herpetic 79
Keratosis
　pilaris 131
　sebaceous 94
Kerion 28, 29, 29*f*
Ketoconazole 46, 54, 152
Kissing chancre 174*f*
Koebnerization, evidence of 191*f*
Koplik's spots 109

L

Labia
　majora 190*f*
　minora 190*f*
Lagophthalmos 119*f*
Lamivudine 183*t*
Langhans giant cell 131*f*, 136
Larva migrans, cutaneous 144
Laser ablation 97
Lazarine leprosy 118
Leech 164
　bite 164*f*
Leg
　bilateral 112*f*
　elephantiasis of 140*f*
　flexor aspect of 132*f*
Leishman–Donovan bodies 151*f*
Leishmania
　amazonensis 148
　braziliensis 147
　chagasi 147
　donovani 147
　　complex 147
　infantum 147
　major 147
　mexicana 147
　tropica 147
Leishmaniasis 116, 129, 147
　cutaneous 58, 60, 116, 147, 151
Lepra reaction 122*f*
Lepromatous leprosy 114, 116, 118, 120*f*, 149*f*
　bilateral symmetrical hypopigmented macules of 116*f*
　leonine facies of 117*f*
Leprosy 60, 114, 120*f*, 121, 123, 185, 186*f*
　diagnosis of 119
　lesions, number of 114
　reactions, management of 123
　spectrum of 114

Index

Lesions 105*f*, 111*f*
Lesions, atypical 80
    bullous 18*f*, 164*f*
    crops of 83*f*
    crusting of 13*f*
    facial 101*f*
    palmar 102*f*
    perianal 103*f*
    recurrent 79*f*, 80
    umbilicated 103*f*
    urticarial 193
Leukemia 85
Lichen
    nitidus 131
    scrofulosorum 130, 131*f*, 185
        follicular papules of 130*f*
        lesions of 131*f*
    spinulosa 131
Linear erosions 50*f*
Linezolid 14, 15
Lipopolysaccharide layer 18
Liposomal amphotericin B 59, 74
    deoxycholate 152
Littritis 169
Livedoid eruption 194
Lobomycosis 56
Loeffler's syndrome 143
Lopinavi 183*t*
Lupus erythematosus 128
    subacute 26
Lupus miliaris disseminatus faciei 160
Lupus profundus 132
Lupus vulgaris 60, 116, 128, 128*f*, 129*f*, 185
    development of 125
    erythematous crusted plaque of 128*f*
    lesion 128*f*, 129*f*
    multifocal lesion of 128*f*
Lyme disease 163
    cutaneous manifestation of 163*f*
Lymph node 73, 119, 135
    clinical assessment of 133
Lymphadenitis, unilateral 171*f*
Lymphadenopathy 101
Lymphangitis, penile 166
Lymphedema
    diagnosis of 139
    lower limb 141*f*
    peripheral 141
Lymphogranuloma venereum 81, 165, 172, 190
Lymphoma 85
Lytic lesions 127*f*

M

Macrolides 24, 138
Macules
    hypopigmented 149*f*, 150*f*
    progressive stages of 105
Maculopapular eruption 192
Madarosis 117, 118, 160
Madura foot 62
Maduramycosis 62
Majocchi's granuloma 27
Malaise 105
Malar rash 37*f*
Malassezia 53
    furfur 53
    globosa 53
    pachydermatis 53
    sympodialis 53
Malathion 159
Malignancy 48
Mantoux testing 185
Maraviroc 183
Mastoiditis 21
Maxillary sinus 196*f*
Measles 103, 108, 113
    encephalitis, subacute 109
    panencephalitis, acute 109
    typical rash of 109*f*
Mebendazole 142
Mediterranean spotted fever 23
Melanocytic nevus 94
Melasma 111*f*
Meningeal signs 23
Meningitis 71, 166
    gonococcal 168
Meningococcemia 18
    acute 18, 19, 19*f*
    chronic 19
Metacarpal bone 127*f*
Metronidazole 160
Miconazole nitrate 54
Micrococcus sedentarius 16
Microfilariae 140
Micropore plaster 98
Microsporum canis 27
Miliaria pustulosa 5
Milker's nodule 107
Miltefosine therapy 152, 152*f*
Minocycline 14, 136
Mites, proliferation of 160
Molecular techniques 72, 151
Molluscipoxvirus 107
Molluscum 191
    contagiosum 67*f*, 107, 187, 187*f*
        papulonodular lesions of 108*f*
        therapeutic modalities for 109*t*
        umbilicated papular lesions of 108*f*
    lesions of 187
Monkeypox 100, 101
    virus 101
Morbillivirus 108
Mouth disease 110, 111*f*
    lesions of 110*f*
Moxifloxacin 137
Mpox 101, 101*f*
    lesions 103*f*
Mucocutaneous leishmaniasis 148, 148*f*, 151
    lesions, resolution of 152*f*

Mucormycosis 56, 74, 75*f*, 196, 196*f*
    cutaneous 75
Mucosal lesions
    benign 93
    oral 101*f*
Multibacillary lepromatous leprosy 114
Multidrug therapy 121*f*
Multiple small
    follicular pustules 184*f*
    vesicular lesions 190*f*
Multiple ulcerated papulovesicular lesions 104*f*
Multisystem inflammatory syndrome 192
Mumps 108
Mupirocin 14
Mus musculus 24
Myalgia 23, 100
Mycetoma 56, 61, 62, 63*f*
    foot 63*f*
Mycobacteria 135
    nontuberculous 135
    rapid-growing 135
    slow-growing 135
Mycobacteriosis, atypical 58
Mycobacterium
    abscessus 135
    avium 127
    bovis 124
    chelonae 135, 137
        infections 137
    fortuitum 135, 137
    leprae 114, 120*f*
    marinum 135
        infection 107, 136*f*
    scrofulaceum 127
    tuberculosis 124, 132, 135
    ulcerans 135, 136, 137*f*
Mycolactone 136
Mycoses, subcutaneous 56, 137
Myeloperoxidase deficiency 48*b*
Myiasis, cutaneous 7
Myocarditis, acute 84
Myrmecia 91, 91*f*

N

Nadifloxacin 14
Nail
    dystrophy, secondary 51*f*
    lacquers 46
    lichen planus 30
    plate
        biopsy 46*f*
        greenish discoloration of 111*f*
        proximal portion of 189*f*
    psoriasis 30
    trauma 21
Nailfold, infection of 13*f*
Nasal septum, destruction of 129*f*
Nasal swabs 7
Nasopharyngeal secretions, microscopy of 109

Index

N-diethyl-M-toluamide 163
Necator americanus 143
Neck
    carbuncle of 8*f*
    lesions 102*f*
    nape of 115*f*
Necrobiosis lipoidica 116
Necrotic herpes zoster ophthalmicus 87*f*
Necrotizing fasciitis 10, 11
Neisseria
    gonorrhoeae 165
    meningitidis 18
Nelfinavir 183*t*
Nemathelminthes 139
Nematodes 139
Neonatal herpes
    prevention of 82
    simplex virus 79, 80*f*
Nephritis 121
Nerve
    peripheral 120*f*
    ultrasound, indications of 121
Nervous system 133
Neuralgia, postherpetic 85
Neurofibromatosis 117, 118
Neuropathy 117
Nevirapine 183
Nevus anemicus 115
Nitrogen oxide 137
Nits 55, 158*f*, 158*t*
Nocardia brasiliensis 62
Nocardiosis 58
Nodular fasciitis 137
Nodular scabies 155, 155*f*, 157
Nodules 27*f*, 150*f*
Nodulocystic acne 7
Noduloulcerative lesions 57*f*, 58*f*
    string of 57*f*
Noma neonatorum 20
Nonbullous impetigo 2*f*
Nondermatophytic mold 31
    onychomycosis 30, 47, 47*f*, 48*f*
Nonnucleoside reverse transcriptase
    inhibitors 183
Nonsteroidal anti-inflammatory drugs
    123
North Asian tick-borne rickettsiosis 23
Norwegian scabies 155, 156*f*
Nose, residual pigmentation of 112*f*
Novy-MacNeal-Nicolle media 150
Nucleic acid amplification
    techniques 167
    test 183
Nucleoside reverse transcriptase
    inhibitors 183
Nutritional deficiencies 117

O

Ocular cavity 196*f*
Old world cutaneous leishmaniasis 147

Onychocola canadensis 47
Onycholysis 21
    proximal jagged edge of 43*f*
Onychomadesis 111*f*
Onychomycosis 42*t*
    candidal 30, 51, 51*f*, 52
    distal and lateral subungual 31, 31*f*, 42
    types of 31*t*, 42, 43
Onychoscopy features 42*t*, 43*t*
Ophthalmia neonatorum 166, 168
Opportunistic mycoses 66
Oral candidiasis, severe 195
Oral thrush 48, 188*f*
Oriental sore 147
Orificial tuberculosis 127
Orolabial herpes 81
    prevention of 81
Oropharyngeal candidiasis 52
Oropharynx 100
Orthopoxvirus 103
    antigens 103
Osteoarticular sporotrichosis 59*t*
Osteomyelitis 21, 68, 137
Otitis externa 20
    malignant 20, 21
    necrotizing 20

P

Pachyonychia congenita 30
Paederus dermatitis 162
Pain
    abdominal 23
    chest 68, 73
    severe 79*f*
Palm 17*f*, 155
Pancreatitis, acute 84
Panencephalitis, subacute sclerosing 109
Panniculitis 67, 137
Papillomaviruses 89
Papular urticaria 161*f*
Papules 105
    hyperpigmented 71*f*
Papulonecrotic tuberculid 130, 131, 185
    lesions of 132*f*
Papulovesicular lesion 104*f*, 105*f*
Paracoccidioides brasiliensis 70
Paracoccidioidomycosis 58, 70
Paramyxoviridae 108
Paravaccinia virus 107
Parkinson's disease 155
Paronychia 21
    acute 12, 12*f*
    candidal 51
Parvovirus 112
Peau d'orange 10
Pediculicides 159
Pediculosis 16
    capitis 159
    corporis 159
Pediculus humanus var. *capitis* 157

Pelvic inflammatory disease 170
Pemphigus 7
    foliaceus 78
    vulgaris 13*f*
Penicilliosis 72
Penicillium marneffei infection 108
Penile squamous cell carcinoma,
    ulcerative lesion of 96*f*
Penis, shaft of 189*f*
Perianal tuberculosis ulcers, painless 127*f*
Perifollicular
    epithelioid cell granulomas 132
    pustules 27*f*
    scale 42*f*
    tissue 7
Perihepatitis 170
Perineal tuberculosis ulcers 127*f*
Periodic acid-Schiff stain 46, 46*f*, 68,
Peripheral blood eosinophilia 143
Peripilar casts 55
Periporitis staphylogenes 12, 12*f*
Periurethral gland 165
Perleche 48
Permethrin 160
Petechiae 112*f*, 194
Phagedenic chancroid 171*f*
Pharyngitis 166
Pharynx, uncomplicated gonococcal
    infections of 167
Pheohyphomycosis 56, 61, 61*f*
Phialophora 61
Photodynamic therapy 98
Phrynoderma 131
Piedra 16, 54, 54*f*
Pigmented Buschke-Löwenstein tumor
    94*f*
Pilonidal cyst 7
Piperacillin 15
Pitted keratolysis 16, 17*f*
Pityriasis
    alba 53, 115
    lichenoid et varioliform acuta 130, 131
    rosea 26, 53
    rubra pilaris 53, 131
    versicolor 15, 25-27, 53, 92, 92*f*, 115
        hyperpigmented 53*f*
        hypopigmented 53*f*
        treatment for 54*t*
Plantar 194*f*
    mosaic warts 17, 91, 91*f*
    warts, myrmecia of 91*f*
Plaques 150*f*
Plasma cells 151*f*
Platyhelminthes 139
Plica polonica 158*f*
Pneumonia 71, 109
Podophyllin 97
    resin 97
Podophyllotoxin 98
Polyarteritis nodosa, cutaneous 132
Polycyclic erosions, multiple 189*f*

Polymerase chain reaction 70, 80, 96, 136, 167
Polymorphic light eruption 115
Polymorphonuclear cells 167*f*
Posaconazole 69, 70
Post-kala-azar dermal leishmaniasis 149
  hypopigmented macules of 150*f*
  lesions of 150*f*
  nodular lesions of 149*f*
  plaques of 149*f*
  sequel of 147
Postmeningococcal reactive disease 19
Postzoster depigmentation 86
Potassium
  hydroxide 45*f*, 52*f*-54*f*, 60*f*, 109
    scrapings 6
  iodide, saturated solution of 59
  permanganate 156
Potent topical steroids, abuse of 40
Poxviruses 100
Prednisolone 123
Pregnancy 97
Prepuce 191*f*
Proctitis 169
Prominent papulonodular lesions 149*f*
Prostatovesiculitis 169
Protease inhibitors 183
Proteinuria 121
Proteus 184
  vulgaris 24
Proximal subungual onychomycosis 31, 31*f*, 43, 189*f*
Prozone phenomenon 190
Pruritus 155
Pseudocowpox 107
Pseudoepitheliomatous hyperplasia 125
Pseudofolliculitis 6
Pseudo-Koebner phenomenon 91
Pseudomembranous candidiasis, oral 49*f*
Pseudomonal infections, spectrum of 20
Pseudomonas 5, 21
  aeruginosa 184
  folliculitis 20, 21
  green nail syndrome 21*f*
  hot-foot syndrome 20
  infections 20
  septicemia 20*f*
Pseudopustular lesions 102*f*
Psoriasiform syphilid 175*f*
Psoriasis 26, 30, 53, 78
  flexural 27, 50
Pthirus pubis 157
Pubic area, infestation of 159*f*
Pubic louse 157, 158*f*, 159
Punctate palmoplantar keratoderma 17
Pure neuritic leprosy 114, 117
Purpuric lesions 194
Purulent cellulitis 11*f*
Pus
  culture 4
  Gram stain of 6

Pustular tinea 36, 36*f*
Pyoderma 20
  gangrenosum 67, 137
  primary 1
  secondary 1, 13
Pyogenic granuloma 107
Pyrizinamide 133

Q

Quadrivalent human papillomavirus vaccine 99
Queensland tick typhus 23*t*
Quinolones 137

R

Radiofrequency ablation 97
Raltegravir 183*t*
Ramam regimen 64
Ramsay Hunt syndrome 85, 87*f*
Rash 22*f*
  urticarial 193*f*
Recalcitrant dermatophytosis 25, 34
  impact of 41
Rectal infection, primary 165
Rectum, uncomplicated gonococcal infections of 167
Red scrotum syndrome 40
Red-half-moon lunula 195*f*
Reiter's syndrome 169
Renal damage 119
Reproductive system 119
Retapamulin 14
Reticuloendothelial system 73
Retroauricular area 58*f*
Retroviruses 182
Reverse cross-blot hybridization assay 136
Reverse transcriptase polymerase chain reaction 194
Rhinitis 166
Rhinocerebral mucormycosis 75
Rhizopus 75
Ribonucleic acid
  single-stranded 108
  virus 100, 182
Rickettsia 21
  akari 24
Rickettsial infections 21, 22, 23*t*
  diagnosis of 24
Rickettsialpox 24, 102
Rifampicin 65, 133, 185
Rilpivirine 183*t*
Ritonavir 183*t*
Ritter's disease 9
Rocky mountain spotted fever 23, 163
Rosacea 28, 160*f*
Rough nail plate 32*f*
Rubella 100, 112, 113
  vaccine 108
Russian vesicular rickettsiosis 23*t*

S

Sabouraud dextrose agar 45
Salicylic acid 97
Salpingitis 170
San Joaquin valley fever 69
Saquinavir 183*t*
Sarcoidosis 116, 118, 128
  cutaneous 116
Sarcoptes scabiei var. *hominis* 154
Scabies 102, 154-156
  bullous 4
  classical 154*f*
    lesions of 155*f*
  clinical variants of 155
  impetiginized lesions of 13*f*
  mite 154*f*
  S-shaped burrows of 155*f*
Scalp
  folliculitis, multiple lesions of 5*f*
  tinea of 38, 38*f*
Scarring 81*f*
Scattered skin lesions 85
Sclerotic bodies 60*f*
Scopulariopsis brevicaulis 47
Scrofuloderma 64, 72, 125, 126, 133, 185, 185*f*
  lesion 127*f*
  widespread lesions of 126*f*
Scrotal erythema, persistent 40
Scrotum 95*f*, 155*f*
Scrub typhus 22
Scytalidium 47
Seizure 23
Selenium sulfide 54
Seminal vesiculitis 166
Sensitivity 4
Sensory neuropathy, hereditary 117
Sepsis 21, 166
Septic arthritis 68
Serological tests 80, 151
Serology 70, 109
Severe acute respiratory syndrome coronavirus-2 (SARS-CoV-2) 192, 192*t*
  infection, cutaneous manifestations of 192*t*
Sexually transmitted
  diseases 189, 191
  infections 165
Sigmoid sinus thrombosis 21
Silver methenamine 67*f*, 68
Single morse code hair 41*f*
Skin 184
  biopsy 120, 135
  colored papules 149*f*
  disease 135
  infections, bacterial 103
  inoculation, direct 67
  involvement 73
  lesions 117

Index

manifestations 1
scraping 156f
surface 154
testing 68
Slit skin smear 120, 120f
Smallpox 100, 102
Sodium stibogluconate
  infusion therapy 152f
  monotherapy 149
Soft tissue
  infections 184
  tumors, benign 64
Soles 155f, 177f
South American blastomycosis 70
Spherulin skin tests 70
Spleen 73
Sporothrix schenckii 58f
Sporotrichoid 135
  lesion 135
  pattern 148f
Sporotrichosis 56, 59, 127
  cutaneous 56, 61
  diagnosis of 58
  disseminated 59
    cutaneous 57
  extracutaneous 57
  fixed cutaneous 56, 57f
  lymphocutaneous 56, 56f
  pulmonary 59
  treatment for 59t
Spotted fever group 22, 23t
Sputum 133
Squamous cell carcinoma 92, 94, 95f, 129
Staphylococcal
  carriage 7
  exfoliative toxin 9
  scalded skin syndrome 9, 9f
Staphylococci 1, 1t, 4, 12
Staphylococcus
  aureus 83
    methicillin-resistant 4, 14, 184
    methicillin-susceptible 14
  epidermidis 184
Stavudine 183t
Stemmer's sign 139
Stevens–Johnson syndrome 81
Stings 161
Streptococcal skin 184
Streptococci 1, 1t, 4, 11, 12, 14
Streptococcus 5
  pyogenes 2, 84
Striae, steroid induced 40f
Strongyloides stercoralis infection 144
Subcorneal pustular dermatosis 5
Submandibular nodes 126
Subungual ruin 43f
Sulfamethoxazole 70, 136, 137
Superficial dermatophytosis 15
  presentation of 34b
Superficial pustules 44f

Superficial white onychomycosis 31, 32f, 43, 44f
Swamps 136
Swelling 11f, 51f
  digital 79f
Swimmer's ear 20
Swollen lymph nodes 121
Sycosis 6
  barbae 6f, 28
Syphilides 174f
Syphilis 64, 102, 173, 178, 190
  congenital 176, 176f, 176t, 177f
  early congenital 176, 176f
  extensive 178f
  late 176
  malignant 190
  primary 173, 190
  secondary 26, 53, 173, 174f, 175f, 179f, 190
Systemic mycoses 66, 66f
  pathogenesis of 66f

T

Tachycardia 11
Taenia
  saginata, life cycle of 145f
  solium
    life cycle of 145f
    tapeworm 144
Taeniasis 145
Talaromyces marneffei 73f, 188
Talaromycosis 72
Tazobactam 15
Tecovirimat 104
Tenofovir
  alafenamide 183
  disoproxil fumarate 183
Terbinafine 30, 46, 59
Tetracyclines 16, 24
Thalidomide 123
Thoracic dermatome 85
Thrombocytopenia 84
Tibia 121
Tick
  bites 163
    prevention of 163
  paralysis 163
Tinea 38f, 39
  auricularis 34, 38, 38f
  barbae 27, 30, 47
  blepharitis 34
  capitis 13f, 28, 28f, 29f, 30, 34, 41t, 47
    inflammatory 29, 29f
    noninflammatory 28
  concentric rings of 27f
  corporis 25, 30, 38f-40f, 44, 47, 116, 188f
    annular plaques of 26f
    diffuse scaly 38, 39f
    extensive 39f, 40f

inflamed lesion of 40f
cruris 27, 36f, 44, 47, 50
  extensive 27f
  inflamed lesion of 40f
faciei 26, 35f, 36, 37f, 47
  atypical lesion of 26f
  extensive 37f
  large annular plaque of 26f
  lesion 39f
genitalis 34
incognito 26, 35, 44
indecisiva 26
infection 27f, 53
  changes of 42f
  pattern of 34
labialis 34
manuum 4, 32, 34, 34f, 36f, 44, 47
pedis 17, 32, 34, 44, 47
  atypical symmetrical 39f
  bullous 4, 33f
  chronic hyperkeratotic 33f
  clinical variants of 32t
  interdigital 33f
  moccasin-type 33f
pseudoimbricata 26, 34, 36f
  extensive 37f
steroid modified 37f, 39f, 44f
tonsurans 28, 30
unguium 30, 43f, 47
versicolor 53
Tingling pain, prodrome of 85
Tipranavir 183t
Tissue edema 9
Toenail 31f
Toe-web infection 20
Tolnaftate 46
Tongue 100
Total dystrophic onychomycosis 31, 32f
Toxins
  bacterial 1
  process of 161
Transepidermal elimination 67
Trematodes 139
Trichloroacetic acid 97
Trichobacteriosis 16
Trichomycosis
  axillaris 16
  concretions of 16f
  nodularis 54
Trichophyton
  concentricum 26
  mentagrophytes 27
  schoenleinii 27
  verrucosum 27
  violaceum 27
Trichosporon 54
Trichotillomania 30
Trigeminal dermatome 85f
Trimethoprim 14, 70, 136, 137
Tubercular chancre 124f

Index

Tuberculides 130, 133
Tuberculoid
  epithelioid granulomas 126f
  leprosy 114, 115
    Hansen, plaques of 115f
Tuberculosis 126f
  acute miliary 125
  cutaneous 61, 124, 185
  cutis orificialis 127
  miliary 130
  primary inoculation 124
  pulmonary 131f
  verrucosa cutis 60, 125, 185
    lesion 125f
Tuberculous gumma 129, 130f
Tularemia 163
Typhus group 21, 22
Tyson's gland inflammation 166
Tzanck smear 80, 87

U

Ulcer
  corneal 74f, 109
  multiple 171f
  nonindurated 171f
  painful 171f
  secondary 40f
  traumatic 81
  trophic 119f
  tuberculous 126f
Ulcerative herpes labialis, severe 81f
Ulcerative lupus vulgaris 125
Universal Immunization Program 133
Upper respiratory tract 118
Urethra, uncomplicated gonococcal infections of 167
Urethral strictures 166
Urethritis 166, 169
  anterior 165
  nongonococcal 169
Urogenital cryptococcosis 72

V

Vaccine-preventable disease 85
Vacuolated epidermal cells, cytoplasm of 106f
Vagabond's disease 159f
Vaginal candidiasis 49
Vaginal discharge 78f
Vaginitis 166
Vaginosis, bacterial 191
Vague hypopigmented macule 115f
Valacyclovir 82, 88
Vancomycin 15
Var duboisii 67
Varicella 82, 82f-84f, 101, 110, 131
  gangrenosa 84
  severe 83f
  zoster virus 76, 186
    infections 82
Variola virus 100
Vascular origin, lesions of 192
Vellus hair, tinea of 34, 38
Venereal diseases 165
Verruca
  multiple 90f
  plana 91, 91f, 92f
  vulgaris 89, 90f
Verrucous papules, multiple hyperpigmented 191f
Vesicles 105
Vesicular eruption 192
Vesicular lesions 194
Viral cutaneous disorders 100
Virucidal therapy 98
Virus isolation 109
Vitiligo 53, 115
Voriconazole 69, 70, 74
Vulvovaginal candidiasis 49, 49f, 52

W

Warthin-starry stain 185
Warts 89, 96
  anogenital 93
  benign cutaneous 89
  common 60
  diagnosis of 96
  flat 91
  genital 191f
  isolated 89
  multiple 90f
  palmar 90f
  penile 93f
  periungual 90f
  pigmented 91, 92f
  regression of 91
  subungual 90f, 97
  treatment of 97b
Warty tuberculosis 125
Web spaces 154f
Weil-Felix test 24
Welsh regimen 64
  modified 65
Western blot assay 183
Whitish pseudomembrane 188f
Wood's lamp 15
  examination 53
Wuchereria bancrofti, life cycle of 140, 140f

Y

Yaws 64, 102
Yucatan spotted fever 23

Z

Zalcitabine 183t
Zidovudine 183t
Ziehl-Neelsen staining 120f, 137
Zinc pyrithione bars 54
Zoonosis 101
Zoonotic orthopoxvirus 101
Zygomycosis, subcutaneous 56

EU GSPR Authorised Reprsentative
Logos Europe, 9 rue Nicolas Poussin
1700, La Rochelle, France
Phone: +33 (0) 6 67 93 73 78
E-mail: contact@logoseurope.eu